Care Planning in Children
and Young People's Nursing

For Breige Morgan, a contributing co-author of Chapter 37, who died suddenly on 12 October 2010. Breige had a huge personality, and she was a great inspiration to her colleagues, and to many sick children and their families.

Care Planning in Children and Young People's Nursing

Edited by

Doris Corkin

Teaching Fellow (Children's Team)
School of Nursing & Midwifery
Queen's University Belfast

Sonya Clarke

Senior Teaching Fellow (Children's & Orthopaedic/Trauma Nursing)
School of Nursing & Midwifery
Queen's University Belfast

Lorna Liggett

Discipline Lead (Children's Nursing)
School of Nursing & Midwifery
Queen's University Belfast

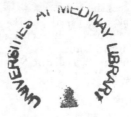

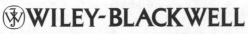WILEY-BLACKWELL

A John Wiley & Sons, Ltd., Publication

This edition first published 2012
© 2012 by Blackwell Publishing Ltd

Blackwell Publishing was acquired by John Wiley & Sons in February 2007. Blackwell's publishing program has been merged with Wiley's global Scientific, Technical and Medical business to form Wiley-Blackwell.

Registered office: John Wiley & Sons, Ltd, The Atrium, Southern Gate, Chichester, West Sussex, PO19 8SQ, UK

Editorial offices: 9600 Garsington Road, Oxford, OX4 2DQ, UK
The Atrium, Southern Gate, Chichester, West Sussex, PO19 8SQ, UK
350 Main Street, Malden, MA 02148-5020, USA

For details of our global editorial offices, for customer services and for information about how to apply for permission to reuse the copyright material in this book please see our website at www.wiley.com/wiley-blackwell.

Library of Congress Cataloging-in-Publication Data

Care planning in children and young people's nursing / edited by Doris Corkin, Sonya Clarke, Lorna Liggett.
    p. ; cm.
  Includes bibliographical references and index.
  ISBN-13: 978-1-4051-9928-5 (pbk. : alk. paper)
  ISBN-10: 1-4051-9928-8 (pbk. : alk. paper) 1. Pediatric nursing. 2. Nursing care plans. I. Corkin, Doris. II. Clarke, Sonya. III. Liggett, Lorna.
  [DNLM: 1. Patient Care Planning. 2. Pediatric Nursing–methods. 3. Adolescent. 4. Child. 5. Nursing Care–methods. 6. Risk Assessment. WY 159]
  RJ245.C368 2011
  618.92'00231–dc23
            2011015846

A catalogue record for this book is available from the British Library.

This book is published in the following electronic formats: ePDF 9781444346039; ePub 9781444346046; Mobi 9781444346053

Set in 10/12 pt Trump Mediaeval by Toppan Best-set Premedia Limited, Hong Kong

Printed and bound in Malaysia by Vivar Printing Sdn Bhd

1 2012

Contents

Foreword

Children's and young people's nursing has a theoretical base which has many elements including physiology, psychology, pathology, pharmacology and sociology. To deliver quality care to children and young people that is focused, safe and organised, it needs to be planned. Documenting the plan of care for a child and the implementation of that plan ensures continuity of care and provides a legal document demonstrating that care has been delivered.

The Nursing and Midwifery Council, the regulator for nursing in the UK, has published policy benchmarks which highlight the importance of nurses making records that are clear, intelligible and accurate, documented in such a way as to ensure that their meaning is clear. The plan of care for an individual child is the cornerstone of their health care journey. This new and exciting textbook is designed to help children's and young people's nurses appreciate the pivotal role that they can play in ensuring that every child receives optimum care based on their assessed needs. This book demonstrates how care can be organised using the nursing process and nursing models to help focus care delivery to meet the specific needs of the child or young person.

The importance of children's and young people's nurses planning and delivering care, underpinned by evidence-based theory, is perhaps best reflected in Nightingale's famous pronouncement articulated in her notes for nursing (1859):

"Children: they are affected by the same things [as adults] but much more quickly and seriously." p. 72

It is because children are different from adults and become sicker much more quickly that children's nurses need a cognitive assessment and care planning toolkit to help them successfully manage the whole care paradigm of sick children and young people. Indeed, it is because sick children need care delivered by well-educated children's nurses that this book has been written by a team of writers dedicated to promoting best practice. Planning and delivering optimum care is the very hallmark and mantra of children's and young people's nurses.

This first edition provides a clear and user-friendly examination of the nursing process, the framework for organising individualised nursing care. Nurses will find the various chapters invaluable in assessing, planning, implementing and evaluating the care that they deliver. Importantly, in the case of children personal injury claims are allowed up to 3 years after their majority, although in all cases an individual judge may lengthen the period allowed. This emphasises the need for nurses to be vigilant in the way that they assess and plan care, as a child's patient record may be called before a judge sometimes decades after the event.

This book also recognizes that the involvement of children, young people and their families in the planning and implementation of care is vital in the formation of effective partnerships with families and children in the provision of care.

However, it is the creation of a care plan that is used to determine the nursing care given to an individual patient using measurable outcomes which are measurable to enable care to be evaluated and then improved upon.

In addition, this book shows the reader the whole purpose of using the nursing process to help assess, plan and deliver care to the child, young person and family which fulfils the whole ethos of nursing, which is 'first to do no harm'.

I commend this book to you.

Dr E.A. Glasper
Professor of Children's and Young People's Nursing
The University of Southampton

Preface

Within this book the editors and contributing authors address a selection of the most common concerns that arise when planning care for infants, children and young people within the hospital and community setting. Discussion within each chapter and scenario will highlight that effective care planning needs to be individualised, yet collaborative, negotiated in partnership with the child or young person and their family in order to meet their many needs. It is hoped the title provides a clear, detailed and comprehensive insight into children's nursing and that this text is appropriate for practitioners throughout the world.

This textbook is mainly aimed at 'child branch' nursing students undertaking undergraduate education, postgraduate programmes and recently qualified children's nurses. It should also be an invaluable resource for the registered nurse (RN), especially when undertaking the dedicated role of mentorship. This text is richly designed with diagrams and photographs to inform the practice of care planning through the report of current research, best available evidence, policy and education, which reflects both the uniqueness and diversity of contemporary children's nursing. The overall intention is that this book will become a core text within children's nursing curricula and serve as a guide when teaching the theoretical foundation and clinical skill of care planning at each stage of the process. Furthermore, it will become an innovative resource for nursing students, nurse educators, practitioners, researchers and carers.

Chapters 1–11 explore central aspects in the rapidly changing field of children's nursing. Key principles are addressed to facilitate children's nurses with the understanding and knowledge that will underpin their care delivery.

The scenarios outlined in Chapters 12–37 provide the link between theory and practice, whilst highlighting the implications for good practice. Proposed questions follow the individual scenarios, offering lists of potential responses with limited rationale; it is therefore recommended that the nursing student/healthcare professional should explore the issues through further reading. Answers are not meant to be definitive or restrictive and may be amended to facilitate changing circumstances at any time. These scenarios will also help develop the fundamental skills of writing competent focused care plans for infants, children and young people. Throughout the scenarios a family-centred partnership has been incorporated within a multidisciplinary and interagency framework. A collective global approach to care planning, whereby the nursing process and a model/models of nursing have been utilised, demonstrates the art and science of individualised care plans. The activities within the scenario chapters are designed to encourage self-directed learning, assimilation of information and searching of literature to stimulate the enquiring mind.

The editors have drawn together a wealth of expertise locally, nationally and internationally from a wide variety of practitioners/nurse specialists, academics and parents and we would like to thank them for their enthusiasm and commitment. Authors have reflected upon their personal/professional experience and in-depth knowledge, whilst respecting confidentiality, to explore important issues that arise when caring for infants, children and young people with a range of conditions some of which could be life-threatening or indeed life-limiting. Outstanding features within this book include contributions from parents and a young person who have shared their 'lived experiences', therefore taking cognisance of the Nursing and Midwifery Council stance on service user involvement. Also highlighted is the uniqueness of the 'practice facilitator' role in supporting mentors and nursing students within practice and the invaluable contribution from the Director of HIV/Aids Programme in Ethiopia.

Having reflected upon the Queen's University Belfast philosophy, which is to 'lead, inspire and deliver', the editors would like to take this opportunity to acknowledge the support from Head of School, Professor Linda Johnston, who has encouraged our learning trajectory.

We would also like to thank Magenta Styles and Alexandra McGregor at Wiley-Blackwell for their editorial assistance and patience throughout this timely editing process.

Doris Corkin
Sonya Clarke
Lorna Liggett

Contributors

Michelle Bennett
Clinical Nurse Specialist, Children's Pain Management, Nottingham University Hospitals NHS Trust: MSc in Pain Management, BSc (Hons) Advanced Nursing Practice, ENB 415, ENB N51, ENB 997, RSCN & RGN

Michelle qualified in Chichester as an RGN in 1989 and then went on to train as a children's nurse at Great Ormond Street Hospital in 1992. After working in London for a short time she moved to Nottingham in 1995 to specialise in paediatric intensive care nursing. Over the following ten years Michelle worked in both paediatric high dependency and paediatric intensive care settings within Nottingham. Michelle has always had an interest in children's pain management, which formed the basis of her BSc Honours degree dissertation, which she undertook whilst working on PICU in Nottingham. During this time Michelle also undertook the role of health lecturer- practitioner in the University of Nottingham, working with undergraduate master's degree child branch student nurses. Michelle was appointed as a Clinical Nurse Specialist in Children's Pain Management almost six years ago and continues to work at Nottingham University Hospitals NHS Trust. In this time Michelle has completed an MSc in pain management. Michelle has presented at several conferences, published articles relating to children's pain management and related topics.

Erica Brown
Vice President of Acorns Children's Hospices, Senior Lecturer at University of Worcester and an Independent Consultant in Children's and Young People's Palliative Care

Erica was formerly Head of Research and Development of Care at Acorns and she worked as Head of Special Education at Oxford University. She has longstanding experience as a senior manager in schools and universities and she has lectured and published nationally and internationally. Erica is a trained bereavement counsellor. Her most recent books include: *Loss, Change and Grief – an Educational Perspective* (1999) London: David Fulton Publishers; *Supporting Children with Post Traumatic Stress Disorder – a Guide for Teachers and Professionals* (2001) London: David Fulton Publishers; *The Death of a Child: Care for the Child, Support for the Family* (2003) Birmingham: Acorns Children's Hospices; *Palliative Care for South Asians – Hindus, Muslims Sikhs* (2008) (2nd edn) London: Quay Books; *Supporting the Child and the Family in Paediatric Palliative Care* (2007) London: Jessica Kingsley; *Supporting Bereaved Children in the Primary School* (2009) London: Help the Hospices; *Life Changes – Loss, Change and Bereavement for Children Aged 3–11 Years Old* (2010) Manchester: Tacade/Lions.

Pauline Cardwell
Teaching Fellow, School of Nursing & Midwifery, Queen's University Belfast, Northern Ireland: MSc in Advanced Nursing; PGCHET, BSc (Hons) Health Sciences, RN (Child Dip) & RGN

Pauline began her nursing career in 1986 and holds qualifications in adult and children's nursing. She has worked in various fields of nursing practice, including adult medical, surgical and general children's nursing in a clinical career which spans over 25 years' experience. Pauline also held a position of practice educator within the university in June 2006 before commencing her current post of teaching fellow in January 2008. Her professional interests and areas of teaching include clinical skills both within the CFP and branch programmes of the undergraduate programmes and simulated learning and practice. She has presented at regional, national and international conferences on a range of topics and has published in books and journals.

Pauline Carson

Teaching Fellow, School of Nursing & Midwifery, Queen's University Belfast, Northern Ireland: MSc Child Health, PG Cert in Learning and Teaching in HE, BSc (Hons) Professional Development in Nursing, RN (Canada), RSCN, RGN

Pauline has both an adult and children's nursing background and has worked in both the UK and Canada. She worked within the field of paediatric cardiology prior to entering into nurse education and is now primarily teaching within pre-registration nurse education. Areas of interest within nursing include adolescent/young people's health care; high dependency care and nurse education.

Julie Chambers

Community Children's Nursing Sister, South Eastern Trust, Health & Social Care, Downpatrick, Co. Down, Northern Ireland: BSc (Hons) Specialist Practice, Teacher Practitioner, Nurse Prescribing, Asthma Diploma, D/N Cert, SCM, RSCN & SRN

Julie commenced her nurse training in 1979 and has worked in community nursing as a District Nursing Midwifery Sister since 1986 specialising in paediatrics. She initiated the setting up of a community paediatric service with her colleague Doris Corkin in 2000. Julie makes every effort to enhance and develop her practice by being a mentor to pre- and postgraduate nursing students and by contributing to and participating in international conferences, book/journal publications and presentations. She also endeavours to ensure that all children and families are nursed to the highest standard and last year was the Well Child's overall winner in the UK Community Practitioner of the Year Award.

Janice Christie

Teaching Fellow, School of Nursing & Midwifery, Queen's University Belfast, Northern Ireland: PhD, MA, BSc, RN & RSCPHN

Janice worked as a health visitor for 15 years and has a special interest in public health and health promotion. She has worked in Queen's since 2005, and teaches from diploma to taught doctorate level (pre- and post-registration nursing across a range of fields).

Sonya Clarke (Editor)

Senior Teaching Fellow, School of Nursing & Midwifery, Queen's University Belfast, Northern Ireland: MSc Nursing; PGCE (Higher Education), PG Cert (Pain Management), BSc (Hons) Specialist Practitioner in Orthopaedic Nursing, RN (diploma/children's nursing) & RGN

Sonya, a nurse for over 20 years, has experience in children's and adult nursing within orthopaedics and as a Marie Curie nurse within palliative care. Her current position encompasses teaching/administration, community outreach and related scholarly activity within the School of Nursing and Midwifery at Queen's University Belfast (QUB). Teaching commitments mainly involve undergraduate children's nursing for the BSc (Hons) Health Studies programme and pathway leader for the registered nurse undertaking orthopaedic and fracture trauma continuing education programmes across the lifespan. Scholarly activity reflects both children's nursing and her specialist subject area of orthopaedics. Prior to her Teaching Fellow position in 2003 she was employed as a Lecturer Practitioner at QUB and Musgrave Park Hospital (MPH, a regional elective orthopaedic unit). Sonya's nursing career commenced in 1988, she qualified as an RGN in 1991 and completed a diploma in Children's Nursing in 1996. Clinical practice was primarily within MPH for the adult and child until 2001, with additional nursing experience (bank position) gained as a Marie Currie nurse until 2009. Sonya continues to actively lead, inspire and deliver evidenced-based education that motivates and develops the Queen's nursing student.

Doris Corkin (Editor)

Teaching Fellow, School of Nursing & Midwifery, Queen's University Belfast, Northern Ireland: MSc in Nursing, PG Dip Nurse Education, BSc (Hons), CCN, RN (Child Dip), ENB904 & RGN

Doris has both adult and children's training, has specialised in neonatology for over 12 years, has worked in an acute medical/surgical ward for six years and was instrumental in establishing a new community children's nursing service before accepting her current teaching position in 2003. Teaching commitments include pre- and post-registration children's nursing, with specific interests in the nursing care of children and young people with complex/palliation needs and encouraging service user involvement within the curriculum. As a module and programme co-ordinator Doris makes every effort to develop her clinical skills within children's nursing through facilitation of interprofessional education, QUB teaching, travel awards and international conference presentations. Doris has contributed to both journal and book publications, external examining and professional committees/ organisations.

Michael Davidson

Practice Education Facilitator, Belfast Health and Social Care Trust, Belfast City Hospital, Belfast, Northern Ireland: MSc Nursing (Cancer), BA (Hons) Nursing Studies, BA Public Administration (with an option in social work), CQSW & RGN

Michael trained initially as a social worker working for the voluntary sector and then latterly in a hospital setting. He went on to train as a registered general nurse, specialising in the field of oncology and haematology nursing. Since qualifying as a registered nurse Michael has worked in a number of cities and towns in Scotland as well as working in Australia. Work roles have included ward manager, specialist nurse, clinical teacher and lecturer. Michael moved to live and work in Belfast, Northern Ireland in 2005, working as a clinical leader within the newly established Northern Ireland Cancer Centre. Most recently he took up a new role as a Practice Education Facilitator within the Belfast HSC Trust. Responsibilities include the support of nurse mentors in practice to ensure that the NMC Standards to Support Learning and Assessment in Practice (2008) are adhered to as well as other professional responsibilities aimed at ensuring a high standard of practice education opportunities exists.

Nuala Devlin

Practice Education Facilitator, Belfast Health and Social Care Trust, Northern Ireland: Postgraduate Certificate in Education (Lecturer/Practice Educator), BSc in Health Studies, Diploma in Nursing Studies & RGN

The initial part of Nuala's career involved working within a nursing home in the private sector before spending time as a theatre nurse. Nuala went on to specialise in intensive care nursing, working for 11 years within a variety of different cities across the UK. On returning to Northern Ireland Nuala worked in several different nursing positions within an ICU/cardiac setting. Following on from this Nuala moved into a teaching position within resuscitation and is a Resuscitation Council (UK) Instructor for Advanced Life Support in both adult and children. In 2009, Nuala accepted her current position as a Practice Education Facilitator, with a remit that includes wards and departments in both the adult and children's hospitals within the Belfast Health and Social Care Trust. Responsibilities include the implementation and adherence to the NMC Standards to Support learning and Assessment in Practice (2008).

Sharon Douglass

Clinical Nurse Specialist, Children's Pain Management, Nottingham University Hospitals NHS Trust; Specialist Practitioner Child Health (2006): BSc (Hons) Health Care Studies (Child Health), B72 NCP, C&G 7307 & RNCB

Sharon qualified in Nottingham as a RNCB in 1999. Since which time she has worked on a variety of children's wards gaining valuable multi-speciality knowledge and expertise. During this time she has undertaken the Managing Children's Pain LBR Module. Sharon has always had an interest in children's pain management, which also formed the basis of her BSc Honours degree dissertation, which she undertook whilst working on a busy surgical and gastroenterology ward in Nottingham. Sharon was appointed as a Clinical Nurse Specialist in Children's Pain Management one year ago and continues to work at Nottingham University Hospitals NHS Trust.

Katie Dowdie

Clinical Educator, Paediatric Intensive Care, Royal Belfast Hospital for Sick Children, Northern Ireland: Cert Intensive Care Nursing for RSCN'S, Diploma module in Principles of Paediatric Intensive Care Nursing, RSCN & RGN

Katie is both adult and children trained. She did her general training in Belfast and children's training in Edinburgh and has also worked in Australia. Katie was a deputy ward manager in paediatric intensive care in Belfast before taking up the post of clinical educator. Her main responsibilities now are practice development, education and training of the intensive care nursing staff. Katie participates, supports and encourages research and evidence-based practice in order to enhance patient care and is at present studying for a degree 'Developing Practice in Healthcare'.

Anne Finnegan

Senior Lecturer, School of Health and Social Care, Teesside University: MSc (Applied Social Science), PGCE, ENB998, BSc (Hons) Nursing Science, RSCN & RGN

Anne has worked in children's services throughout her nursing career, with posts in orthopaedics, cardiac and ENT areas. Teaching interests relate to physical assessment, acute illness in children, service improvement and skills delivery, working with pre- and post-registration students, and she is currently a pathway leader for a children's nursing degree. Anne has published journal articles, contributed to publications, has experience as an external examiner and external reviewer.

Alan Forster

Head of Unit (Adult Nursing), School of Nursing & Midwifery, Queen's University of Belfast, Northern Ireland: BSc (Biological Sciences), PG Dip (Biomedical Sciences), RN (Learning Disabilities), RN (Adult), RCNT & RNT

Alan is qualified in both learning disability and adult nursing. After registration he worked with adults with severe learning disabilities before becoming ward manager in a unit for children with profound learning disabilities. In 1978 he became a clinical teacher in learning disability nursing before transferring to adult nursing as a tutor in 1982, gaining experience in pre- and post-registration education. Alan became a senior tutor in 1992; he had responsibility for both the Common Foundation Course and Learning Disability branch, was also module leader for the Life Sciences module. Following integration into higher education in 1997, Alan taught on child, adult and learning disability programmes, with a special interest in biomedical sciences. As Head of Unit for Adult Nursing he had responsibility for the day-to-day management of the programme. At the same time he maintained his involvement in teaching the biomedical aspects of nursing to both learning disability and adult students. Throughout his career he has been fortunate to maintain his clinical involvement in both adult and learning disability nursing. Alan has recently retired.

Idy Fu
Teaching Consultant, School of Nursing, the University of Hong Kong: DNc, MPHC, BN, RN & RTN

Idy has had eight years of clinical experience in paediatric haematology and oncology, adult oncology and palliative care and three years in medical and geriatric nursing. She had worked as a registered nurse in both Hong Kong and Australia before she joined the School of Nursing in 1999 and accepted her current teaching position in 2006. Her teaching commitments include adult care, children care, health promotion and education and fundamental nursing. As a course and year co-ordinator for the undergraduate nursing programmes, Idy is also involved in curriculum planning and development, teaching and learning innovations, assessment and evaluation, etc. Her research interests are public health and nursing education and her current research projects include smoking cessation, scoliosis screening and breastfeeding.

Hazel Gibson
Paediatric Renal Nurse Co-ordinator, Royal Belfast Hospital for Sick Children, Northern Ireland: BSc (Hons) Health Studies, RN (Child Diploma), ENB136, RMN & RGN

Hazel's nursing career has included general adult nursing, psychiatry and adult renal nursing, which lead her into children's renal care in 1996. Initially she was involved in delivering haemodialysis to children with acute and end-stage renal failure, until she took up her current position in 2003. As well as co-ordinating a clinical caseload for pre-dialysis, dialysis and post-transplant care, her role involves teaching programmes for parents, in-house training, plus pre- and post-registration student education. Community commitments further demand educational input in schools, nurseries and community nursing teams, together with home visits to prepare children and their families for renal replacement therapies. Hazel was involved in the adaptation of the haemodialysis module at QUB within the adult renal course leading to a paediatric module. She has presented and had poster presentations at local forums and national conferences.

Diane Gow
Lecturer in Child Health, University of Southampton, Faculty of Health Sciences: MSc, BA (Hons), RGN, RSCN, RNT & RCNT

Diane completed a combined programme in Children and Adult Nursing at Westminster Hospitals. She held posts in a range of paediatric settings within the UK, USA and Australia before she became a Clinical Teacher at Westminster Children's Hospital, prior to becoming a lecturer in Child Health at the University of Southampton. Her research interests lie in exploring the impact of nut allergy on families. She has led a range of programmes within pre-and post-qualifying curricula, and is now specialising in professional law and ethics, and is currently studying for her LLM in Medical Law.

Gloria Hook
Paediatric Renal Nurse, Royal Belfast Hospital for Sick Children, Northern Ireland: RMN, ENB 136 & RSCN

Gloria trained in adult psychiatry before moving to the Royal Belfast Hospital for Sick Children in 1991. After training she worked in medicine, before going to the Nightingale Institute at the University of London; then returning to her current position. Her role includes providing care for all children requiring intervention from the renal multidisciplinary team. She is a member of the Paediatric Irish Nephrology Group, helping to maintain standards of renal care throughout Ireland.

Una Hughes
Children's Nursing Services Training Co-ordinator, Southern Trust, Northern Ireland: RGN, ENB 415, ENB998 & RSCN

Una has both adult and children's training; she specialised in paediatric intensive care over ten years and has taught in a college of further and higher education and worked in the community children's nursing team before accepting current training co-ordinator position in 2010. Teaching and training commitments include NVQ Level 3 for paediatric community healthcare workers, paediatric ward-based nursing auxiliaries and training for classroom assistants in special schools. Una has recently completed a paediatric palliative care module and develops her clinical and teaching skills through ongoing study.

Janet Kelsey
Associate Professor (Senior Lecturer) in Health Studies (Paediatric), School of Nursing & Community Studies, University of Plymouth: MSc Health Psychology, BSc (Hons) Psychology, Adv Dip Ed, PGCE, RSCN, RGN & RNT

Janet has contributed to journal and book publications, presented at regional, national and international conferences on a range of topics and is an external examiner. She has managed both diploma and BSc child nursing programmes and teaches both acute care of the child and family and clinical skills in children's nursing. Her particular interests lie in the care of young people within the acute health care environment.

Gilli Lewis
Child Health Nurse Lecturer, Capital & Coast District Health Board Wellington, New Zealand: MPH (Public Health), PG Cert Health Education, Diploma in Asthma Care, BN & RN (General and Child)

Gilli is an experienced educator and children's nurse. She began her career with the Wellington Asthma Research Group, where she developed research skills as well as a foundational knowledge and interest in asthma. She worked with both adults and children in this role and fostered a particular interest in children with atopic disease. She has collaborated on a number of scientific papers, and has attended and presented research at conferences nationally and internationally. In 2002 she completed a Master's in Public Health from Otago University NZ. A position at Queen's University Belfast School of Nursing and

Midwifery provided Gilli with experience in tertiary education, from which she gained a PG certificate in Tertiary Health Education. Since her return to New Zealand, Gilli has worked in both undergraduate, post-registration and post-graduate nursing education, with a focus on children's nursing. Gilli has maintained her clinical skills throughout her career, working in a variety of paediatric wards in New Zealand and in Northern Ireland. She is a member of the Paediatric Society of New Zealand and a member of the Nurses for Children & Young People of Aotearoa, New Zealand Nurses Organisation (NZNO) Section committee.

Lorna Liggett (Editor)
Discipline Lead – Children's Nursing, School of Nursing & Midwifery, Queen's University Belfast, Northern Ireland: BSc (Hons), RNT, RCNT, DASE, SRN & RSCN

Lorna completed her RSCN programme at the Royal Belfast Hospital for Sick Children and staffed in a children's medical ward for a short time. She then undertook her SRN programme at Craigavon School of Nursing. Following a one-year staffing experience in a gynaecological ward in Craigavon Area Hospital Lorna transferred to staff in a general children's ward. Several years later she became a clinical teacher and was attached to the children's ward and general adult wards. Lorna then completed the tutor's course and was employed at the Southern College of Nursing. At integration into Queen's University Belfast in 1997 she became Course Director and had ongoing responsibility for pre-registration education. In 2008 she was appointed Head of Unit for Children's nursing at QUB. Her main interests are children's rights, children and young people's health and safeguarding to protect children.

Mary Macfarlane
Regional Paediatric Cystic Fibrosis Centre, Allen Ward, Royal Belfast Hospital for Sick Children, Northern Ireland: RSCN & RGN

Mary has both adult and children's training. After qualifying she was staff nurse on a busy paediatric ward. Her interest in children with cystic fibrosis (CF) began at this time and she took the post as a staff nurse dedicated to CF and held this position for four years. After one year as a Hospital Medical Representative, she was successful in her application to become the Community Cystic Fibrosis Nurse for all children with CF in Northern Ireland. This was a new post and Mary was instrumental in establishing this role, to ensure all children with CF were followed out into the community, providing healthcare at home, advice and support from diagnosis through transfer to adult services, liaising with other health providers to ensure a seamless web of care. Mary also facilitates a lecture in Queen's University Belfast for pre- and post-registration nursing students in the care and management of children with CF.

Nicola Markwell
Registered General Nurse

Nicola commenced her nurse training in 1986 and qualified as a Registered General Nurse in December 1989. She took up a staffing post in the diabetic unit until 1994 and then transferred to the acute stroke unit where she worked until 2000, when Ryan was born. Since then Nicola has given up her nursing career to look after Ryan on a full-time basis. As a service user, she has become involved in a Queen's University Belfast module for child branch nursing students, by presenting on the challenges of caring for a child with complex needs in the community.

Barbara Maxwell

Staff Nurse, Allen Ward, Royal Belfast Hospital for Sick Children, Northern Ireland: Cert in care of child with CF, Asthma Dip, RSCN & RGN

Barbara qualified as a general nurse in 1991, at Royal Victoria Hospital Belfast, then she completed her post-registration children's nursing in Great Ormond Street Children's Hospital in 1994. For over 15 years Barbara has staffed in Allen ward (Royal Belfast Hospital for Sick Children, Belfast). Her specialist skills include caring for children with acute and chronic respiratory conditions such as cystic fibrosis, acute or brittle asthmatics, pleural effusions/empyemas, which require chest drains and patients with neuromuscular conditions who require a tracheostomy +/– non-invasive ventilation. Barbara has now taken up a post as the Regional Respiratory Paediatric Nurse Specialist and will be undertaking further study in relation to allergies.

Orla McAlinden

Nurse Lecturer, School of Nursing & Midwifery, Queen's University Belfast, Northern Ireland: MPhil (Medical Ethics and Law): BSc (Hons), ENB 415, Advanced Diploma in Education, Certs in: Palliative Care, Counselling and Child and Adolescent Interventions, RSCN & RN

Orla has extensive adult and children's training and experience, and specialised in paediatric and neonatal intensive care nursing at Guy's Hospital, London, before returning to her native Northern Ireland for further studies. She has been in nursing education for over eighteen years and has been teaching on pre- and post-registration nursing programmes at Queen's University Belfast since 1997. Orla's academic and clinical interests include general children's nursing, infant/child and adolescent mental health, ethics and law in healthcare and issues around suicide and mental health in society. She is also an ASIST and Safetalk Trainer helping to equip local community/education providers with immediate skills for suicide awareness and intervention.

Carol McCormick

Ward Manager, Paediatric Intensive Care, Royal Belfast Hospital for Sick Children, Northern Ireland: Paediatric Intensive Care Course, RSCN & RGN

Carol has experience in adult critical care, thoracic and vascular surgery. She has also worked in a variety of specialties within paediatrics. However, critical care is where she has spent many years of her nursing career and what she finds most challenging and rewarding. Carol has a special interest in transfer and retrieval of the critically ill child and is currently developing her clinical skills in this area following completion of the relevant short courses.

Gill McEwing

Lecturer in Nursing, School of Nursing & Midwifery, Faculty of Health, University of Plymouth: MSc, Diploma Nursing, Certificate of Education, RGN, RSCN & RNT

Gill has gained experience caring for children with a variety of clinical conditions in both specialised children's and district general hospitals. Gill has been a lecturer in child health since 1987, co-ordinating and teaching pre- and post-registration courses at degree and diploma level. She has edited several books, published journal articles and presented at national and international conferences.

Heather McKee

Teaching Fellow, School of Nursing & Midwifery, Queen's University Belfast, Northern Ireland: Bsc (Hons) in Nursing, Advanced Diploma in Educational Studies, PGCE, RSCN & RGN

Heather qualified as an adult and children's nurse and has gained experience in children's medical, ENT and ophthalmology surgery before commencing her current teaching post in 1997. Teaching commitments are within the common foundation and child branch programmes. Specific interests include care planning, health promotion and the incorporation of uni-professional and interprofessional simulation in the development of clinical skills. Heather has continued to update her clinical skills and knowledge base within her role as a programme co-ordinator for the child branch programme.

Hazel Mills

Cystic Fibrosis Nurse Specialist, Royal Belfast Hospital Sick Children, Northern Ireland: Advanced Diploma in Health Care at QUB, Management of CF Patients Course, (Brompton, London), RSCN & RGN

Hazel has over 12 years' experience working with CF patients. Currently she works as part of the multidisciplinary team facilitating the provision of a high standard of hospital and domiciliary care to children and adults with CF in Northern Ireland. This involves developing clinical policies and providing expert advice and support to patients and their families. Before specialising in CF, Hazel gained experience nursing patients in adult neurosurgery and paediatric general surgery and cardiology.

Catherine Monaghan

Teaching Fellow, School of Nursing & Midwifery, Queen's University Belfast, Northern Ireland: MSc in Nursing, Postgraduate Certificate in Education for the Health Care Professionals, BSc (Hons) Specialist Practice in Nursing, Dip in Community Nursing, RGN & RMN

Catherine is both adult and mental health trained and has worked in a variety of hospital settings throughout her career. Prior to taking up her appointment within nurse education, Catherine worked in the community where she was community team leader and worked within a multidisciplinary team. At present Catherine is an MSc programme co-ordinator and is also involved in teaching in both the undergraduate and post-graduate programmes, which include community nursing and research in practice. As part of the Erasmus exchange programme she has been involved in the delivery of the International Community Nursing/Community Assessment (Global Health) module in Mikkelin University, Finland. Catherine works in collaboration with her colleagues to promote research-focused teaching and she has had the opportunity to present areas of her work in journal publications and at conferences.

Clare Morfoot

Neonatal Clinical Practice Educator, Trevor Mann Baby Unit, Royal Sussex County Hospital, Brighton: PgCert, ENB 405, BSc (Hons), RN & Dip Nursing Studies

Clare completed a degree in anatomy and developmental biology at University College London, before undertaking her nurse training at St Bartholomew's Hospital in London and has worked in adult oncology prior to specialising in neonatology for the last 11 years. Currently Clare works on a neonatal intensive care unit, delivering medical and surgical nursing care to premature and sick infants and their families. As the clinical practice educator, Clare facilitates the professional development and education of neonatal nursing staff. Having successfully completed her post-graduate Certificate in Health and Social Care Education, Clare also teaches pre- and post-registration nurses at the School of Nursing and Midwifery, University of Brighton.

Breige Morgan
Children's Discharge & Transition Coordinator SHSCT & Acting Senior Community Children's Nurse SHSCT: BSc (Hons) CCN & RN (Child Dip)

Breige was a registered children's nurse and worked in numerous settings, including a general paediatric ward gaining both medical/surgical experience, the regional paediatric intensive care unit and the children's hospice, which enhanced her experience of caring for children with palliative needs. She then moved to the ENT setting as a charge nurse. In June 2004 she took up a post as a community children's nurse and was instrumental in establishing the new community children's nursing service in the locality. In September 2009 she took up post as the Discharge & Transition Co-ordinator and was influential at a regional level to improve services for children with complex healthcare needs.

Philomena Morrow
Nurse Lecturer in Children's Nursing, School of Nursing & Midwifery, Queen's University Belfast, Northern Ireland: MSc & BSc in Nursing

Philomena undertook a four-year integrated nursing course to gain registration as an adult and children's nurse. Following a clinical career she entered nurse education initially as a clinical teacher and then a nurse tutor. At integration into Queen's University Belfast in 1997 Philomena became engaged in developing pre- and post-education for children's nursing. Her interests include cardiology, respiratory care, diabetic and burns/plastic surgery in children and publications relate to subject areas. Philomena has been involved in leading and developing IPE within children's nursing and medical education.

Kathryn O'Hara
Staff Nurse, Craig Ward, Ulster Hospital, Dundonald, Northern Ireland: PG Dip Organisation Management, PG Certificate Nurse Education, BSc (Hons) Nursing, RGN & RSCN

Kathryn is currently a staff nurse on a children's surgical ward specialising in ENT, plastics, maxillofacial and orthopaedic surgery. The ward has a five-bedded unit for adolescents. She is both adult and children trained and has spent more than twenty years nursing sick children and their families, mainly in the acute medical and surgical setting. She has worked as a ward sister and taught for one year in Our Lady's Hospital for Sick Children, Dublin, implementing the nursing process into all wards and departments and teaching undergraduate student nurses. She worked for six years as a patient advocate for the Eastern Health and Social Services Council, advocating for patients and their carers in all trusts throughout the Eastern Health and Social Services Board. Kathryn does occasional lecturing to undergraduate student nurses (children's branch) at Queen's University, Belfast.

Catherine Paxton
Nutrition Nurse Specialist, Royal Hospital for Sick Children, Edinburgh: BN, RN (Child Health), ENB N15, DipHE Nursing & RGN

Catherine graduated from Glasgow University with a Bachelor of Nursing degree and RGN qualification in 1994. After working in adult orthopaedics in Cambridge she moved to Edinburgh to do her paediatric training at Lothian College of Health Studies. While staffing on a general surgical, GI and ENT ward, at the Royal Hospital for Sick Children

Edinburgh, she developed her interest in complex nutrition. She was appointed Paediatric Nutrition Nurse Specialist in 2003. As a member of the multidisciplinary nutrition support team, she provides care, advice and support to children requiring enteral and parenteral nutrition, and their families. She has presented locally and nationally on enteral feeding tubes and been on the review group for both the Lothian Enteral Tube Feeding Best Practice Statement for Adults and Children and the NHS, and also Quality Improvement Scotland Best Practice Statement, Caring for Children and Young People in the Community Receiving Enteral Tube Feeding.

Jim Richardson
Head of Division (Family Care), Faculty of Health, Sport & Science, University of Glamorgan, Pontypridd, Wales: PhD, PGCE, RSCN, RGN & BA

Jim undertook a Bachelor of Arts (Humanities) at the University of Strathclyde, Glasgow, before completing general nurse training in Aberdeen, Scotland. He then worked in neurology, anaesthetics and paediatrics at the Oulu University Central Hospital in Finland for a period of eight years. He obtained a specialist paediatric nursing qualification from Great Ormond Street Hospital in London and took up the position of head nurse in the paediatric medical unit at the University Hospital of Wales in Cardiff.Jim took up the post of lecturer in children's nursing at the University of Wales College of Medicine in Cardiff, a post he occupied for nine years. He was also awarded a PhD during this period. He took a position in 1999 at the University of Glamorgan as Principal Lecturer in Children's Nursing and a year later took the role of Field Leader (Head of Division) of Family Care. This division encompasses all aspects of educational provision and research in the field of maternal and child health within the faculty. Jim has a role within the faculty to promote international activity and has participated in work with the World Health Organisation. Current activity includes working with Bulgarian colleagues to establish a nursing workforce development unit in Bulgaria. This has involved collaboration with a wide range of agencies and individuals, including the Ministry of Health, in Bulgaria.

Debbie Rickard
Child Health Nurse Practitioner Candidate, Capital & Coast District Health Board Wellington, New Zealand: MN (Child & Family, Hons), Cert in Community Child Health, Cert in Allergy Nursing, BN & RN (comp)

Debbie has been nursing in child health for 18 years. After three years in acute paediatric nursing, a clinical move to the community setting provided Debbie with many opportunities to evolve her specialist paediatric practice. Over the last ten years Debbie has also held a management role in the paediatric community team service. However, the management focus has recently changed, with Debbie becoming the first Nurse Practitioner Candidate in Child Health and this role has a DHB wide focus. Debbie's interest in working with children and their families, especially those living with chronic and/or complex conditions, is to support their empowerment to meet care needs. Her interest has lead to improved nursing services for managing complex skin conditions. Debbie's work began after gaining a Margaret May Blackwell Travel Study Fellowship award to visit child health services in the United Kingdom and Australia in 1999. This experience helped consolidate her vision for improved outcomes for children and families through proactive nursing services. The success of increased community services lead to starting the first Nurse Eczema Clinics in New Zealand. Fourteen years later clinics held at all the hospitals in the Wellington region and in outreach clinics held with Maori and Pacific Services are meeting the population needs. In addition, practice nurses who have undertaken training with Debbie now provide nurse eczema services within their primary health practices. Wellington provides the most comprehensive nurse eczema service in New Zealand. Debbie provides teaching, training and ongoing professional support in optimal eczema management to doctors and nurses working in the secondary and primary health sector and this has enabled a more consistent and collaborative approach to care. Since 2002, Debbie has actively been involved in childhood eczema research projects.

Karen Salmon

HIV/AIDS Programme Director, Crosslinks' Mission Partner, Mekelle Youth Centre, Mekelle, Ethiopia: MSc in Nursing, Health Visitor & RGN

Karen has both adult and public health training, worked in community health in West Belfast for five years, and in nurse education in Ethiopia over ten years, before accepting her current position in 2004. Teaching commitments focus on prevention through formal and informal HIV/AIDS awareness classes and clubs, peer education and training of trainers. HIV/AIDS care is implemented among orphans and prisoners living with HIV. As programme director Karen works with children and youth of all backgrounds, with special involvement among vulnerable children, including orphans, blind and deaf children, and youth.

Susanne Simmons

Senior Lecturer, University of Brighton: MSc Nursing Research and Practice Development: BSc (Hons) (Open) Applied Social Sciences, RNT, ENB 405, RSCN & RGN

Susanne is qualified in children's and adult nursing, specialising in neonatal surgery and medicine. Following three years as a lecturer/practitioner, she became a full-time senior lecturer in 2000. During her time in education, Susanne has had experience co-ordinating the child branch diploma programme, second registration (child) programme and neonatal pathway. Teaching commitments include: pre-registration teaching of clinical skills to child diploma and degree students; and post-registration teaching on the neonatal pathway. Susanne endeavours to maintain links with clinical practice and is committed to facilitating service user engagement and interprofessional learning within the curriculum.

Rosi Simpson

Paediatric Renal Nurse, Royal Belfast Hospital for Sick Children, Northern Ireland: RSCN, ENB 147 & RGN

Rosi trained in both adult and children's nursing at the Ulster Hospital, Dundonald. After working in the Isle of Man, she returned initially to work in the regional cardiac surgery intensive care unit, before moving to the Royal Belfast Hospital for Sick Children. She completed her ENB 147 Paediatric Nephro-urology course at the University of Central England and Birmingham Children's Hospital before taking up her current position. Her role includes providing clinical care for pre-dialysis, dialysis and post-transplant children and families, supporting the role of renal nurse co-ordinator, and is involved in parental teaching programmes and in-house training. She is also secretary of the Paediatric Irish Nephrology Nurse's Group, liaising with and standardising renal nursing care between paediatric renal units in the North and South of Ireland.

Acknowledgements

The editors would like to express their appreciation to the contributing authors and publishers for their kind permission to reproduce photographs and copyright material. Thanks also to Paul Morris and Kevin Campbell, clinical skills technicians, School of Nursing and Midwifery, Queen's University Belfast for their photographic support.

Every effort will have been made to contact all copyright holders. However, if any have inadvertently been omitted the contributing authors/editors or publishers will be pleased to make the necessary arrangements at the earliest opportunity.

Section 1

Principles of Care Planning

1

The Nature of Care Planning and Nursing Delivery for Infants, Children and Young People

Doris Corkin and Pauline Cardwell (contribution from Lisa Hughes)

Introduction

As a healthcare professional caring for children, young people and their families we are accountable for our individual practice. Therefore we must strive to deliver high quality care, acknowledging evidence-based practice and recognising finite resources within contemporary healthcare systems. In order to achieve success, care planning and delivery of individualised care must encompass multiprofessional collaboration, involving service users and carers as essential contributors to the overall process.

Within this introductory chapter the children's nurse will be provided with an overview of the nursing process, its components and how these assist in organising and prioritising care delivery to the child and family. Philosophical perspectives of care will also be discussed and how this impacts on care delivery in the clinical setting. In conjunction with these aspects of care planning, several models of nursing will be explored, and their contribution in the planning and delivery of care will be illustrated within the scenarios in the second section of this book.

Nursing process – what is the nursing process?

The nursing process is a logical, structured approach, which promotes the nurse's critical thinking in a dynamic manner. This process is used to identify and deliver individualised family-centred care, supported by nursing models and philosophies. Yura and Walsh (1978) identified this process, consisting of four interrelated stages (see Figure 1.1):

Care Planning in Children and Young People's Nursing, First Edition.
Edited by Doris Corkin, Sonya Clarke, Lorna Liggett.
© 2012 Blackwell Publishing Ltd. Published 2012 by Blackwell Publishing Ltd.

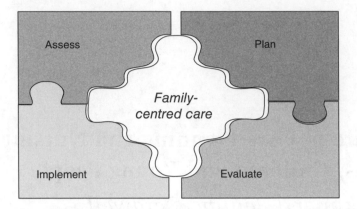

Figure 1.1   The nursing process.

- Assess
- Plan
- Implement
- Evaluate

More recently, Castledine (2011) has acknowledged the evolvement of the nursing process to be a methodical way of thinking that guides care delivery; whilst focusing on the patient the nurse should base best practice on available evidence with artistic interpretation.

More recently, however, this process has sometimes included a fifth stage relating to 'nursing diagnosis'. For example, a six-week-old infant has been brought to the hospital with a history of breathlessness and poor colour, especially during feeds, who tires easily and poor weight gain has been noted. Upon examination, heart rate and respiratory rate are both increased and this may lead the nurse to consider a possible cardiac related diagnosis. In utilising the nursing process a problem-solving approach is applied to the management of individualised patient care. The application of the process is continuous and cyclical in nature and commences with the assessment stage.

Assessment

This important stage of the care planning process aims to collect and record information pertaining to the health status of the individual child and its effect on the family unit. This phase of the nursing process should provide a comprehensive insight into the needs of the child and their impact on the integrity of the family. The children's nurse must consider not only the physical needs of the child but address the social, emotional and spiritual needs of the child and entire family. In order to achieve a comprehensive assessment the children's nurse must utilise a range of proficiencies, including theoretical knowledge and interpersonal skills. Matousova-Done and Gates (2006) highlight the need to both observe and listen to the child and family, utilising verbal and non-verbal communication with the use of appropriate questioning skills to ensure an accurate nursing assessment.

A precise and comprehensive assessment is vital to identify the problems which are currently encroaching on the child's health status and ultimately will ensure safe, effective and efficient nursing care for the child. This stage of the process links closely with the discrete fifth stage identified earlier as nursing diagnosis, which is supported by an accurate and comprehensive assessment of the child's health needs. During the assessment stage the children's nurse is also involved in analysing and interpreting the information collected, thus contributing to the formulation of a care plan.

A very good example of assessment is the ABCDE (airway, breathing, circulation, disability, exposure) systematic approach to assessing the acutely ill child, as recommended by Dieckmann *et al.* (2000) and the Resuscitation Council UK (2005). This approach aims to enable healthcare staff to recognise when they need additional support from the interprofessional team (see Chapter 8). Furthermore, this systematic process helps guide the healthcare professional in planning the frequency of ongoing assessment, especially in the paediatric intensive care setting (see Chapter 16).

Planning

During the essential second stage of the process, a plan of care is developed aimed at addressing the problems identified in the assessment phase. This phase of the process involves cognitive and written elements in identifying goals to meet the child's needs. The children's nurse develops mutually agreed goals which endeavour to address the child's problems through the provision of nursing care. These goals are then further developed within the plan, in a sequence of interventions aimed at resolving, controlling or preventing escalation of the problem. In creating these goals, Wright (2005) proposes they should be SMART: specific, measurable, achievable/agreed, realistic and time-limited. The care plan is developed to guide the nursing interventions in a timely manner to meet the needs of the child and family.

The children's nurse must be able to clearly articulate and document priorities of care, tailored to meeting the individual needs of the child and family, and easily understood by all members of the interdisciplinary team.

Effective communication with the child and family are integral to this stage of the nursing process, as the children's nurse must work collaboratively to ensure the care plan is dynamic in meeting the needs of the child and family. In developing the care plan the children's nurse must engage in developing a partnership with the child and family in which they are active partners in the decision-making processes and their involvement in care provision is recognised. This partnership requires empowerment and negotiated involvement of the child and family, which requires skilled children's nurses who are able to ensure children and their families are at the centre of effective care planning (Corlett & Twycross 2006). Having identified, agreed and set short and long-term goals specific to the child's needs, these must be regularly evaluated during implementation to ensure they remain responsive to the individual's requirements.

Implementation

This penultimate stage of the nursing process relates to the delivery of care, which has been planned based on the needs of the child and family. Nursing interventions should aim to achieve the goals identified in the care plan and these should clearly identify the actions to be undertaken by the children's nurse. The children's nurse must possess the knowledge, skills and abilities to deliver the care to the child and assess the appropriateness of planned interventions (Alfaro-LeFevre 2006). Effective communication with the child and family is central to the success of implementing the care plan, which may require adjustment in response to changing needs.

The cooperation and involvement of the child and family is a pre-requisite in this phase of the nursing process. Children and their families must be given choices and involved in decisions regarding nursing interventions, and their participation will personalise their own care implementation. All goals set must be clear and agreed by the child, family and other carers, including health professionals. Identifiable goals should be achievable, within a realistic timeframe for those involved in care delivery, whilst recognising their continued appropriateness for the child.

Evaluation

The fourth and final stage of the nursing process, requires the children's nurse to consider the impact of the preceding three stages on the child's care trajectory. However, it is essential that the children's nurse continually evaluates the child's response to interventions and modifies planned care to meet the individual's needs and their response to previously identified goals. Overall, this evaluation process aims to recognise changes in the child's condition and identify the need for modification. Analysis of the care delivered by the children's nurse requires critical thinking in order to consider its effectiveness and other possible required interventions to meet the changing needs of the child. The frequency of evaluation may vary depending on the acuity of the child's condition.

This evaluative stage of the nursing process links closely with the assessment phase of the cycle, assessing the attainment of previously identified priorities of care and goals (Heath 2005). Documentation and reporting in this phase of the nursing process is critical in accurately measuring and recording the child's response to planned interventions and to support the continuity of care delivery. Furthermore, this assists in information sharing between healthcare professionals and identification of progress towards goal attainment and also the continued relevance of previously identified goals.

Nursing diagnoses

The North American Nursing Diagnosis Association (NANDA International) is the clearing house for nursing diagnosis work both within the United States of America and internationally (Carpenito-Moyet 2010). This association was initially established in 1973, and later recognised worldwide as NANDA-I in 1982 and is committed to developing the nursing contribution to patient care through 'nursing diagnoses' which informs the creation of care plans (NANDA International 2008). Those care plans approved by NANDA International are rigorously tested and refined in line with current best practice and evidence-based guidelines in clinical settings. Within the NANDA International system, five levels of nursing diagnoses are identified:

- Actual
- Risk
- Possible
- Syndrome
- Wellness

What is a nursing diagnosis?

This is a professional judgement relating to the health problems of the individual or family, which is used to identify appropriate goals and interventions in nursing plans of care, based on a holistic nursing assessment (see Chapter 34).

Nursing Process in Practice

Overall, this nursing process provides a flexible framework to organise and deliver care of a high standard to the child and family in a holistic manner (NMC 2008). This facilitates recognition of the individual's contribution, their consent to care, whilst acknowledging organisational quality initiatives, such as policies, procedures and clinical audit (Holland et al. 2008). This nursing process framework assists the children's nurse in documenting care assessment, planning, implementation and evaluation, whilst recognising the legal responsibility and professional accountability aspects of accurate record keeping.

In order to apply the nursing process, the children's nurse requires knowledge, skills and attributes which will only develop over time with practice and experience. Therefore, the nursing student will initially require direct supervision and mentor support (see Chapter 9) in applying the nursing process to their clinical practice, ensuring care planning and delivery is safe, competent and effective in meeting the child and family's needs (NMC 2010).

Planning of care – what is a care plan?

A care plan is a comprehensive record (handwritten, pre-printed or electronic) of essential information which is created following discussions between the child, family and the children's nurse, detailing priorities of care aimed at meeting the individual's needs. This record consists of a table featuring problem identification, patient goals and nursing intervention, alongside day-to-day living activities affected (see Appendix 1). This is a legal document which is managed and stored in accordance with legislative and professional guidelines, whilst still being accessible to the individual patient and other healthcare professionals with responsibility for care delivery, whether in the hospital or community setting (NMC 2009).

Activity 1.1

Look at these practice-based questions.

1. Identify which care planning documentation is currently being used in your clinical placement:
   (a) Hospital
   (b) Community

2. Discuss with your clinical mentor which nursing model is being utilised to support care delivery:
   (a) Has the model been adapted for children's nursing?
   (b) How does the model ensure individualised care of the child and family?

In addition to the framework provided by the nursing process, care plans are normally developed with the support of a nursing model, which assists in managing and enhancing effective, high quality care delivery. The development of nursing models attempts to link nursing theory to clinical practice and indirectly informs the growing body of nursing knowledge. Various models of nursing are available and utilised, for example Roper, Logan and Tierney (1985), Casey (1988; 1995), Mead (McClune & Franklin 1987), Orem (1995) and Neuman's system model (Neuman & Fawcett 2002), as well as chapters within this book that demonstrate the application of these models to clinical practice. These models are flexible structures that can be easily adapted to incorporate elements from other models in order to address individual care needs, encouraging the children's nurse to think creatively about the holistic care of the infant, child or young person and their family.

Increasingly, evidence-based practice is advocated globally as effectively delivering quality care, and thus must be integrated within care plans for the individual (Parsley & Corrigan 1999). The children's nurse must be able to appraise nursing research critically and use this up-to-date knowledge to underpin their clinical judgement and practice, and promote efficiency within healthcare systems. Whilst aiming to provide contemporary high quality care, the children's nurse should reflect upon his/her knowledge and experiential learning, which are key requisites to ensuring best practice as identified in professional regulatory guidelines (NMC 2008).

The nursing care plan is also supportive of engaging and sustaining interdisciplinary collaboration with the child, family and other health professionals involved in their care. Children's nurses do not work in isolation, instead care delivery is organised around a team approach and in collaboration with other members of the multiprofessional team. More recently, integrated care pathways have evolved, supporting the development of a multiprofessional document, to which the nursing care plan is integral. These multiprofessional documents are supported by clinical governance and quality agendas within healthcare organisations in delivering effective outcomes (DH 1998).

✎ Activity 1.2

Using the template below, identify concepts related to care planning. We have given you some ideas for the first letter of each word.

Child-centred care

A_____

R_____

E_____

Process guided by model(s) of care

L_____

A_____

N_____

Philosophy of care

This aspect of professional practice relates to the expectation of service users and nursing staff in a particular clinical environment of how care and services will be organised and delivered. A philosophy of care helps nurses to define their role and guide practice, within a growing diversity of roles in the clinical environment. Children's nursing, as a distinct field of practice, may relate to a philosophy of care that recognises the individuality of each child and their family, understanding their unique needs in relation to healthcare provision and ensuring their involvement in decisions about their care. The child's needs must be paramount, whether physical, psychological, social, cultural or spiritual, as well as those of their family, and these should be embedded in the philosophy of care within the clinical environment (RCN 2003).

Activity 1.3

Seek out the philosophy of care in your clinical placement:

* Enquire from ward manager how this ward philosophy was created.
* Does it identify what children and their families can expect from the service?

What are nursing models?

Nursing models, which are also known as grand theories, attempt to illustrate the theory of nursing practice and facilitate the children's nurse to organise and deliver care. When applied to practice these models of care influence the performance of the nurse and the experience for the child and family (McGee 1998; Pearson *et al.* 2005). The construction and application of nursing models support the development of nursing practice, whilst recognising the values, beliefs and culture of the individual and the changing clinical environment.

Since early work by Fawcett in 1984, numerous nursing models identify the four components of a model as:

* The person
* Their environment
* Health
* Nursing

Care is organised and delivered around identified deficits relating to these components. The development of nursing models, aims to enhance the delivery of family-centred care whilst facilitating the experienced children's nurse to practice autonomously. Through engagement with the child and family the children's nurse is able to identify needs and create a plan of care for the individual and their family, when employing the nursing process in conjunction with a model/s of care.

Table 1.1   An adaptation of the Roper, Logan and Tierney Model of Nursing (1985).

1. Maintaining a safe environment	2. Communication	3. Breathing	4. Eating and drinking
• Risk management • Medications • Infectious diseases	• Difficulties with hearing, sight or speech • Cognitive disability • Interpreter services required	• Respiratory problems • Cardiac conditions • Compromised airway	• Special diets • Alternative feeding methods • Swallowing difficulties
5. Elimination	6. Personal cleansing and dressing	7. Controlling body temperature	8. Mobilising
• Altered function of bowel/bladder • Infections • Structural anomalies	• Level of dependence • Skin integrity • Personal preferences	• Abnormal body temperature • Regulatory disorders • Environmental factors	• Level of independence • Mobilising disabilities • Use of aids
9. Working and playing	10. Expressing sexuality	11. Sleeping	12. Dying
• Relevant to age • Effects of hospitalisation/illness • Hobbies/interests	• Stage of development • Altered body image • Sexual preferences	• Altered sleep patterns • Sleeping aids • Environmental factors	• Relevance to illness • Fear of dying • Spiritual needs

Roper, Logan and Tierney – the 12 activities of living model

This conceptual model of nursing was devised by three United Kingdom-based nurses and is widely recognised both nationally and internationally. The model is practice orientated whilst incorporating a theoretical framework for care delivery. The model relates to the lifespan of the individual, identifying twelve activities of living (see Table 1.1), which are considered in relation to the continuum of dependence to independence throughout life, appreciating aspects of age, environment and circumstances which may impinge on this continuum. Each activity of living is influenced by five identified factors, which are biological, psychological, socio-cultural, environmental and politico-economic (Roper *et al.* 1985). This model is used in conjunction with the nursing process to identify actual and potential problems for the individual and how nursing care can advance the patient along the dependence to independence continuum. This model of care will be utilised in subsequent chapters such as Chapter 22, illustrating its application in care planning.

Family-centred care

Child and family-centred care has become a central tenet of children's nursing and other health professionals' practice, it is viewed as a multifaceted concept that has evolved over the last 60 years (Coleman 2010). Various attributes of family-centred care are identified in the nursing literature, and include collaborative working, partnerships, respect and involvement of family, negotiation, empowerment/engagement and provision of a family friendly environment (see Figure 1.2). Whilst there is no clear definition, this concept of family-centred care (FCC) has continued to grow and develop a body of evidence to support its utilisation in contemporary children's nursing practice, since the earlier work of Casey (1988, 1995). The evolvement of the concept FCC and its theoretical underpinnings can be sourced in early work by psychologists Bowlby (1953) and Robertson (1958) who recognised the damaging effects of maternal deprivation and separation caused by hospitalisation, on

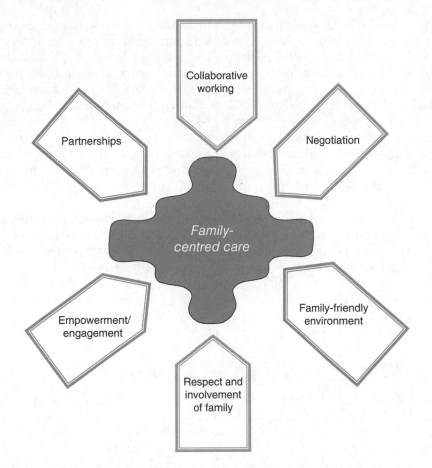

Figure 1.2   Attributes of family-centred care.

children. These important findings were later endorsed and supported in the findings and recommendations presented by the Platt Report (Ministry of Health 1959).

The development of a national association by parents in 1961 (National Association for the Welfare of Sick Children in Hospital (NAWCH): http://www.nch.org.uk/ourservices/index) gave parents a voice to demand services which recognised them as central caregivers to their children. This further supported and challenged the need for healthcare delivery for children and their families, to change from a medically dominated service to a service responsive to the needs of children and their families, which provided facilities for parents to remain with their hospitalised child. Recognising and supporting the family as central care providers alongside children's nurses, requires respect for the integrity of the family unit, whatever its structure, with the provision of services which are responsive to the needs of the child and family (United Nations (UN) 1989; Department of Health (DH) 2003). The notion of children, families and children's nurses as partners in care delivery is integral to achieving the best plan of care and promotes functioning at the highest possible level (Gance-Cleveland 2006). Indeed, Shields *et al.* (2006) suggest FCC aims to plan and deliver care not just to the child but to the family as a whole, and all family members are recognised as care recipients.

Governmental policies have identified the importance of involving parents in the care of their children and identified this as a major theme in the development of services (Audit Commission 1993; DH 1991; 1996). Further progress has led to the demand for service users, including parents and children, to have a greater voice in shaping future services as identified in more recent literature (DHPSSPS 2005; Noyes 2000). Conversely, Bradshaw *et al.* (2000/2001) suggest delivering FCC is challenging and demanding, requiring the children's nurse to possess a range of complex skills to ensure its implementation in practice is effective, whilst proposing the theory of FCC has advanced ahead of clinical practice to the detriment of its operationalisation. The lack of a nursing model to support the implementation of this concept in children's nursing is identified by Coleman (2002) as a contributory factor in the difficult translation of the concept from theory to clinical practice.

The lack of involvement of children and their families in the decision-making process regarding their care provision, as perceived by children and their parents, has been identified within nursing literature (Kawik 1996; Noyes 2000). To address this issue children's nursing must relinquish power in relation to the service they provide and embrace parents as partners in care provision, through the recognition of children and their parents as service users (Cardwell 2006). Their involvement in the design and development of services to meet their individual needs is vital in ensuring an equitable service irrespective of regional, cultural or socio-economical status.

The Mead model

This model was developed for the intensive care setting and for practical use at the bedside. Mead's framework was adapted from the Roper *et al.* (1985) nursing model, with which it shares some of its attributes. In addition to knowledge and experience of the intensive care environment, the nurse must be familiar with Roper's model, to ensure care planned is delivered in an effective manner. This adapted model identifies the individuality, lifespan (age), dependence/independence and needs of the patient as the aspects to be assessed when planning care. Factors which impact on the health and wellbeing of the individual are similar to those identified by Roper *et al.*, namely physical, psychological, environmental, socio-cultural and politico-economical. Additionally, within the dependent/independent continuum on the nurse, Mead (McClune and Franklin 1987) identifies five stages:

1. Total dependence
2. Intervention
3. Intervention with some prevention
4. Prevention
5. Total independence

Each patient is continuously evaluated within the continuum in relation to the five factors highlighted above, identifying appropriate goals for the patient and progression towards independence, with cognisance of the patient's lifespan position. In conjunction with the nursing process the nurse is able to devise a plan of care unique to the needs of the individual patient. In devising a care plan, physical care needs are subdivided into elements specific to the intensive care environment. These include: respiratory, cardiovascular, pain sedation, neurology, nutrition, elimination, skin care, mobility, psychological and social/cultural and circumstantial (Viney 1996). To illustrate the

Table 1.2   Stages on the neurology dependence/independence continuum.

Criteria for stages on neurology continuum
1. Unstable neurological state, requiring continuous monitoring.
2. Potentially unstable neurological state, requiring frequent monitoring.
3. Potentially unstable neurological state, requiring monitoring.
4. Stable neurological state, requiring monitoring to detect/prevent deterioration.
5. No assistance required to maintain neurological state.

Table 1.3   Self-care requisites (Orem 1995).

Universal self-care requisites

Universal self-care requisites are associated with the maintenance of human functioning and serve as a framework for assessment (Cutliff *et al.* 2010):

- The maintenance of a sufficient intake of air.
- The maintenance of a sufficient intake of water.
- The maintenance of a sufficient intake of food.
- The provision of care associated with elimination processes and excrements.
- The maintenance of a balance between activity and rest.
- The maintenance of a balance between solitude and social interaction.
- The prevention of hazards to human life, human functioning and human wellbeing.
- The promotion of human functioning and development within social groups in accordance with human potential, known human limitations and the human desire to be 'normal'. Orem calls this 'normalcy' (see Chapter 21).

Developmental self-care requisites

Developmental self-care requisites are related to developmental processes throughout the life cycle and can include physical, social or psychological changes, i.e. adolescence or social life changes such as bereavement.

Health deviation self-care requisites

Arise out of ill health or injury and are associated with the effect and changes of disease or trauma on the individual.

stages on the dependence/independence continuum, which are relevant to the neurology element as identified in the Mead model, see Table 1.2 which is linked to care planning in Chapter 16.

Orem's self-care model

The self-care model of nursing was developed by Dorothea Orem (between 1959 and 2001) with the aim of helping the patient and family achieve self-care (Walsh 1998). The Orem model is based on the premise that individuals have self-care needs which they themselves have an ability and right to meet except when their ability to do so has been compromised (Pearson *et al.* 2005). When undertaking a comprehensive assessment this self-care model identifies what care the patient or family can do for themselves (Nevin *et al.* 2010). The model has three key concepts: self-care, self-care deficit and nursing systems. Self-care concerns the various activities individuals carry out on their own behalf in maintaining life, health and wellbeing, which Orem (1995) categorises as universal self-care requisites, developmental self-care requisites and health deviation self-care requisites (Table 1.3), and also identifies actions for meeting the universal self-care requisites. According to Orem the person best placed to meet these requisites is the individual themselves, whom she calls the self-care agent. In the case of an infant and child this would be the parents; Orem calls this dependent care (Orem 1995). When in an individual or, in the case of a child, a parent the demand for self-care is greater than the individual or parent's ability to meet it then a self-care deficit occurs and nursing may then be required.

Orem (1991) identifies four goals of nursing:

- Reducing the self-care demand to a level whereby the individual or parent is able to meet the demand independently.
- Increasing the individual or parent's capacity or ability to meet the demand independently.
- Enabling the individual or parents (or significant others) to give dependent care when self-care is impossible for the individual or parent.
- The nurse meets the individual or parent's self-care demand directly.

Orem (1995) also refers to the role of the nurse within nursing systems, which are carried out on one of three levels:

- Total compensatory system – the nurse provides all the patient care.
- Partial compensatory system – nurse assists with care of patient.
- Educative/supportive system – patient has control over their health.

Although the children's nurse may find this self-care theory process time consuming, the overall aim is that the young person or parent is able to meet most of their needs with supportive education. Therefore the nurse's role is one of teaching and supporting in order to meet the self-care need.

Activity 1.4

To read more on Orem's self-care model, please review the following texts:
Cutliff, J., McKenna, H. & Hyrkas, K. (2010) *Nursing Models: Application to Practice*. London: Quay Books.
Pearson, A., Vaughan, B. & FitzGerald, M. (2005) *Nursing Models for Practice*, 3rd edn. Edinburgh: Elsevier.

Neuman's systems model

Betty Neuman, an American nurse devised this theoretical model of nursing which places great emphasis on prevention (primary, secondary and tertiary), interventions and a systems approach to holistic wellness (Neuman & Young 1972). The overall focus of this model is the total wellness of the person in attaining and maintaining health to a maximum level. Neuman's model identifies three types of stressors (intrapersonal, interpersonal and extrapersonal) that act on five individual variables, namely physiological, psychological, socio-cultural, spiritual and developmental aspects, which interrelate with each other. This model is easily adapted to the community setting where the wider contextual (environmental) factors affecting individual health need consideration, and are fundamental to service provision. When used in conjunction with the nursing process this model aims to support the stability of the person. For further discussion please see Chapter 17.

Summary

This chapter has attempted to outline some of the nursing models in contemporary practice within children's nursing, which will be applied to clinically based care planning scenarios within this book. These nursing models have been summarised in Chapters 1–10 and then analysed within care planning scenarios (Chapters 12–37) with emphasis on assessing the individual needs of infants, children and young people. The children's nurse has also been introduced to several reflective activities. An appreciation of other nursing models such as the Nottingham model (Smith 1995) and its application in clinical practice is also encouraged, to help enhance knowledge and understanding of care planning.

Care of the child and family during illness: student perspective

Scenario

Oliver Love (a pseudonym), aged four months, was taken this afternoon to his GP by his parents with a history of being unwell for the past 24 hours with a troublesome cough and difficulty with breathing. The GP diagnosed Oliver as suffering from croup, so he was quickly referred to the children's medical ward for admission and further management. On arrival at hospital, Oliver was accompanied by his six-year-old sister and anxious parents. Whilst establishing Oliver's clinical observations the children's nurse noted sudden deterioration in his condition.

Proposed care plan

Using the care plan sheets provided, *two* key activities of living (A/L) requiring *immediate* attention were selected by the nursing student and goals identified. A plan of care for Oliver and his family was constructed, supported with rationale, relating to the nursing process and Roper *et al.* (1985) model of nursing, incorporating a family-centred approach to care and reference to literature.

Sample care plan

Child's Name: Oliver Love   DOB: 8 December 2010

continued

Date and time	A/L No	Potential/ actual problems	Nursing objectives/ outcomes/ goals	Nursing care plan (actions with rationale)	Review dates	Nurse's signature
9/12/2011 16.00hrs	No.3	Oliver has been admitted to the ward with a troublesome cough and difficulty with his breathing – differential diagnosis is croup.	Ensure Oliver is nursed safely and effectively to maintain patency of his airway, relieve cough and return breathing pattern to within normal limits.	Approach Oliver and his family in a calm and friendly manner; introduce them to the ward, try to reassure parents and keep them informed. Nurse Oliver upright, prop with pillows to increase his lung capacity and beside working oxygen and suction in case of an emergency situation. If Oliver is unsettled his mum may nurse him on her lap, though handling should be avoided. Use the ABC approach (Resuscitation Council UK 2010). Assess Oliver's respiratory function – initially assess patency of his airway using look, listen and feel approach; gently check for any obstruction or signs of inflammation and distress. Next assess Oliver's breathing – record and monitor his respiratory rate, rhythm and depth of breaths; note respiratory effort, e.g. if indrawing, nasal flaring or tracheal tug. Important to assess Oliver's cough, recording frequency and effects it has on Oliver's breathing (Holland et al. 2008).		Std Nurse L. Hughes

Date/time	No.	Problem	Goal	Nursing action	Signature
				Check Oliver's oxygen saturations – if less than 92% consult doctor and administer humidified oxygen at a rate of 5 litres per minute initially, record response and adjust accordingly (BNFC 2010–2011).	Std Nurse L. Hughes
				Assess Oliver's circulation – check and monitor his capillary refill time. Note any signs of cyanosis, e.g. mottled skin appearance and check body temperature. Record and report accordingly (NMC 2008).	
				Administer medication (e.g. adrenaline or steriod via nebuliser) as prescribed by doctor and as per ward policy – check against six rights of administration (Olsen *et al.* 2010) and medicine guidelines.	Std Nurse L. Hughes
				Carry out oral and nasal hygiene as and when required – should Oliver produce secretions obtain a specimen and send to laboratory for culture and sensitivity.	
9/12/2011 16.00hrs	No.2	Oliver's parents are very anxious about his condition.	Ensure Oliver's parents are well informed about his condition, in order to reduce their fears and anxieties.	Welcome Oliver and his parents to the ward. Introduce Oliver and his parents to their primary nurse who will show them the facilities available and inform them of visiting times for extended family.	Std Nurse L. Hughes
				Accompany doctor when he explains to parents the effects croup will have on Oliver and be aware that his parents may want answers to questions.	

Date and time	A/L No	Potential/ actual problems	Nursing objectives/ outcomes/ goals	Nursing care plan (actions with rationale)	Review dates	Nurse's signature
				Provide Oliver's parents with both written and verbal information on croup – encourage parents to participate in Oliver's care. Establish a therapeutic relationship with Oliver and his parents, work in partnership to help meet holistic needs (Casey 1995). Oliver is in the sensorimotor stage of development, so the children's nurse needs to be aware of his needs throughout hospitalisation (Bee & Boyd 2007). Contact play therapist who can provide suitable toys for Oliver during his stay in hospital. Complete a detailed history from Oliver's parents, in order to accurately assess and develop a plan of care and aid diagnosis.		Std Nurse L. Hughes

Care plan by second year Child branch Nursing Student, Lisa Hughes.

References

Alfaro-LeFevre, R. (2006) *Applying Nursing Process – a Tool for Critical Thinking*, 6th edn. Philadelphia: Lippincott Williams and Wilkins.

Audit Commission (1993) *Children First: a Study of Hospital Services*. London: HMSO.

Bee, H. & Boyd, D. (2007) *The Developing Child*, 11th edn. Boston: Allyn and Bacon.

BNF for Children (2010–2011) *BNF for Children*. London: BMJ Publishing Group.

Bowlby, J. (1953) *Child Care and the Growth of Love*. Harmondsworth: Penguin.

Bradshaw, M., Coleman, V., Cutts, S., Guest, C. & Twigg, J. (2000/2001) Family-centred care: A step too far? *Paediatric Nursing*, **12**(10), 6–7.

Cardwell, P.B.M. (2006) *Family-Centred Care: the Northern Ireland Experience*. Unpublished MSc dissertation.

Carpenito-Moyet, L.J. (2010) *Nursing Diagnosis: Application to Clinical Practice*, 13th edn. Philadelphia: Wolters Kluwer/Lippincott Williams & Wilkins.

Casey, A. (1988) A partnership with child and family. *Senior Nurse*, **8**(4), 8–9.

Casey, A. (1995) Partnership nursing: Influences on involvement of informal carers. *Journal of Advanced Nursing*, **22**, 1058–62.

Castledine, G. (2011) Updating the nursing process. *British Journal of Nursing*, **20**(2), 131.

Coleman, V. (2002) The evolving concept of family-centred care, Chapter 1. In: Smith, L., Coleman, V., Bradshaw, M. *Family-centred Care – Concept, Theory and Practice*. Basingstoke: Palgrave.

Coleman, V. (2010) The evolving concept of child and family-centred healthcare, Chapter 1. In: Smith, L. and Coleman, V. *Child and Family-centred Healthcare – Concept, Theory and Practice* 2nd edn. Basingstoke: Palgrave Macmillan.

Corlett, J. & Twycross, A. (2006) Negotiation of parental roles within family-centred care: a review of the research. *Journal of Clinical Nursing*, **15**(10), 1308–16.

Cutliff, J., McKenna, H. & Hyrkas, K. (2010) *Nursing Models Application to Practice*. London: Quay Books.

Department of Health (1991) *Welfare of Children and Young People in Hospital*. London: HMSO.

Department of Health (1996) *The Patient's Charter: Services for Children and Young People*. London: DH.

Department of Health (1998) *A First Class Service: Quality in the New NHS*. London: The Stationery Office.

Department of Health (2003) *Getting the Right Start: the National Service Framework for Children, Young People and Maternity Services – Standard for Hospital Services*. London: DH.

Department of Health, Social Services and Public Safety (DHSSPS) (2005) *A Healthier Future: a Twenty-year Vision for Health and Wellbeing in Northern Ireland 2005–2025*. Belfast: DHSSPS.

Dieckmann, R., Brownstein, D. & Gausche-Hill, M. (2000) *Pediatric Education for Prehospital Professionals* (PEPP), (Chapter 4). Sudbury, MA: American Academy of Paediatrics, Jones & Barlett Publishers.

Fawcett, J. (1984) The metaparadigam of nursing: current status and future refinements. *Journal of Nursing Scholarship*, **16**, 84–7.

Gance-Cleveland, B. (2006) Family-centred care, decreasing health disparities. *Journal of Specialist Pediatric Nurses*, **11**(1), 72–6.

Heath, H.B.M. (2005) *Potter and Perry's Foundations in Nursing Theory and Practice*. London: Mosby.

Holland, K., Jenkins, J., Solomon, J. & Whittam, S. (2008) *Applying the Roper, Logan, Tierney Model in Practice*, 2nd edn. Edinburgh: Churchill Livingstone.

Kawik, L. (1996) Nurses attitudes and perceptions of parental participation. *British Journal of Nursing*, **5**(7), 430–4.

Matousova-Done, Z. & Gates, B. (2006) The nature of care planning and delivery in intellectual disability nursing, Chapter 1. In: *Care Planning and Delivery in Intellectual Disability Nursing*. Oxford: Blackwell Publishing.

McClune, B. & Franklin, K. (1987) The Mead model for nursing – adapted from the Roper/Logan/ Tierney model for nursing. *Intensive Care Nursing*, 3(3), 97–105, cited in Viney, C. (1996) *Nursing the Critically Ill*. Edinburgh: Baillière Tindall.

McGee, P (1998) *Models of Nursing in Practice: a Pattern for Practical Care*. Cheltenham: Stanley Thornes.

Ministry of Health and Central Health Services Council (1959) *The Welfare of Children in Hospital – Platt Report*. London: HMSO.

Neuman, B. & Young, R.J. (1972) A model for teaching person approach to patient problems. *Nursing Research*, **21**(3), 264.

Nevin, M., Mulkerrins, J. & Driffield, A. (2010) Essential skills. In: Coyne, I., Neill, F. & Timmins, F. (eds). *Clinical Skills in Children's Nursing*. Oxford: Oxford University Press.

Newman, B. & Fawcett, J. (2002) *The Neuman Systems Model*, 4th edn. Upper Saddle River, NJ.

North American Nursing Diagnosis Association International (NANDA-I) (2008) *Nursing Diagnoses: Definitions and Classification*, 2009–2011 edition. Indianapolis: Wiley-Blackwell.

Noyes, J. (2000) Are nurses respecting and upholding the rights of children and young people in their care? *Paediatric Nursing*, **12**(2), 23–7.

Nursing and Midwifery Council (2008) *The Code – Standards of Conduct, Performance and Ethics for Nurses and Midwives*. London: NMC.

Nursing and Midwifery Council (2009) *Record keeping: Guidance for Nurses and Midwives*. London: NMC.

Nursing & Midwifery Council (2010) *Standards for Pre-registration Nursing Education*. London: NMC.

Olsen, J., Giangrasso, A., Shrimpton, D. & Cunningham, S. (2010) *Dosage Calculations for Nurses*. Harlow: Pearson Higher Education.

Orem, D.E (1991) *Nursing: Concepts of Practice*, 4th edn. St Louis: Mosby.

Orem, D.E (1995) *Nursing: Concepts of Practice*, 5th edn. St Louis: Mosby.

Parsley, K. & Corrigan, P. (1999) *Quality Improvement in Healthcare – Putting Evidence into Practice*, 2nd edn. Cheltenham: Stanley Thornes.

Pearson, A., Vaughan, B. & FitzGerald, M. (2005) *Nursing Models for Practice*, 3rd edn. Edinburgh: Butterworth Heinemann.

Resuscitation Council (UK) (2005) *Resuscitation Guideline 2005*. London: RCUK.

Robertson, J. (1958) *Going to Hospital with Mother*. London: Tavistock.

Roper, N., Logan, W. & Tierney, A. (1985) *The Elements of Nursing*, 2nd edn. Edinburgh: Churchill Livingstone.

Royal College of Nursing (2003) *Children and Young Peoples Nursing: a Philosophy of Care, Guidance for Nursing Staff*. London: RCN.

Shields, L., Pratt, J. & Hunter, J. (2006) Family-centred care: a review of qualitative studies. *Journal of Clinical Nursing*, **15**, 1317–23.

Smith, F. (1995) *Children's Nursing in Practice: the Nottingham Model*. Oxford: Blackwell Science.

United Nations (1989) *The Declaration of The Rights of the Child*. New York: United Nations.

Viney, C. (1996) *Nursing the Critically Ill*. Edinburgh: Ballière Tindall.

Walsh, M. (1998) *Models and Critical Pathways in Clinical Nursing. Conceptual Frameworks for Care Planning*, 2nd edn. Edinburgh: Baillière Tindall.

Wright, K. (2005) Care Planning: an easy guide for nurses. *Nursing and Residential Care*, **7**, 71–3.

Yura, D. & Walsh, M.B. (1978) *The Nursing Process: Assessing, Planning, Implementing and Evaluating*. New York: Appleton Century Crofts.

2

Risk Assessment and Management
Sonya Clarke and Doris Corkin

Introduction

Risk assessment and management is everybody's business, a major component of daily living and nursing practice. In 1995, Russell defined risk as 'the potential for an unexpected or unwanted outcome' (p607). As healthcare professionals we come across difficult and challenging moments that are often unexpected each and every day, as patient care is individual and unpredictable on occasions. Therefore, when the unexpected happens, making time to learn from the experience is essential, as learning after the event may be the single most powerful insight into any healthcare organisation.

Risk assessment

Risk assessment is simply 'an assessment or calculation of risk or potential risk of an issue which cannot be easily rectified' (Stower 2000, p42). Assessing risk factors and establishing that a patient is at risk should be part of the initial assessment and care planning for any patient who is entering the healthcare system. As children's nurses our behaviours become as important as our technical skill and knowledge when serving the best interests of sick children, their families and our colleagues. Nurses monitor risk each time they meet patients; it may be through experience and intuition or through application of a valid and reliable risk assessment tool. Indeed, a student or staff nurse can often walk onto a ward

Care Planning in Children and Young People's Nursing, First Edition.
Edited by Doris Corkin, Sonya Clarke, Lorna Liggett.
© 2012 Blackwell Publishing Ltd. Published 2012 by Blackwell Publishing Ltd.

and know when something is 'just not right'; such an emotion can be described as a 'gut feeling'. We must, however, question the weight that the nursing profession gives to a decision based on intuition, as opposed to those who follow best practice, national standards or clinical guidelines.

Main sources of risk

- Poor communication pathways
- Lack of clear up-to-date policies/procedures/guidelines
- Poorly defined responsibilities
- Staff working beyond their level of competence (Bowden 1996)

Nonetheless, a *Nursing Times* reporter (Lomas 2009) on behalf of Professor Peter Griffiths warns that risk assessment tools are not always backed by evidence. He has suggested that: 'tools should be used as a baseline, but they also need to be reused when it is clinically indicated or in line with NICE guidelines. It must not be a paper filing exercise.'

A recent article by Griffiths and Jull (2010) proposes pressure ulcer guidelines, suggesting that risk assessment tools must be used collectively with clinical judgement (RCN 2005), primarily because the tools may not be accurate and reliably predict which patients are at risk. The article concludes that formal assessment tools may or may not have a place within risk assessment with good clinical judgement and appropriate intervention, but does not advocate the 'use of a tool' as the vital indicator to produce the absence of a pressure ulcer.

Studies published in the early 1990s found that nurses base decision making on experience (Luker & Kenrick 1992), with intuition being described as the process of instant understanding of a situation (Miller 1993). There is limited empirical evidence that examines how risk is actually assessed within clinical practices. Trenoweth's limited small study in 2003 suggests that in a crisis situation risk assessment may be based on intuition. Even though risk assessment has been around for decades we are often unaware of how 'we do it' and most often do not realise we are undertaking 'risk assessment'. Brunton (2005) suggests the method for making a decision regarding risk is situation dependent, where the nurse will in the first instance use a risk assessment tool to aid in a scientific manner. The tool's high inter-rater reliability may reduce the risk to patients from an individual nurse's lack of experience and ability. They may be of comfort to the nurse, but if time consuming they may not always be practical for every patient/nurse contact.

Healthcare professionals undertake risk assessments to identify problem areas so that risk management measures can be put in place to make a situation as safe as possible for all concerned. Risk assessments are carried out on a daily basis, sometimes without nurses even realising it, such as checking the emergency trolley every morning. Renowned risk assessment tools such as Waterlow (1997), Braden (1987) and Norton (1962) are used to predict a patient's high profile areas such as patient falls, malnutrition, moving and handling and pressure ulcers. Such tools have been widely used by nurses in clinical practice for many years. Sadly, nurses can be put in difficult situations when staffing levels are stretched. For example, the moving and handling of patients continues to cause nursing staff to have back injuries, and to suffer severe pain for weeks and ongoing pain for years.

Categories of risk

- Risks for the nurse (Chadwick & Tadd 1992)
- Risks for the child and parents
- Risks arising from research (Coyne 1998)

More tools are currently being developed for the child and young person, as highlighted by Willock *et al.* (2007), who have found that the Glamorgan scale for pressure ulcer prevention in children may give a more accurate estimate of risk than other scales. However, it is important to note no risk assessment tool is 100% accurate. The study noted nurses should examine and try to resolve the individual problems that contribute to the 'total risk'.

Shields and Clarke (2010) have also explored 'reducing the risk' through the use of a validated tool for children. The paper suggests that children who require orthopaedic surgery or who have casts or fixation devices applied will require ongoing neurovascular monitoring as they will have a restriction of movement. The paper found Wright (2007) to have used evaluation research to evaluate and validate the Wessex Paediatric Neurovascular Assessment Tool (WPNA). The main consensus in the literature showed that the basis for any neurovascular assessment should be based on Dykes (1993) '5 Ps' (pain, pulses, pallor, paraesthesia and paralysis). This consists of an assessment of vascular status, movement, sensation and pain. Pain assessment was the second area that warranted special attention in the literature, as it is offered as 'the most reliable indicator of neurovascular impairment'. Shields and Clarke (2010) clearly promote the use of a valid tool when trying to reduce the risk of neurovascular injury.

Brunton (2005) alternatively suggests that nurses should use 'decision trees' which assess risk using a systematic approach. The decision trees can be presented as a flow chart or algorithm. Good examples of decision-making trees are generated by the NHS National Patient Safety Agency, which aims to reduce risks to patients receiving NHS care and improve safety. NPSA developed *How to Confirm the Correct Position of Nasogastric Feeding Tubes* for the adult, child and infant in 2005 (view via Activity 2.1).

✎ Activity 2.1

View decision making trees at:
http://www.nrls.npsa.nhs.uk/resources/type/alerts/?entryid45=59794&p=3

Back in 1994 Ainsworth and Wilson recognised that tools are based around the probable outcomes of specifications, which should be evidenced based. A significant advantage of the decision tree is that they are seen to offer choices, highlight the strengths and weakness of those choices and give evidence on them (Monkey-Poole 1998). Strategies such as clinical assessment tools and decision trees involve employing formal methods to assess risk. However, the majority of risk assessments carried out by nurses are based on decisions made by the individual nurse (Doyle & Dolan 2002).

Risk management

Risk management is linked with clinical governance, a framework which helps all clinicians to practice safely, deliver effective care and improve quality of clinical services (RCN 2003). The NHS is committed to management of risk and has operational systems in place to identify, analyse and control risks, resulting in changes within practice. A risk management consideration is avoiding hyponatraemia in acutely ill hospitalised children, which may occur during inappropriate rehydration or with maintenance fluids (see Chapter 16). Although the majority of healthcare trusts have structures in place for addressing clinical risk, reducing litigation is an ongoing problem for management as clinical negligence claims appear to cost the NHS millions of pounds each year (NEWS 1999).

Examples of risk

- Prevention of fire/noise in the hospital
- Security of children on the ward
- The play environment (Stower 2000)
- Pharmacological side-effects
- Breach in nurse's 'duty to care'

A study by Verdu (2003) investigated whether a decision tree can aid pressure ulcer management. It hypothesised that nurses who use a decision tree in pressure ulcer care assess wound grade more accurately and select more appropriate dressings. Sixty-six nurses were randomly assigned to two groups. Each nurse reviewed written information and pictures of three cases of pressure ulceration, and then graded and selected a dressing for the lesions. The absence or presence of a decision tree was used as an independent variable and the results found baseline characteristics were comparable for both groups. There was no statistically significant difference between the grades selected by the two groups. But significantly more of the decision tree users selected an appropriate dressing ($p < 0.02$). The study concluded that decision trees could help nurses to make complex clinical decisions and that further studies undertaken in a clinical setting are needed.

Following an incident

Upon reflection (Johns 1995), should an incident occur, it is important that professional discussion following the incident takes place, to enable the individuals involved to learn for themselves what happened, why it happened, what needs to be improved and the lessons learnt. According to Vincent (2001) 'when a patient safety incident occurs, the issue is not who is to blame, but how and why did it occur', because it would appear that when blame comes into the room truth may leave it. Indeed, handling the truth takes courage: sharing it and learning from it takes leadership.

Furthermore, decisions cannot always wait for senior staff, for example when dealing with verbal complaints from parents. Children's nurses need to become empowered and confident leaders in order to make decisions on a daily basis.

Summary

Within this chapter risk assessment and management have been explored, highlighting the need to prevent or minimise risks within the nursing process of providing care. However, clear communication pathways and interdisciplinary working is essential if risks are to be minimised. Everyday incidents in clinical practice occur; therefore children's nurses should not become complacent, instead assertive with clinical judgement, encouraging discussion about their concerns.

References

Ainsworth, J. & Wilson, P. (1994) Would your judgement stand up to scrutiny? *British Journal of Nursing*, **3**(19), 1023–8.

Bowden, D. (1996) Calculate the risk. *Nursing Management*, **3**(4), 10–11.

Braden, B. & Bergstrom, N. (1987) A conceptual schema for the study of the etiology of pressure sores. *Rehabilitation Nursing*, **12**(1), 8–12.

Brunton, K. (2005) The evidence on how nurses approach risk assessment. *Nursing Times*, **101**(28), 38.

Chadwick, R. & Tadd, W. (1992) *Ethics and Nursing Practice*. London: Macmillan Education.

Coyne, I.T. (1998) Researching children: some methodological and ethical considerations. *Journal of Clinical Nursing*, **7**(5), 409–16.

Doyle, M. & Dolan, M. (2002) Violence risk assessment: combining actuarial and clinical information to structure clinical judgements for the formulation and management of risk. *Journal of Psychiatric and Mental Health Nursing*, **9**(6), 649–57.

Dykes, C. (1993) Minding the five Ps of neurovascular assessment. *American Journal of Nursing*, **193**(6), 38–9.

Griffiths, P. & Jull, A. (2010) How good is the evidence for using risk assessment to prevent pressure ulcers? *Nursing Times*, **106**, 14.

Johns, C. (1995) Framing learning through reflection within Carper's fundamental ways of knowing in nursing. *Journal of Advanced Nursing*, **22**(2), 226–34.

Lomas, C. (2009) Top nurse warns risk assessment tools are not backed by evidence. www.nursingtimes.net/whats-new-in-nursing/acute-care/top-nurse-warns-risk-assessment-tools-are-not-backed-by-evidence/5009295.article (accessed 14 June 2010).

Luker, K.A. & Kendrick, M. (1992) An exploratory study of the sources of influence on the clinical decisions of community nurses. *Journal of Advanced Nursing*, **17**(1), 108–112.

Miller, V.G. (1993) Measurement of self perception of intuitiveness. *Western Journal of Nursing Research*, **15**(5), 595–606.

Monkey-Poole, S. (1998) Calculating risk community mental health nursing: the decision analysis approach. *Mental Health Care*, **21**(92), 56–9.

NEWS (1999) *Journal of Advanced Nursing*, **29**(1), 4–8.

Norton, D., Exon-Smith, A. N. & McLaren, R. (1962) *An Investigation of Geriatric Nursing Problems in Hospital*. Edinburgh: Churchill Livingstone.

Royal College of Nursing (2003) *Clinical Governance: an RCN Resource Guide*. London: RCN

Royal College of Nursing (2005) *The Nursing Management of Pressure Ulcers in Primary and Secondary Care: A Clinical Practice Guideline*. London: RCN.

Russell, S. (1995) Risk management. *British Journal of Nursing*, **4**(10), 607.

Shields, C. & Clarke, S. (2010) Using neurovascular assessment tool within children's A&E. *International Journal of Orthopaedic and Trauma Nursing*. doi:10.1016/j.ijotn.2010.04.002.

Stower, S (2000) Keeping the hospital environment safe for children. *Paediatric Nursing*, **12**(6), 37–42.

Trenoweth, S. (2003) Perceiving risk in dangerous situations: risks of violence among mental health inpatients. *Journal of Advanced Nursing*, **42**(3), 278–87.

Verdu J. (2003) Can a decision tree help nurses to grade and treat pressure ulcers? *Journal of Wound Care*, **12**(2), 45–50.

Vincent, C. (2001) *Clinical Risk Management, Enhancing Patient Safety*, 2nd edn. London: BMJ Publishing Group.

Waterlow, J.A. (1997) Pressure sore risk assessment in children. *Paediatric Nursing*, **9**(6), 21–4.

Willock, J., Baharestani, M & Anthony, A. (2007) A risk assessment scale for pressure ulcers in children. *Nursing Times*, **103**(14), 32–3.

Wright, E. (2007) Evaluating a paediatric neurovascular assessment tool. *Journal of Orthopaedic Nursing*, **11**, 20–29.

3

Safeguarding to Protect Children, Young People and Their Families

Lorna Liggett

Introduction

The term child protection was predominately concerned with protection from abuse and neglect, whereas the term 'safeguarding' is a much broader term which encompasses vulnerable children in need of safeguarding from mental and physical ill health, which could arise from educational failure, crime or antisocial behaviour (DfES 2007). Safeguarding children is everyone's business and to that end we must accept our mutual responsibility as citizens to safeguard the vulnerable, to be aware of the danger signs and to act on concerns by referring these to the appropriate agency or police. It will mean ensuring that organisational boundaries between professions and agencies do not act as barriers to meeting the safeguarding needs of children or in the delivery of their right to safety.

Inquiry into Victoria Climbié

This inquiry, which was reported in the Laming Report (2003), described the shocking maltreatment of Victoria at the hands of her great aunt and her partner. During the period from 1998 to 2000 there were twelve occasions when opportunities to detect the maltreatment and protect Victoria were overlooked. These missed opportunities in the system were described by Lord Laming as 'lamentable' and he said that it must never happen again.

A range of key agencies all failed in their duty to protect Victoria and within the report a series of recommendations were set out for all the agencies involved.

Care Planning in Children and Young People's Nursing, First Edition.
Edited by Doris Corkin, Sonya Clarke, Lorna Liggett.
© 2012 Blackwell Publishing Ltd. Published 2012 by Blackwell Publishing Ltd.

The inquiry acknowledged that there were omissions and failures in the healthcare professionals' documentation and in their reporting mechanisms. It also reported that the 'failure of nursing staff ' to record their observations in the notes, and the consequent discrepancy between the levels of concern they expressed in their oral evidence and that reflected in the records made at the time, was a matter which arose with depressing regularity' (Laming 2003). This would indicate that essential principles of assessment, record-keeping and care planning were not what they should have been for whatever reason.

Following the death of Victoria Climbié in 2000 and the subsequent report in 2003 the Government produced new guidance on child protection processes and systems. This guidance is contained in *What to do if You are Worried a Child is Being Abused*, published in 2003 and updated in 2006. The Laming Inquiry also lead to the revised Children Act (2004) which sets out the process for integrating services to children so that every child can achieve the five outcomes as laid out in the *Every Child Matters* (2003).

Recognition of child abuse and neglect

Access this site for further information www.safeguardingchildren.co.uk/recognising.

All health professionals need to be aware of the signs and symptoms of child abuse and neglect and act accordingly. There is no one definitive sign, symptoms or injury and also a series of seemingly minor incidents can be just as damaging as any one incident. Health professionals must place the interests of children at the core of their practice and share their concerns with other health professionals.

Physical abuse

Physical abuse may involve hitting, shaking, throwing, poisoning, burning or scalding, drowning, suffocating or otherwise causing physical harm to a child. Physical harm may also be caused when a parent or carer feigns the symptoms of or deliberately causes ill health to a child whom they are looking after.

Signs and symptoms include:

- Bruising
- Black eyes
- Burns and scalds
- Bites and scratches
- Lesions and cuts

Other indicators of physical abuse include:

- Delay in seeking medical attention
- No explanation or inadequate explanation of injuries
- Changing explanation of injuries
- Recurrent injuries – particularly if forming a pattern
- Inadequate parental concern
- Multiple injuries that occurred at different dates

Sexual abuse

These symptoms can present singly or in clusters of behaviours, depending on each child's environment and specific situation. It is crucial for the health professional to recognise the behaviours exhibited in the child according to their stage of development, for example the pre-school child, the 6–12-year-old and the older child.

Emotional abuse

Emotional abuse is the persistent emotional ill-treatment of a child such as to cause severe and continuing adverse effects on the child's emotional development. It may involve conveying to children that they are worthless or unloved, inadequate or valued only insofar as they meet the needs of another person. Furthermore, emotional abuse may involve inappropriate age or developmental expectations being imposed on children and could cause a child to feel frightened or in danger and can lead to the exploitation or corruption of children.

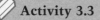 **Activity 3.3**

Write 250 words on the effects of emotional abuse on a pre-school child.

Neglect

This area can be sub-divided into the following:

• Medical neglect
• Physical neglect
• Educational neglect
• Stimulation neglect
• Nutritional neglect
• Environmental neglect

Activity 3.4

A three-year-old child is admitted to the ward with a failure to gain weight.

• What concerns would you have?
• What questions would you ask to gain a comprehensive picture?
• Who might you discuss your concerns with?

Vulnerable child

Protecting vulnerable children in specific circumstances is particularly important to health professionals in that they need to know which children are deemed to be high risk in either a community, hospital or residential setting. All health professionals need to have a working knowledge of the interagency arrangements and support mechanisms to be put in place in these circumstances.

The following is a list of the different types of vulnerable children:

• Children who have been sexually abused
• Children who have been physically abused
• Children who have been emotionally abused
• Children who have been neglected
• Children who present with faltering growth/failure to thrive
• Children who present with fabricated or induced illness
• Children who present with high-risk and challenging behaviour, self-injurious behaviour and suicidal ideation
• Children living away from home and children placed outside the trust's area
• Children with ill health or who have a disability
• Children with significant language, speech and communication impairment
• Children in need of Child and Adolescent Mental Health Service (CAMHS) and psychological support services
• Children who are homeless
• Children who are exploited, including those exposed to child/human trafficking

- Children who abuse others
- Children who are bullied
- Children who are under-age parents
- Children who are carers
- Children whose parents/carers have a disability
- Children who are victims of domestic violence
- Children whose parents/carers have a mental illness
- Children whose parents/carers misuse drugs/alcohol
- Children who live with or have contact with families or individuals who may expose a risk to children, including persons where there is risk of sexual and/or violent behaviour
- Children who are exposed to potential abuse on the Internet
- Children from black and minority ethnic groups and from the travelling community
- Unborn children, where risks are posed by parents

DHSSPS (2008)

Policies and procedures

The Children Act 1989, revised in 2004, legislates for England and Wales. The Children (Northern Ireland) Order 1995 and the Children (Scotland) Act 1995 share the same principles and have their own guidance.

Local Safeguarding Children Boards (LSCBs) in England and Wales, and the Safeguarding Board Northern Ireland (SBNI) replace the Area Child Protection Committees. These are local interagency forums that bring together the local authorities, police and health professionals to work more effectively in safeguarding children.

Safeguarding is concerned with child protection, multidisciplinary working and creating a broader understanding of child protection to include prevention and family support. The scope of the LSCBs and SBNI aims to protect all children from maltreatment, to target specific groups in a proactive manner, to safeguard and promote the welfare of chidren potentially more vulnerable and to protect children who are suffering from significant harm.

The key principles are:

- Best outcomes achieved through collaborative working
- Value each other's contributions
- Sharing information
- Sharing commitments
- Understanding each other's roles and responsibilities
- Collaborative at all levels
- Agencies encouraging and promoting safeguarding
- Voice of the child
- Joint training

There are a range of strategic documents published to inform nursing and midwifery services across the UK in order to secure the continued development of effective services which safeguard children, young people and their families. These legislative and policy frameworks provide guidance and clear direction, including specific detail of the roles and responsibilities of all those involved in the care and delivery of services to children.

> ### Activity 3.5
>
> List the range of policies and procedures in your region that you must be aware of.

All healthcare professionals are responsible for ensuring timely and appropriate responses to safeguard children regardless of the setting or speciality. Safeguarding children is everyone's business; therefore all health professionals must be competent and knowledgeable in order to safeguard and promote the welfare of children. The Royal College of Paediatrics and Child Health (RCPCH) (2006) sets out clearly the knowledge, skills and competencies required of all nurses, and other health professionals and the need for regular updating to ensure safe and effective practice.

Working together to Safeguard Children (Department of Health (DH) (2006) and *Co-operating to Safeguard Children* Department of Health, Social Services and Public Safety (DHSSPS Northern Ireland) (2003) sets out the roles and responsibilities of different agencies and practitioners and outlines the way in which joint working arrangements should be agreed, implemented and reviewed.

It followed closely the *Protection of Children and Vulnerable Adults (NI) Order* (POCVA) Department of Health and Social Services and Public Services Northern Ireland (DHSSPS 2003), which aims to improve existing safeguards for children and vulnerable adults by preventing unsuitable people working with them in paid or voluntary positions. POCVA is designed to augment the protection of children and vulnerable adults and is not a substitute for a robust recruitment and selection process within an organisation, which should include employment history, interviewing candidates and taking up references.

The children's *National Services Framework* (NSF) (DH 2004) is a ten-year programme intended to stimulate long-term and sustained improvement in children's health. Setting standards for health and social services for children, young people and pregnant women, the NSF aims to ensure fair, high quality and integrated health and social care from pregnancy, right through to adulthood.

At the heart of the Children's NSF is a fundamental change in thinking about health and social care services. It is intended to lead to a cultural shift, resulting in services being designed and delivered around the needs of children and families. The Children's NSF is aimed at everyone who comes into contact with, or delivers services to children, young people or pregnant women.

Standards six to ten address children and young people and their parents who have particular needs, and should be implemented in conjunction with the standards in the document:

- Children and young people who are ill
- Children in hospital
- Disabled children and young people and those with complex health needs

- The mental health and psychological wellbeing of children and young people
- Medicines for children and young people

http://www.dh.gov.uk/en/Healthcare/NationalServiceFrameworks/Children/DH_4089111

This document clearly states that all staff should understand their roles and responsibilities in safeguarding children and also promote the welfare of children and young people. In order to do this all staff will need training, updating and support to function effectively. This was echoed in the Laming Inquiry (2003) which states that 'all staff appointed to any of the services where they will be working with children and families must have adequate training for the positions they will fill.' The RCN (2007) endorses this statement and includes the need for all nurses, midwives and health visitors to receive training in recognising child abuse. The RCN further recommends that a senior lecturer should be appointed within university nursing and midwifery education programmes to ensure the teaching of this subject. The following key areas are suggested by the RCN to be included as a minimum in the undergraduate programmes:

- Nurse's role and accountability
- Policies and procedures
- Record-keeping
- Use of case studies
- Reference documents to highlight key issues
- Ways to achieve effective interagency and multidisciplinary working

The *Standards for Child Protection Services* (DHSSPS 2008) and the *Children's National Service Framework* (DH 2004) for England and Wales set national standards for children's health and social care. They aim to promote high quality women and child-centred services and individualised care that meets the needs of parents, children and their families. Standards will be used to promote the planning, delivery, audit, review and inspection of child protection services across Northern Ireland and provide the foundation for informing practice and improving the services to children, young people and their families. To that end the standards are to be used by all health and social care commissioners, organisations and professionals who provide statutory services to children, representative groups who speak for children, practitioners, regulatory bodies, training providers and members of the public.

Health professionals working with ill adults, or children who are misusing drugs or alcohol, must recognise the risk to all children. They must assess the effects of illness or lifestyle and habits on the children and if a risk assessment is required they should work in collaboration with social services and the police.

Within the adult mental health field, professionals should also be aware of the need to consider the risk to children from patients who are paedophiles or known to be perpetrators of abuse towards children. Mental health issues or a psychiatric disorder can affect a parent's ability to safeguard their child, resulting in various degrees of abuse, neglect and emotional deprivation. Again, a risk assessment may have to be carried out in consultation with social services, the probation service and the police.

However, there will always be a potential area of sensitivity for health professionals working in adult mental health services when confidential information has to be shared with another agency. Confidential information should be shared on a 'need to know' basis. The main consideration here is to act in the best interests of the child. The nurse in this particular setting must express their concern immediately to a line manager and the doctor responsible for the patient's care and consider what appropriate action to take in line with procedures.

Likewise, where a child who is the subject of concern has a parent with a learning disability the health professionals in this situation are well placed to identify and respond to the increased vulnerability and potential risk of abuse to children with special needs. The health professionals involved must act in the best interests of the child and discuss such concerns with other agencies.

All professionals must be mindful that the protection of the child is of paramount importance and where there are concerns they should follow agreed procedures. These concerns or referrals must be shared and discussed with the line manager, named doctor or child protection nurse.

Activity 3.6

Find out who is the named doctor and the child protection nurse in your area.
  Discuss what you should do when you have a concern.
  Discuss the key stages of the referral process.

Safeguarding children is a complex aspect of practice; therefore nurses will require support through effective supervision and this should be available to nurses at a level that reflects their involvement with children and families. Indeed, a quality supervision process should result in a more efficient and confident nursing workforce.

Assessment

The lives of disadvantaged and vulnerable children cannot be improved unless their needs are identified and appropriate action taken. The Government's objective has been to develop a framework for assessing children in need and their families to ensure a timely response and effective provision of services (DHSSPS 2007; DH 2000).

The key emphasis of these frameworks places the child centre-stage within the assessment process. Family health needs assessment is a holistic approach to identify the health needs of individuals, family and communities in order to provide a client-centred service. The framework was introduced following a strategic review in 2003. It includes a full assessment of the child's developmental needs, parenting capacity, family health and environmental factors which impact on the child's health and wellbeing, in order to identify children and families who may require additional support to achieve the five outcomes identified in *Every Child Matters* (DfES 2004). The benefit of having this process will be to promote best practice and a standardised approach to assessment of children throughout the UK.

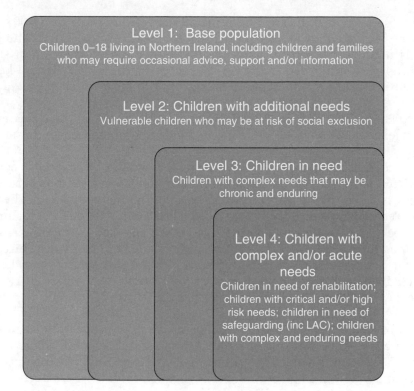

Figure 3.1   Threshold of needs model.

To assist with this framework, a model of the levels of need was conceptualised – www.dhsspsni.gov.uk/threshold (see Figure 3.1).

The framework provides a systematic way of analysing, understanding and recording what is happening to children, young people and their families within their communities. From this, clear professional judgements can be made, which may include whether the child being assessed is in need, or suffering or likely to suffer significant harm. This then leads to what actions must be taken and which services would best meet the needs of this child and family.

Record-keeping

Record-keeping is an integral part of nursing and to that end all health professionals must adhere to the principles of good record-keeping (NMC 2008). It is a process and not an optional extra to be fitted in if and when convenient. The best record remains one that is the product of collaboration between all members of the health professional team and the child/parent. It is one that is reviewed and adapted in response to the needs of the child. The record should enable any nurse to care for the child, regardless of where they are within the care process or care environment. It is an invaluable way of promoting communication between those involved in the care of the child and with the parents themselves. Good record-keeping is, therefore, the product of good teamwork and an important tool in promoting high quality health care. The principles set out by the NMC (2008) apply across all care settings and to both written and electronic held records. The NMC accepts that, until there is national agreement between all healthcare professionals on standards and format, records may differ depending on the needs of the child. Record-keeping must, however, follow a logical and methodical sequence with clear milestones and goals for the process.

Laming (2003) stated: 'I regard the keeping of proper notes and the accurate recording of concerns felt about a child as being a fundamental aspect of basic professional competence.'

Effective record-keeping means that the record should be factual, consistent and accurate, written in a way that the meaning is clear and always written as soon as possible after an event has occurred with, wherever possible, the involvement of the child and/or parent. The records should also be recorded clearly and in such a manner that the text cannot be erased or deleted without a record of such a change. Any justifiable alterations or additions should be dated, timed and signed or clearly attributed to a named person so that the original entry can still be read. All information should be accurately dated, timed and signed, with the signature printed alongside the first entry where this is a written record, and attributed to a named person in an identifiable role for electronic records.

The subject of a record does have the right in law to request access to their record at any stage. Therefore it is important that all information regarding a child should be collated in one set of notes, as recommended by Laming (2003). They should also be in chronological order and demonstrate the collaboration between professionals where decisions were made and actions taken.

In 2009 the Nursing and Midwifery Council undertook a review of pre-registration education (RPNE) which focused on the future and how nursing programmes across the UK would need to look in order to enable nurses to meet the needs of patients safely and effectively. Under the domain of communication and interpersonal skills the draft domain states:

'All nurses must maintain accurate, clear and complete written or electronic records using the right kind of language, avoiding jargon and use plain English so that everyone involved in the care process understands the meaning' and 'all nurses must keep information secure and confidential in accordance with the law and ethical and regulatory frameworks, taking account of local protocols'.

www.nmc.uk.org

These statements clearly indicate how crucial communication is for nurses in their day-to-day work and the importance to the safety of the patient and protection of nurses.

Roles and responsibilities

Health professionals need to understand the importance of their role and responsibilities in safeguarding children. As Laming (2003) reported, there was poor communication, disjointed lines of accountability and inadequate exchange of information between agencies. The report also highlighted the need to work in a collaborative manner, which is why it is crucial to have effective systems in place for information sharing and understanding between agencies and health professionals.

Therefore, health professionals must:

- Be familiar with recent policies and procedures within their area of work
- Know who to contact if they have a concern regarding a child
- Act in the best interests of the child
- Be able to assess the needs of the child and capacity of the parents to meet their child's needs
- Plan and respond to the needs of the child/parent, particularly those who are vulnerable
- Understand the risk factors and recognise children in need of support/safeguarding
- Be alert to the signs of abuse/neglect
- Be aware of the stages of the referral process
- Record all communication accurately
- Have a knowledge of child development
- Ensure that the child receives appropriate and timely interventions
- Share information with other professionals/agencies
- Attend update sessions/training

Health professionals have a key part to play in safeguarding and promoting the welfare of children and must be clear about their own roles and responsibilities and be aware of the roles and responsibilities of other professionals. They must also be confident about their own standards, respectful of others and be mindful of the attitudes required for effective collaboration and negotiation. Good communication skills are also essential in order to contribute to the assessment and investigations of concerns about a child. They must also demonstrate skills in engaging children, parents and other professionals and actively seek knowledge to deliver improved services to children and young people, and comply with statutory requirements regarding training and working together.

In the aftermath of the Laming Inquiry it can be seen that the Government reacted with a plethora of policies and procedures to strengthen child protection to ensure improved and consistent quality of service and better standards across all agencies. However, in August 2007 a seventeen-month-old baby boy (baby P) suffered fatal injuries despite being seen by social workers and other professionals on 60 occasions. This case raised concerns again and Lord Laming was asked by the Government to carry out a review which was published in 2009 (Lord Laming 2009). In this he stated there were still significant failings, and progress on key reforms that should have been instituted after his landmark report into the case of tortured Victoria Climbié had yet to be properly implemented. In 2008, 55 children were killed by their parents/carers, making it imperative that the key reforms are taken seriously so no more children die.

Summary

Safeguarding children and promoting their wellbeing is the responsibility of us all and we must strive for best possible practice so that vulnerable children receive the protection they need. All nurses must remember that they have a duty to care, safeguard and promote the welfare of children and young people at all times (NMC 2008).

References

Department for Education and Skills (2004) *Every Child Matters: Change for Children*. London: Stationery Office.

Department for Education and Skills (2007) *Statutory Guidance on Making Arrangements to Safeguard and Promote the Welfare of Children Under Section 11 of the Children Act (2004)* London: Stationery Office.

Department of Health (2000) *Framework for Assessment of Children in Need and their Families*. London: HMSO.

Department of Health (2004) *National Service Framework for Children*. London: Stationery Office.

Department of Health (2006) *Working Together to Safeguard Children: a Guide to Interagency Working to Safeguard Children and Promote the Welfare of Children*. London: Her Majesty's Government.

Department of Health, Social Services and Public Safety in Northern Ireland (2003) *Co-operating to Safeguard Children*. Belfast: Stationery Office.

Department of Health Social Services and Public Safety in Northern Ireland (2008) *Standards for Child Protection Services*. Belfast: Stationery Office.

Department of Health and Social Services and Public Services Northern Ireland (2003) *The Protection of Children and Vulnerable Adults (Northern Ireland) Order*. Belfast: Stationery Office.

Department of Health and Social Services and Public Services in Northern Ireland (2007) *Understanding the Needs of Children in Northern Ireland (UNOCINI)*. Belfast: DHSSPSNI.

HMSO (1989) *The Children Act*. London: HMSO.

HMSO (1995) *Children (Northern Ireland) Order*. Belfast: HMSO.

HMSO (1995) *Children (Scotland) Act*. Scotland: HMSO.

Laming Report (2003) *The Victoria Climbié Inquiry: Report of an Inquiry by Lord Laming*. Norwich: the Stationery Office (TSO).

Lord Laming (2009) *The Protection of Children in England: A Progress Report*. HC330. London: Stationery Office.

Nursing and Midwifery Council (2008) *Standards of Conduct, Performance and Ethics for Nurses and Midwives*. London: NMC.

Royal College of Nursing (2007) *Safeguarding Children and Young People: Every Nurse's Responsibility*. London: RCN.

Royal College of Paediatrics and Child Health (2006) *Safeguarding Children and Young people: Roles and Competencies for Healthcare Staff*. Intercollegiate document. London: RCPCH.

4

Ethical and Legal Implications When Planning Care for Children and Young People

Orla McAlinden

Introduction

According to the Nursing and Midwifery Council (NMC 2008) children's nurses are required to safeguard the interests of infants, children and young people at all times. When planning care children's nurses must practice in an anti-discriminatory way, remaining alert to the legal, moral and ethical implications of their practice. This chapter should enable the children's nurse to recognise and meet the professional and ethical imperatives expected from the registered nurse working with children, young people and their families.

Where exactly in a nursing curriculum ethics and law should be introduced is arguably a matter for those who are involved in the consultation, design and delivery, and evaluation of that higher education programme. The central issue is that all nurses seeking to register with the NMC as a Registered Nurse (RN Child) must show that they have achieved all the proficiencies required by the NMC in order to do so. Their programme will have met the initial and ongoing scrutiny of the NMC and the individual academic institutions and, thereafter, the respective auditing teams such as internal audits by Northern Ireland Practice Education Committee (NIPEC) or similar statutory bodies throughout the UK.

The clear intention of these scrutineers is that those exiting from a higher educational nursing programme will be:

- Fit for practice
- Fit for purpose

Care Planning in Children and Young People's Nursing, First Edition.
Edited by Doris Corkin, Sonya Clarke, Lorna Liggett.
© 2012 Blackwell Publishing Ltd. Published 2012 by Blackwell Publishing Ltd.

- Fit for award
- Fit for professional standing

These recommendations were highlighted in the United Kingdom Central Council Peach Report (UKCC 1999).

A nursing student (and the RN subsequently) needs to demonstrate that *academically and clinically* they can meet the requirements of NMC (http://www.nmc-uk.org). The addition of a 'Declaration of good character' is another requirement which clearly indicates that there is a need to use fundamental skills and knowledge in a way that is morally acceptable.

It is therefore, not sufficient to just 'know' and 'do or not do'. The registered children's nurse must be able at all times to demonstrate that the knowledge underpinning action or omission is based on the best available contemporary evidence and is also mindful of the imperatives of current legislation and ethical behaviours. Indeed, it follows from this that the children's nurse needs to be aware of what role ethical action and legislation has upon all dimensions of practice – and the nurse should then be seen to practice consistently in a way that shows internalisation and commitment to those principles.

Activity 4.1

List below some of the reasons why a children's nurse would need to be informed about the *law* and *ethical actions*.
  Why law?
  Why ethical actions?

Ethics and morality

Principles or virtues?

Quite commonly in practice, children and young people's nurses are in a position of uncertainty. Arguably, ethical thinking and moral reasoning has the effect of making those involved more empowered to take an effective course of action, more able to articulate what their concerns are and why they deserve consideration or action. Unease or uncertainty about a certain action or situation prompts us to reflect upon what the correct response should be in any given situation. This reflection is a *moral* reflection because it is about the notion that something is important and it is therefore worth worrying about the 'rightness' or 'wrongness' of a particular course of action (Beauchamp & Childress 2001; Brown *et al.* 1992).

Decision making

There are different models for ethical decision making described in the literature (Beauchamp & Childress 2001; Thompson *et al.* 2006) and choosing is usually a matter of personal preference or ease of understanding. All of them begin with identifying an issue and end with taking a decision of some sort. What happens in between the beginning and end steps will influence the end decision.

Example: Brown et al. (1992) – five stages of moral deliberation

Principles approach:

- Appreciation of the situation (what is happening and going to happen)
- Review the possible courses of action (review them all, whether good, bad or indifferent)
- Selection and application of principles
- Weigh up the practicalities of all actions
- Decision (or choosing one of the practical possibilities on offer)

The principles referred to in the model above are:

- *Beneficence* (doing good or correct things)
- *Non-maleficence* (not doing bad or wrong things)
- *Respect/autonomy* (recognise that individuals should be able to make their own decisions)
- *Justice* (treat all cases alike unless they differ in some relevant respect)

Hardly a day goes by without these principles being played out in public view in healthcare settings. The media, and in particular the 'soaps', are a case in point and are viewed nationally and globally by millions of people daily. This means that the 'users' of health and social care hold their own perceptions and expectations of these services and the public servants (for we are public servants) who manage and deliver that care.

This public accountability is one compelling reason why we, as healthcare professionals in a multi- and interdisciplinary setting need to ensure that we can justify our actions and decisions on both *ethical* and *clinical* grounds. It should be noted that holding ethical views or being aware of ethical principles is not enough in itself – we need to demonstrate ability to apply this knowledge to our clinical practice. This means inclusion of ethical policies, procedures and standards as well as clarifying what goals and values we uphold as children's nurses.

Some issues are more topical than others, some change and recede or magnify over time, but the fact remains that we need to constantly ensure that our practices can always be justified as *moral* as well as 'scientific' and within the law, including employment law. Thompson *et al.* (2006) classify succinctly the types of moral theories and explore these in relation to ethical decision making. These theories are identified as:

- Deontological (causes and related to 'duty', including deontological ethics)
- Pragmatic/axiological (means and the moral agent, including virtue ethics)
- Teleological (end or goal outcomes, including utilitarianism and consequentialism)

The law

Griffith and Tengnah (2010) remind us of the NMC Standards of Proficiency (2008) for entry to the register (http://www.nmc-uk.org): 'Practice in accordance with an ethical and legal framework which ensures the primacy of patient and client interest and well being and respects confidentiality'. This emphasises that the *accountable* practitioner is one who recognises that law underpins practice and is therefore fundamental to the theory and practice of nursing.

The NMC Code (2008) uses the 'principles' based approach to the care of patients and clients and also indicates how law intertwines and informs healthcare practices.

The NMC Code is a combination of rules; some are positive rules (legally binding) and some normative rules (what a person 'should ' do rather than what legislation imposes). This is because it reflects the reality of what happens in life and in health and social care.

A simple way to view this is perhaps:

- The law spells out the *minimum* acceptable standard of care expected.
- The code sets out the *best possible standard* of care expected.

So together:

> Law + code = protection of the interests of the public by enshrining law as well as the highest aspirations for the health and welfare of individuals.

Duty of care, accountability and negligence

As an RN you are *accountable* for your actions and omissions to society in general *and* your individual patient/family in particular. You have a 'duty to care' for patients, which can be challenged by those in your care or your employers if they believe that you as an RN have *not* fulfilled that duty. If a patient/family/employer considers that this is the case then they may claim negligence, which is where harm occurs as a result of a nurse's carelessness.

The three aspects of *negligence* which must be proved in law are that:

- There was a duty of care *owed*
- That this duty of care was *breached* and
- As a result the patient suffered *harm* (physical or psychological)

De Cruz (2005)

Note: all three elements must be proven in law and following from this the nurse is liable to be sued for compensation for the consequential harm. At this point it is also important to realise that the requirements of the Code will have been infringed and so the RN will also come under the scrutiny of the NMC and also their employer. This is a very clear example of where the Code not only meets but extends beyond the standards expected in law.

De Cruz (2005) provides an excellent brief introduction to relevant issues in healthcare law. This also provides an overview of the UK NHS and ethical as well as legal frameworks to guide the competent practitioner. As ever, Dimond (2008) and Tingle and Cribb (2007) are excellent resources for all nurses in relation to current legal and contemporary ethical issues in healthcare practice. McHale *et al.* (2004) provide an excellent insight into the matters involving human rights and nursing and healthcare issues.

What is advocacy?

'A simple definition of advocacy is helping and supporting someone else to speak up for what they want. This can involve expressing their views or acting on their behalf to secure services that they require or rights to which they are entitled. Key concepts in advocacy are: equality, inclusion, empowerment and rights.'

(Newport Mind Advocacy 2010)

Boylan and Dalrymple (2009) describe the antecedents of advocacy for children as stemming from the nineteenth and early twentieth century. A timeline can be used to demonstrate development of what was essentially a paternalistic concern for children in the earlier years.

✎ Activity 4.2

For all relevant reports and legislation *specific to your country* visit the appropriate governmental websites and make a note of pertinent material.

England: www.dh.gov.uk/en/Publications
Northern Ireland: www.dhsspsni.gov.uk
Scotland: www.scotland.gov.uk
Wales: www.new.wales.gov.uk
Republic of Ireland: www.gov.ie
Irish Health Reports: www.mater.ie/depts./library/health-reports.htm

---

From 1970 onward concerns took the shape of a more inclusive view of the health and social welfare of children and young people. This development recognised importantly that this group of individuals need to have a voice of their own and their rights extended beyond the purely paternalistic concerns of previous years. Legislation and governmental reports such as Platt (Committee of the Central Health Services Council 1959), Court (Committee on Child Health Services 1976), up to Kennedy (DH 2001) urged advocacy and listening to and learning from the voice and developmental needs of children and families. The advent of pressure groups such as the National Association for the Welfare of Children in Hospital (NAWCH) slowly pushed back the boundaries of care for this group and influenced the development of advocacy in the wider social context. By the early 1990s NAWCH changed its name to Action for Sick Children. This change of name highlighted the need for a more encompassing focus for children and young people who were ill but were not necessarily hospitalised; this better reflects the contemporary needs of children and young people.

Boylan and Dalrymple (2009) have noted that the growth of advocacy for children and young people has been slow and has a tendency to remain adult-led rather than focused on the needs of the child or young person. England and Wales were ahead of Scotland and Northern Ireland in the landmark establishment of independent advocacy positions for children, with the appointment in 1987 of the first UK Children's Rights Officer and the development of the first national advocacy service to cover England and Wales in 1992.

A Children's Commissioner was appointed in Wales in 2001, in Northern Ireland in 2003 and in Scotland in 2004. England appointed their Children's Commissioner in 2005 under the provisions of the Children Act (HMSO 2004). Unlike the other countries mentioned, the English Commissioner must consult with the Secretary of State before it is possible to hold an independent inquiry.

Although undoubtedly welcome there is still a large discrepancy between the dates in the timeline and the actual appointment of the UK Children's Commissioners. Advocacy exists but there are differing levels, definition models and also a recognised limitation to the advocacy role that some nurses and healthcare professionals can uphold in certain situations (Boylan & Dalrymple 2009).

The rights of the child

The concept of children's rights emerged in the 1920s, with one of the earliest pioneers Janusz Korczak (*holocaustresearchproject.org*) and then with the Declaration of Geneva in 1924. The Declaration on the Rights of the Child followed in 1959, although it should be noted that this declaration *was not legally binding*. The 1970s saw a further development in the interest of children's rights.

The United Nations Convention on the Rights of the Child (adopted by the UN General Assembly in 1989 was ratified by the UK in 1991 and came into legal force in 1992 in the UK) saw the first *legally binding* legislation in relation to the rights of children and young people. This convention was also to be the most universally ratified of all the UN instruments, showing 'intent' at least of member states to recognise and uphold the rights of children and young persons.

Children and young persons have differing needs and perspectives at various stages of their social, cultural and developmental continuum (Bee & Boyd 2007). Dependence upon others is normal at the beginning of the lifespan and this tends to decrease with developmental progress and move towards a more independent lifestyle. At all early stages children require nurture, care and protection and are 'socialised' throughout their early childhood by the dominant culture of their community/society and the specific manner of their parenting. Others, often parents or the law bring influence to bear which is claimed to be in the 'best interests' of the child. Whilst this is considered acceptable in the early years of childhood it is increasingly less acceptable as children and young people become seen as social entities in their own right.

Some categories of children and young people will require particular or increased attention. These include: transitional care, children going into or leaving the care system, fostering and adoption, entering or leaving the prison or young offender's system, refugees and asylum seekers from political and conflict situations.

James and Prout (1990) developed a framework which supported the idea that children's views and opinions should underpin what happens to them and thus have an important role in shaping their lives as active rather than passive recipients of health, education and social care. More traditionalist theorists may disagree with this competence approach, preferring an age-based model with increasing competence as a result. Wherever we stand in this discussion it is clear that there continues to be a move towards *inclusion of the views and opinions of children and young people of all ages* which will influence how we as adults react to their perceived needs. This can be seen as a conflict in approach by some, between a 'rights based' approach to care as opposed to a 'needs' or 'welfare' based approach. Lundy (2007) notes that those involved in developing children's services may need reminded that the UNCRC (1989) is a universal legal imperative and not a just a 'nicety' (Soderback., 2011).

The same should be true for health and social care policy, education, research and practice. This is and will continue to be a central consideration expected in law, of all nurse practitioners in proving that the best interests of the child or young person were taken into consideration. The voice of the child and young person *must* be heard and consideration given to the implications of all our actions (Article 12, UNCRC 1989).

Consent

Competence of children in giving consent is another notable advance which supports the value of listening to what children say and experience. Gillick *vs.* West Norfolk & Wisbech Area Health Authority (1985) enabled minors under 16 to consent if the doctor is satisfied with the criteria as follows:

- Capacity of child to consent
- Voluntariness of child to consent
- Understanding of risks and benefits (informed consent)

Importantly in the eyes of the law, this 'Gillick competence' can be applied to other medical/surgical/dental treatment if in the opinion of the treating doctor the child can be said to have sufficient understanding and intelligence and is capable of making a 'reasonable' assessment of the advantages and disadvantages of proposed treatment, with sufficient discretion to make a choice in his or her own interest. Furthermore, it is important to remember that informed consent is a process and not a one-off event and that doctors and healthcare professionals sometimes influence parent/child consent either way.

The Courts can overrule a child's refusal to consent in cases which are life threatening, but all cases *should be considered on their own merits* in accordance with the principle of justice (treating each case the same unless there is a significant difference). It is very important that all health professionals act at all times in such a way as to help *build a child's capacity* to understand what they are involved in, and not to exert undue influence upon their decision making (UNCRC 1989 and http://capacityltd.org.uk http://www.unicef.org/adolescence/cypguide).

View this online tutorial for more information and a self-test on consent: http://www.mediator.qub.ac.uk/ms/nursingconsent/index.htm

Challenges to healthcare decisions and actions

There continue to be many challenges under the Human Rights Act (1998) and the UNCRC (1989). This is due to a number of factors, including more awareness by the public of their perceived 'rights' and retribution, but also because of the competing complexity of meeting healthcare needs which may indeed infringe some aspects of human rights.

As the care of children and young people involves other practitioners and therapists, not only nurses, there is a clear implication here in relation to how multidisciplinary teams (MDT) and interdisciplinary teams should work. There should be a shared understanding of the complexities of ethical, legal and professional imperatives and guidelines, and legislation should be observed to the letter. All multidisciplinary working practices, particularly the assessment and referral processes are an essential element of the communication process when dealing with the care of children and young persons. This is particularly important where the care management and delivery crosses the interfaces.

Evidence-based practice

In the quest for underpinning evidence it would seem to be easy to fall foul of the belief that evidence is the 'be all and end all' of care interventions. Rolfe (2006) reminds us that just as there are different 'hierarchies' of evidence so, too, different clinical issues may be best served by differing 'kinds' of evidence, and explores the notion that in some cases clinical judgement and expertise is more important, as external evidence can inform practice but never totally replace individual clinical expertise. This is an important distinction because it recognises the value of individual professional judgement in the decision-making process.

In general it is accepted that the safe and competent practitioner should always seek out an action which is in the best interests of the child and family and is also the best from the available current evidence. It should go without saying that in order to meet the requirements of the law, as well as ethical practice, the nurse must keep their knowledge, skills and competence up to date and relevant to their field of practice throughout their working life (http://www.nmc-uk.org).

Documentation within care planning

Good record-keeping, whether at an individual, team or organisational level, has many important functions. These include a range of clinical, administrative and educational uses (Douglas & Ruddle 2009; McGeehan 2007; NMC 2010; NPSA 2007; Oliver 2010; Scovell 2010; Woodward 2007) such as:

- Showing how decisions related to patient care were made
- Supporting the delivery of services
- Supporting effective clinical judgements and decisions
- Supporting patient care and communications
- Making continuity of care easier
- Providing documentary evidence of services delivered
- Promoting better communication and sharing of information between members of the multiprofessional healthcare team
- Helping to identify risks and enabling early detection of complications
- Supporting clinical audit, research, allocation of resources and performance planning
- Helping to address complaints or legal processes

Essential to the provision of good care, record-keeping is a very high-risk activity. Different contexts of care and different systems for record-keeping are used from country to country and in different organisations. Challenges include the move from written paper-based reports to electronic systems and issues around confidentiality and disclosure. Hinchcliff and Rogers (2008) note that the burden to respect the confidentiality of our patients is considerable and point out that in community settings the issue of confidentiality of record-keeping may require more rigor in protection than is automatically available in an acute care setting. The NHS Confidentiality Code of Practice (DH 2003) provides further guidance on record-keeping and confidentiality to that issued by the NMC. NHS employees will be expected to understand and follow the NHS code.

The NMC Code (2008) states that records should show effective communication within the MDT; they must be an accurate record of care planning, treatment and delivery for the individual. Records should be consecutive and completed as soon as possible after the event. They should also show clear evidence of decisions taken and that the information was shared appropriately. Recording and documenting for assessment, intervention and referral processes should follow best practice guidelines to ensure transparency of all interventions and consultations and the informed consent of those involved as clients. Despite this clear directive there are many instances year on year, of incomplete care plans, poor or absent documentation or records which have a disproportionate lean towards physical care and medical problems rather than the holistic needs of a patient care plan. Documentation should, according to the Patient Health Service Ombudsman (2005) include the items of *information and education* provided to patients in the clinical setting to assure effective communication between healthcare professionals. This author asserts that this should also include any developmentally appropriate comfort and communication methods used in family-centred care delivery within the context of the rights of the child.

Social networking sites have widespread usage today. Technology facilitates the spread of information in an instant and with a global reach. The implication for nurses is significant; remember that anything written, uploaded, transmitted or otherwise broadcast is in the public domain. What one individual sees as venting their emotions after a stressful day can be seen by others as offensive, libellous or as whistle-blowing. Material or media considered explicit or inappropriate will result in a nurse putting their registration at risk. The Code states that you are accountable for your actions at all times and for upholding the Code in your personal life as well as your professional activities (RCN 2009).

So, exercise caution before you hit that post/send button on your PC or mobile device (Cain, 2008).

Summary

The need to exercise great *conscience* (accountability) in nursing and social care practice, with particular relevance to the care of children and young people has been identified in this chapter. Acting *ethically or doing the right thing* can be fraught with difficulties. It will be necessary to seek guidance and clarity in all deliberations and actions. Advocacy is an *ethical stance* which should be enshrined in all heath and social care enquiry and action. Each individual children's nurse should be aware of the contents and meaning of the NMC Code, both in their personal and professional life. The nurse should be aware that the standard expected in professional practice is at least that expected in law and indeed *often exceeds the legal expectation.* All nurses should be able to demonstrate that they are practising with due regard for the benefit of, and in the *best interests* of their clients. Record-keeping and care delivery are very high-risk activities in which all healthcare professionals must follow the standards set by professional bodies. Accountability of the practitioner is essential and a *secure knowledge and skills* base must be constantly updated according to need and within the guidance of current NMC Code, the employment contract and that country's legislation. A *children's rights* based approach is *a legal imperative*, not an optional extra in the planning, delivery and evaluation of all education practice and research involving children, young people and their families. Capacity building should be an informed approach *embedded in all aspects of our practice* and communication as children's nurses.

References

Beauchamp, T.L. & Childress, J.F. (2001) *Principles of Biomedical Ethics*, 5th edn. Oxford: Oxford University Press.

Bee, H. & Boyd, D. (2007) *The Developing Child*, 11th edn. Boston: Allyn and Bacon.

Boylan, J. & Dalrymple, J. (2009) *Understanding Advocacy for Children & Young People*. Maidenhead: McGraw Hill, Open University Press.

Brown, J.L., Kitson, A.L. & McKnight, T.J. (1992) *Challenges in Caring: Explorations in Nursing Ethics*. London: Nelson Thornes.

Cain, J. (2008) On-line social networking issues within academia and pharmacy Editorial. *American Journal of Pharmacy Education*. **72**, 10.

Committee of the Central Health Services Council (1959) *The Welfare of Children in Hospital (Platt Report)*. London: HMSO.

Committee on Child Health Services (1976) *Fit for the Future (Court Report)*. London: HMSO.

De Cruz, P. (2005) *Nutshells: Medical law*, 2nd edn. London: Sweet & Maxwell.

Department of Health (2001) *The Kennedy Report: Learning From Bristol. The Report of the Public Inquiry into Children's Heart Surgery at the Bristol Royal Infirmary 1984–1995*, Cm 5207 (1).

Department of Health (2003) *Confidentiality Code of Practice*. London: DH.

Department of Health and Social Services (1995) *The Children Order (NI)*. Belfast: DHSS.

Dimond, B. (2008) *Legal Aspects of Nursing*, 5th edn. Essex: Pearson Education.

Douglas, E. & Ruddle, G. (2009) Implementation of the NHS Knowledge and Skills Framework. *Nursing Standard*, **24**(1), 42–8.

Gillick *vs.* Wisbech & West Norfolk AHA (1985) House of Lords. London: All ER 402.423.

Griffith, R. & Tengnah, C. (2010) *Law and Professional Issues in Nursing*, 3rd edn. Exeter: Learning Matters. www.learningmatters.co.uk.

HMSO (1959) *The Welfare of Children in Hospital*. London: HMSO (Platt Report).

HMSO (1976) *Court Report: Fit for the Future: Report of the Committee on Child Health Services* (Cmnd. 6684). London: HMSO.

HMSO (1989) *The Children Act*. London: HMSO.

Hinchcliff S. & Rogers, R. (2008) *Competencies for Advanced Nursing Practice*. London: Edward Arnold.

Human Rights Act 1998 (1998) Chapter 42. *Elizabeth II*. London: Stationery Office.

James, A. & Prout, A. (1990) Re-presenting childhood: time and transition in the study of childhood. In: *Constructing and Reconstructing Childhood: Contemporary issues in the Sociological study of Childhood*. Basingstoke: Falmer Press.

Lundy, L. (2007) Voice is not enough: conceptualising Article 12 of the United Nations Convention on the Rights of the Child. *British Educational Research Journal*, **33**(6), 927–42.

McGeehan, R. (2007) Best practice in recordkeeping. *Nursing Standard*, **21**(17), 51–5.

McHale, J., Gallagher, A. & Gallagher, N. (2004) *Nursing and Human Rights*. London: Butterworth Heinmann.

National Patient Safety Agency (NPSA) (2007) www.npsa.nhs.uk

Newport Mind Advocacy. www.newport-mind.org (accessed 30 July 2010).

Nursing and Midwifery Council (2008) *The Code: Standards of Conduct, Performance and Ethics for Nurses and Midwives*. London: NMC.

Nursing and Midwifery Council (2010) *Record-keeping: Guidance for Nurses and Midwives*. London: NMC.

Oliver, A. (2010) Observations and monitoring: routine practices on the ward. *Paediatric Nursing*, **22**(4), 28–32.

Patient Health Service Ombudsman (2005) *Making an Impact*. Annual Report 2009–10. www.ombudsman.org.uk.

Rolfe, G. (2006) Evidence based practice (Chapter 5). In: Jasper, M. (ed.) *Professional Development, Reflection and Decision-making*. Oxford: Blackwell Publishing.

Royal College of Nursing (2009) *Legal Advice for RCN Members Using the Internet*. London: RCN.

Scovell, S. (2010) Role of the nurse-to-nurse handover in patient care. *Nursing Standard*, **24**(20), 35–9.

Soderback, M., Coyne, I. & Harder, M. (2011) Importance of including both a child perspective and the child's perspective within health care settings to provide truly health child centred care. *Journal of Child Health Care* **15**, 95–106.

Thompson, I.E., Melia, K.M., Boyd, K.M. & Horsburgh, D. (2006) *Nursing Ethics*, 5th edn. Edinburgh: Churchill Livingstone, Elsevier Ltd.

Tingle, J. & Cribb, A. (2007) *Nursing Law and Ethics*, 3rd edn. Oxford: Blackwell Publishing.

United Kingdom Central Council (UKCC) (1999) *The Peach Report*. UKCC Commission for Nursing and Midwifery and Education Fitness for Practice. London: UKCC.

United Nations Convention on the Rights of the Child (UNCRC) (1989) UNCRC.

Woodward, S. (2007) Learning and sharing safety lessons to improve patient care. *Nursing Standard*, **20**(18), 49–53.

5

Young People and Truth Telling
Catherine Monaghan

Introduction

Having open, honest and clear communication channels with a patient is what is viewed as the 'gold standard' for patient-centred care, which can in turn help facilitate proper assessment and planning of high quality care for the individual (Dawood 2005). Providing young people with the correct information about their diagnosis can help maximise the person's autonomy; however, there are times where it is less straightforward for the whole truth to be disclosed to the patient. Ethical issues arise on a daily basis and Butts and Rich (2005; Goethals et al. 2010) challenge nurses to think critically about the ethics of our day-to-day practice.

Ethical issues will be analysed from traditional perspectives: deontology and utilitarianism, and in addition to this a virtue-based approach will be explored. Begley (2008) suggests that the process of telling the individual about his/her diagnosis should not be based on ethical principles/theories alone and asserts that the nurse must consider virtues such as honesty and compassion.

It is not the intention of this chapter to address in detail whether it is right or wrong to disclose the truth about the individual's diagnosis. The aim is to explore what good practice is and how the children's nurse can enhance best practice by examining key points which should be considered when caring for a young person with a terminal illness.

A framework is useful in assessing the nature of a dilemma, for example the DECIDE model (for further reading see Thompson *et al.* 2000). In this chapter the framework will reflect the steps in the nursing process: assess, plan, implement and evaluate. A scenario and guidance notes are used to illustrate and explore crucial ethical points. This chapter will be useful for educational purposes when used as a framework for discussion in student nurse education.

Care Planning in Children and Young People's Nursing, First Edition.
Edited by Doris Corkin, Sonya Clarke, Lorna Liggett.
© 2012 Blackwell Publishing Ltd. Published 2012 by Blackwell Publishing Ltd.

Case study 5.1

Sara was 16 years old and she had sailed with her father for many years. Even though the boat was small it still needed a crew of two to sail comfortably. A year ago the boat had been a place of fun and sport where both of them enjoyed the thrill of sailing. Today, however, it had become a place of quiet reflection for Tom, her father. So much had changed within the last ten months.

Sara had been diagnosed with myelodysplastic syndrome, a defect in stem cells leading to bone marrow failure, involving red and white cells plus platelets (Kumar and Clark, 2005). Both Tom and his wife were fraught with anxiety about what lay ahead for their daughter. Tom approached the children's nurse who had been involved in Sara's care and asked how best to disclose this news with his daughter (see guidance note 1, Assess).

Their initial reaction was to protect their daughter from pain arising from being told that her condition had become worse (see guidance note 2, Plan). On the other hand, they knew that their daughter would want to know and have the right to know. Both parents considered who would share this information with Sara. The team of healthcare professionals who were caring for Sara were asked to tell Sara about her situation (see guidance note 3, Implement). The children's nurse involved in Sara's care planning reflected on the situation (see guidance note 4, Evaluate).

Assess

Throughout the assessment phase, consider the following questions which the children's nurse might want to address in Sara's case:

- What different ethical approaches might be employed?
- What are the ethical principles that need to be explored?
- Can a virtue ethics approach offer guidance in Sara's situation?

Guidance note 1

The children's nurse will begin by assessing the situation, the context and the individuals involved. By reflecting on the situation and approaching it from a deontological perspective, the nurse will ascertain that she has a professional duty and obligation to tell the truth to Sara. The nurse is less concerned with the consequences and it is more her belief that it is her duty to adhere to the principle of veracity at all times. She believes that it is morally indefensible to engage in any act of lying or deceit (Monaghan and Begley 2004). Furthermore, the nurse feels bound by her *Code of Professional Conduct* (NMC 2008), which reminds us that all actions are performed in the patient's best interest. The nurse believes that as an individual Sara has the right to be told the truth regardless of the consequences of telling her. Such an approach reflects Kant's duty-based moral theory, which demands an absolute adherence to rules and duties and respect for autonomy (Kendrick 1994). The children's nurse is concerned that Sara will not be able to exercise autonomy if she is not informed of her diagnosis.

In contrast, if the nurse believes that Sara should be told the truth but at the same time takes a utilitarian approach, she will be concerned that the consequences of the truth may

Table 5.1 A summary of the ethical principles, ethical approaches and virtues relevant to Sara's situation.

Ethical principles	Ethical approaches	Virtues
Veracity	Deontology/duty – obligation	Compassion
Beneficence	Utilitarianism	Honesty
Non-maleficence	Virtue-based approach	Integrity
Justice		Kindness
Confidentiality		Understanding
Autonomy		

cause more harm rather than 'good'. This is where a conflict of principles can arise. The nurse is motivated to do 'good' (principle of beneficence) and avoid harm which is the principle of non-maleficence (Monaghan and Begley 2004).

Utilitarians appraise the moral worth of an act by considering the consequences or end result; the act should bring about the greatest good for the greatest number and result in more happiness than pain (Edwards 1996). The children's nurse will also know that Sara already has insight into her condition and suspects that something has changed. Feelings of fear and uncertainty may be expressed by the patient and according to Fallowfield *et al.* (2002) usually the individual will have some insight into their condition and know that something is wrong. Traditional objective moral theories such as deontology and utilitarianism may not be appropriate alone, and virtue ethics, which includes virtues such as compassion and integrity, should be considered. For further reading and discussion of virtue ethics, refer to Hodkinson (2008). See Table 5.1.

Plan

Throughout the planning phase, consider the following questions which the children's nurse might want to address in Sara's case:

- What options does the children's nurse have when planning to share the information about her condition with Sara?
- What consequences are likely to occur?

Guidance note 2

In order for the children's nurse to make effective planning, issues such as when this information will be shared with Sara, who will disclose such information and where the is best venue for this to take place need to be decided. The children's nurse needs to consider first of all who will be best placed to give this information. In general, a member from the healthcare profession tends to adopt the role of informing the patient about his/her diagnosis. According to Parsons *et al.* (2007) direct communication with adults about their diagnosis has become more apparent over the last 50 years. However, when it comes to communicating a cancer diagnosis with a young person it is not without great difficulty. Sometimes a family member may feel they are best placed to impart such information, but this can prove to be an immense emotional challenge for the parent/guardian and there should always be support for the individual and patient. Rowlands (2005) points out that the nurse must strive to explore what normal practice is for individuals from different cultural backgrounds when sharing a diagnosis. For further reading and discussion refer to Karim (2003) and Rowlands (2005).

Initially, Sara's parents did not want Sara to be told about the change in her condition. The issue of paternalism versus autonomy arose here. Her father felt that if Sara heard such information she would not be able to cope and that the truth could possibly destroy any hope that his daughter had. If the children's nurse agreed with Sara's parents and they had decided to withhold such information, then both the nurse and parents would have been exercising paternalism. Monaghan and Begley (2004) point out that it can present a challenge for the healthcare professional when there is a decision to withhold the information from the patient and to consider a decision based on 'the professional knows best' or respect for the patient's autonomy.

On the other hand, let us consider at how non-disclosure of the truth/information might affect the patient. Limited information sharing can lead to the patient not possessing important information which can affect the ability to make sound decisions about his/her care and future treatment plans. Charles-Edwards & Brotchie (2005) suggest that by keeping the younger person informed you are treating him/her with the utmost respect. They further assert that in order for the young person to be able to make informed decisions, the truth needs to be disclosed and answers to questions asked need to be given in a meaningful and sensitive manner. Miller (2001) reminds us that the correct amount of information must be shared with young people at the right level for his/her current understanding. Therefore each situation must be carefully assessed and planned on an individual basis and the interests of the young person must remain the focus and central in the decision-making process.

If the information is shared with Sara then she can make informed choices in partnership with the healthcare professional and her parents. According to Parsons *et al.* (2007) autonomy has become the prevailing ethical principle. All parties can then engage with Sara in decision making about the right care for her. This reflects a more family-centred approach. See Table 5.2.

Implement

Consider the following questions which the children's nurse might want to address once an action plan has been established as to who will share Sara's information with her.

Table 5.2   Possible outcomes if the truth is shared with the young person or if information is withheld.

Positive aspects: telling truth	Negative aspects: not telling truth
Patient autonomy	Paternalism
Compliance	Patient non-compliance
Trust	Issue of deceit
Informed choices	Decreased sense of security
Hope	Despair
Open communication	Secrecy
Engagement	Exclusion
Family-centred approach	Isolation

- How will this information be shared with Sara?
- In addition to the virtues highlighted below what other virtues might the children's nurse posses?
- What important aspects of communication must be considered?

Guidance note 3

Careful thought must be given to how information is imparted. A virtue ethics approach is appropriate here and in Sara's situation the nurse must be able to demonstrate compassion, a friendly and caring approach, sensitivity and respect. When any aspect of care is being implemented the young person needs to feel valued and meaningful communication must take place. This can be facilitated in a venue where the individual is able to discuss any fears and worries. The children's nurse needs to take into consideration what has already been communicated to Sara, what she has already heard or not heard and indeed misunderstood. Thought must be given to the choice of words and terminology used when communicating with Sara about her situation. Explanations should not be misleading and time needs to be afforded so that Sara is able to express her feelings.

In order for the nurse and Sara's parents to be able to communicate effectively with Sara there needs to be trust and this trust will only develop and be therapeutic whenever the children's nurse/patient relationship embraces truth telling. As Rockwell (2007) points out, if the professional is striving to achieve being honest with the individual, then truth is the vehicle that surely facilitates us reaching that goal. Whenever the individual knows the truth about his/her illness this can help with the psychological and emotional adjustment (Pinner 2000). This allows for proper support services to be implemented into Sara's treatment plan.

At this point let us consider possible reasons why the truth may not be communicated (see Box 5.1).

Evaluate

Consider the following questions which the children's nurse might want to address in the process of evaluation:

- What needs to be evaluated in relation to Sara, her parents, the nurse and practice?
- What important aspects of evaluation need to be considered?

Box 5.1 Possible reasons why the truth may not be communicated with the young person

The young person clearly states that she does not wish to receive this information at present. This situation, however, must be continually assessed as this may change.
Medical staff may not always be in a position to know the truth about the individual's condition.
Consideration must be given to the development level of the child/young person as well as cultural background.

Guidance note 4

In Sara's situation there are four areas that need to be evaluated throughout the disclosure process. Evaluation is an ongoing process; therefore the children's nurse will continually need to assess what the impact of revealing the truth has on Sara. The nurse must continuously assess for any signs of distress that Sara may experience and monitor how she copes with this. The diagnosis and deterioration in her condition is Sara's information and needs to be shared with her as opposed to Sara being told. This, however, must be communicated in a sensitive and caring approach.

Sara's parents have engaged in a family-centred approach rather than adopting a paternalistic view. If a partnership approach is adopted and implemented it helps facilitate a more open channel for Sara's parents to approach the children's nurse and, where appropriate, seek support services which they may require, such as advice and counselling. Appropriate and timely information throughout all aspects of Sara's care is paramount for both Sara and her parents. As a result they will feel empowered to be able to make informed choices and be able to take an active role and fully engage in decisions being made about Sara's situation and treatment plan. This must be continuously monitored and ways to enhance this partnership must be explored.

The children's nurse must equally evaluate his/her own involvement in the process of truth telling. Being involved in facilitating the truth being shared with a young person can be viewed as extremely difficult and cognisance must be taken of the impact it can have on the children's nurse. Reflection on how the children's nurse can manage and cope in such delicate and emotional situations must be encouraged and promoted. Dunlop (2008) advocates that the nurse reflects on his/her own emotions and how any reluctance to engage in the process of truth telling may be as a result of avoiding confronting a difficult emotional responsibility. The children's nurse needs to be knowledgeable and well equipped to deal with situations such as these. Best practice in this area, which can be an ethical minefield, requires proper training and support. Good education and mentoring of staff is, therefore, essential in achieving a positive outcome for patient, family and professional. Dunlop (2008) stresses that training needs should address and include the nurse becoming skilled in developing effective and meaningful communication skills and in developing a reflective approach. See Table 5.3.

Summary

As Butts and Rich (2005) point out, the nurse must think critically about the ethics of day-to-day practice. Harvey and Stobbart (2006) stress the importance of the nurse ensuring that a clear date for a review of all agreed actions in the patient's care plan is set and reviewed. In addition, all documentation throughout the process must be accurately recorded. In

Table 5.3 Four areas which need to be evaluated throughout the disclosure process and possible issues arising in each.

Young person	Parent/guardian	Nurse	Practice
Coping	Partnership	Reflection	Guidelines
Central to decision-making process	Support and advice	Critical thinking	Research focused
Approach		Training needs	Cultural needs

Sara's situation, it would appear to be morally indefensible to withhold the information from the patient (Monaghan and Begley 2004). Furthermore, they assert that each situation is fluid; the children's nurse must take into consideration what is happening with the young person, what the parent/guardian is experiencing and what different views and ethical principles each professional holds. Consideration must also be afforded to different cultural backgrounds and different beliefs.

References

Begley, A. (2008) Truth-telling, honesty and compassion: a virtue-based exploration of a dilemma in practice. *International Journal of Nursing Practice*, **14**, 336–41.

Butts, J.B. & Rich, K.L. (2005) *Nursing Ethics. Across the Curriculum and into Practice*, 2nd edn. London: Jones and Bartlett Publishers.

Charles-Edwards, I. & Brotchie, J. (2005) Privacy: what does it mean for children's nurses? *Paediatric Nursing*, **17**(5), 36–43.

Dawood, M. (2005) Patient-centred care: lessons from the medical profession. *Emergency Nurse*, **13**(1), 22–7.

Dunlop, S. (2008) The dying child: should we tell the truth? *Paediatric Nursing*, **20**(6), 28–31.

Edwards, S.D. (1996) *Nursing Ethics. A Principle-Based Approach*. London: Macmillan Press.

Fallowfield, L.F., Jenkins, V.A. & Beveridge, H.A. (2002) Truth may hurt but deceit hurts more: communication in palliative care. *Palliative Medicine*, **16**, 297–303.

Goethals, S., Gastmans, C. & Dierckx de Casterle, B. (2010) Nurses' ethical reasoning and behaviour: A literature review. *International Journal of Nursing Studies* **47**(5), 635–650.

Harvey, S. & Stobbart, V. (2006) The legal and ethical implications of care planning and delivery for intellectual disability nursing. In: Gates, B. *Care Planning and Delivery in Intellectual Disability Nursing*. London: Blackwell Publishing.

Hodkinson, K. (2008) How should a nurse approach truth-telling? A virtue ethics perspective. *Nursing Philosophy* **9**(4), 248–256.

Karim, K. (2003) Informing cancer patients: truth telling and culture. *Cancer Nursing Practice*, **2**(3), 23–31.

Kendrick, K. (1994) Tools which aid the decision-making process: addressing moral dilemmas in nursing practice. *Professional Nurse*, **9**, 739–42.

Kumar, P. & Clark, M. (2005) *Clinical Medicine*, 6th edn. Edinburgh: Elsevier Saunders.

Miller, S. (2001) Facilitating decision-making in young people. *Paediatric Nursing*, **13**(5), 31–5.

Monaghan, C. & Begley, A. (2004) Dementia diagnosis and disclosure: a dilemma in practice. *International Journal of Older People Nursing* in association with *Journal of Clinical Nursing*, **13**(3a), 1–8.

Nursing and Midwifery Council (2008) *The Code – Standards of Conduct, Performance and Ethics for Nurses and Midwives*. London: NMC.

Parsons, S.K., Saiki-Craig, S. & Mayer, D.K. (2007) Telling children and adolescents about their cancer diagnosis: cross-cultural comparisons between paediatric oncologists in the US and Japan. *Psycho-Oncology*, **16**, 60–68.

Pinner, G. (2000) Truth-telling and the diagnosis of dementia. *British Journal of Psychiatry*, **176**, 514–15.

Rockwell, L.E. (2007) Truthtelling. *Journal of Clinical Oncology*, **25**(4), 454–5.

Rowlands, J. (2005) To tell the truth. *Cancer Nursing Practice*, **4**(5), 16–21.

Thompson, I.E., Melia, K.M. & Boyd, K.M. (2000) *Nursing Ethics*. Edinburgh: Churchill Livingstone.

6

Sexual Health
Jim Richardson

Introduction

When addressing nursing considerations the issues identified through considering the case study and the questions posed will help to identify those aspects of the situation which will require further nursing assessment, planning and, ultimately, the nursing interventions which will help to address Kylie's needs (see case study below).

Case study 6.1

Kylie is a 16-year-old girl who lives with her parents and younger sister. She attends school enthusiastically and plans to study to become a primary schoolteacher.

Kylie has a 24-year-old boyfriend of two months and although she is sexually active, she has not sought advice about contraception.

She now wants to speak to a nurse as she thinks she may be pregnant.

 Questions

1. What constitutes good sexual health?
2. What do young people need to promote their own sexual health?
3. What problems might young people experience in maintaining their sexual health and wellbeing?

Care Planning in Children and Young People's Nursing, First Edition.
Edited by Doris Corkin, Sonya Clarke, Lorna Liggett.
© 2012 Blackwell Publishing Ltd. Published 2012 by Blackwell Publishing Ltd.

Answers to questions

Question 1. What constitutes good sexual health?

Good sexual health can be defined by concrete factors such as the absence of sexually transmissible disease. However, there are more abstract perspectives too, such as freedom of expression of sexual self.

It is worth considering the definition of sexual health to ensure that all dimensions are identified. The World Health Organisation (WHO 2002) defined sexual health as:

> 'A state of physical, emotional, mental and social wellbeing related to sexuality. It is not merely the absence of disease, dysfunction or infirmity. Sexual health requires a positive and respectful approach to sexuality and sexual relationships, as well as the possibility of having pleasurable and safe sexual experiences, free of coercion, discrimination and violence. For sexual health to be attained and maintained, the sexual rights of all persons must be respected, protected and fulfilled.'.

This rather long statement serves to highlight the complexity of sexual health. Some of the key ideas from a nursing perspective include:

- Sometimes we think of sexual health rather narrowly in terms of sexually transmissible infection and unintended pregnancy. While these factors are important, they are not the whole story.
- People may need help to achieve the sexual life they want, free of social pressures (such as the peer group for young people), coercion (such as being pushed into engaging in sexual activity against their better judgement or before they feel ready to do so).
- Sexual bullying and violence are too common and young people need to be equipped with the skills to protect themselves.
- Sexual health is not merely a matter of physiological or mechanical issues. It is important that young people learn how to conduct their sexual lives in a way that is emotionally and psychologically rewarding and satisfying.
- Sexually transmissible infections are prevalent among young people and there is evidence that they are rather taken for granted by this age group. However, the long-term consequences of some of these can be severe, for example chlamydia and HIV (see Chapter 36). Misinformation about these infections is widespread among young people
- Some young people actively opt for early parenthood. However, the UK has among the highest rates of teenage pregnancy in the Western world and this is even more marked in areas of relative deprivation. Many of these pregnancies will be unintended and have the potential to limit the life opportunities of these young parents.

In the light of these factors, it is important for nurses working with children and young people to consider what young people need to be able to protect and improve their own sexual health and wellbeing. Equally significant will be a consideration of factors which serve as barriers to young people being able to act in their own best interests in this central facet of their health. Exploration of these issues will allow the children and young people's (CYP) nurse to identify their learning needs so that they are equipped with the knowledge and skills necessary to help young people meet their health needs.

Some facts

In Scotland during 2008, 16% of 15–24-year-old men who were tested for chlamydia proved to be infected (NHS National Services Scotland 2010).

In Wales, between 2005 and 2008, 44 per 1000 young women between the ages of 15 and 17 became pregnant (Welsh Assembly Government 2010).

In England during 2009, 4249 young men between the ages of 16 and 19 were diagnosed as having genital warts (Health Protection Agency 2010).

In Northern Ireland in 2000, the average age of first heterosexual intercourse was 14.9 years for young men and 15.9 for young women. The age of consent for all in Northern Ireland is 16 (Family Planning Association 2009).

All of these indicators are significantly more negative than those found among our Western European neighbours (UNICEF 2004). These facts indicate rather starkly the need for improvement in sexual health promotion among our young people.

Question 2. What do young people need to promote their own sexual health?

The first and most obvious need is for accurate and constructive information in relation to sex. Young people readily identify this need but often have difficulty accessing this information:

- While many young people get their sex-related information at home, many parents find it difficult to discuss sex with their children, often because they feel ill-equipped themselves to discuss this matter. This attitude can also lead to young people feeling unable to bring their sexual concerns to their parents (Rhondda Cynon Taff Fframwaith 2009).
- The school can play an important role in ensuring the sex education of young people. However, this provision is patchy and variable in quality. Sometimes sex-related information offered is excellent and versatile, tailored to the needs of the young people and covering all aspects of sexuality. On the other hand, some young people receive information relating to the biology of sex with little reference to relationship aspects of a healthy sexual life. Excluded and hard-to-reach young people suffer a further disadvantage in this respect.
- For many young people, the principal source of sex-related information is the peer group. This may be unhelpful and inaccurate and lead to negative feelings about sex and sexuality and risky behaviour.
- Young people who are gay, lesbian, bisexual or transgendered can be particularly disadvantaged in this key element of their lives. Their particular needs must be identified and respected, although currently that generally is not the case for most.
- The media offer distorted images of sexuality in our sexualised society. Young people can be led to believe that this is reliable and dependable information and may base their expectations on this.
- Expectations of sexuality and sexual health can vary between ethnic, religious and cultural groups. Sex-related information will have to be couched in formats which are sensitive to these expectations.

Young people need access to services which exist to promote their sexual health:

- Contraceptive and sexual health (CASH) services need to be orientated towards the needs of young people and specifically address the needs of this age group.

- Sexual health services which offer diagnosis and treatment of sex-related disorders need to be readily available and accessible as well as youth-friendly.
- Counselling in relation to sexual wellbeing needs to be available. This is particularly important for those who have experienced sexual coercion or exploitation (Scottish Government 2010).
- Dedicated facilities for the support of victims of sexual violence are particularly crucial.

CYP nurses and other professionals who work with young people are in a position to help this group with their informational needs. There are a number of approaches to this (NICE 2007) and might include:

- Drop-in services offered by specifically prepared professionals. Young people particularly value the services of groups such as school nurses and youth workers.
- Educational programmes delivered by specially prepared peer educators can be effective.
- Mass health education campaigns can be effective, especially when channelled through media and platforms used by young people.
- Projects designed to improve access to contraception services can be very useful (Health Development Agency 2004).

On occasion, the most important role of the CYP nurse is, having assessed sexual health-related needs, being aware of appropriate local services and being able to refer to these effectively.

Question 3. What problems might young people experience in maintaining their sexual health and wellbeing?

- Being unaware of what good sexual health is and how this can be achieved is the first and most obvious need and can be answered by good educational provision.
- Young people sometimes meet professionals and others who have negative, judgemental, flawed and damaging attitudes and assumptions. This, in place of a proper and comprehensive assessment of need, constitutes a real barrier.
- Young people have a real concern for confidentiality in relation to their sexual health needs and can be impeded from accessing services. This can naturally be particularly marked in rural and remote settings. There is some evidence that young people perceive health professionals as being sensitive to confidentiality needs.
- Assertiveness and negotiation skills within relationships, is something many young people find difficult to achieve.
- If an atmosphere conducive to open discussion and questioning is not created, embarrassment can be a real hurdle to communication.
- A lack of awareness that substance and alcohol use can lead to errors of judgement and risky behaviour.
- Victimisation, exploitation and abusive relationships are sources of substantial damage to sexual health in every respect.

From consideration of this range of factors, it begins to become evident how care in relation to sexual health for Kylie might be approached. The first step to care will always be to assess need.

> ✏ **Activity 6.1**
>
> Draft an assessment approach to establishing Kylie's sexual health needs. You may find Mitchell and Wellings (1998) helpful in doing this.
>
> Once you have done this, it will be straightforward to draft a plan of care which will address Kylie's sexual health needs. Bear in mind that the plan will be drafted in negotiation with Kylie and will fully take into account Kylie's perceptions of her needs in this respect.

Summary

The sexual health of young people in the UK could be improved in every dimension. Sexual wellbeing is an important part of people's lives and is a significant determinant of perceptions of quality of life. Children's and young people's nurses can contribute to this aspect of their patients' care needs but need the appropriate knowledge and skills to be able to do this effectively and in an appropriate manner.

References

Family Planning Association (2009) *Teenagers: Sexual Health and Behaviour.* London: Family Planning Association.

Health Development Agency (2004) *Teenage Pregnancy and Sexual Health Interventions.* London: Health Development Agency.

Health Protection Agency (2010) *STI Diagnoses Made at Genitourinary Medicine Clinics in England: 2009.* London: Health Protection Agency.

Mitchell, K. & Wellings, K. (1998) *Talking about Sexual Health.* London: Health Education Authority.

National Institute for Health and Clinical Excellence (2007) *One-to-one Interventions to Reduce the Transmission of Sexually Transmitted Infections (STIs) Including HIV, and to Reduce the Rate of Under 18 Conceptions, Especially Among Vulnerable and at Risk Groups.* London: National Institute for Health and Clinical Excellence.

NHS National Services Scotland (2010) *Key Clinical Indicators for Sexual Health.* Glasgow: NHS National Services Scotland.

Rhondda Cynon Taff Fframwaith (2009) *Developing a Strategy for Preventing Teenage Pregnancy, Supporting Teenage Parents and Meeting Sexual Health Needs.* Pontypridd: Rhondda Cynon Taff Fframwaith.

Scottish Government (2010) *Draft National Guidance: Under-age Sexual Activity – Meeting the Needs of Children and Young People and Identifying Child Protection Concerns.* Edinburgh: Scottish Government.

UNICEF (2004) *A League Table of Teenage Births in Rich Nations.* Florence: UNICEF.

Welsh Assembly Government (2010) *Sexual Health and Wellbeing Action Plan for Wales, 2010–2015.* Cardiff: Welsh Assembly Government.

World Health Organisation (2002) *Definition of Sexual Health.* www2.hu-berlin.de/sexology/ECE5/definition_4.html (accessed 15 November 2010).

7

Integrated Care Pathways

Pauline Cardwell and Philomena Morrow

Introduction

In Chapter 1 a review of the development of the nursing process and several models of nursing were presented in relation to children's nursing. In more recent times healthcare delivery has focused on developing services which are inclusive of patient and health professionals' views and flexible to ensure evidence-based practice is supported within the finite resources of service provision. Thus, the goals of planning and delivering patient focused and effective care and services which meet the needs of patients has been developed and supported by the use of integrated care pathways. Health delivery systems globally are under increasing pressure to provide effective services to meet the increasing needs of society, whilst working with finite resources in aiming to do so (National Council for the Professional Development of Nursing and Midwifery (NCNM) 2006). Whilst family-centred care has developed within the field of children's nursing and is utilised alongside the nursing process to organise and aid care delivery, there is an increasing acknowledgement and development of integrated care pathways (ICP). Such developments are purported to support interprofessional working and improve the effectiveness of care delivery in mapping patients' journeys and predicting care trajectories (Allen *et al.* 2009). These pathways are increasingly used in care planning and delivering patient care relevant to various conditions and settings, whilst also aiding practitioners in making timely decisions, alongside other health professionals, which are appropriate to the needs of the child and family.

Within this chapter, the origin and elements of ICPs will be discussed and consideration will be given to the development of ICPs for specific patient groups within a clinical environment. The chapter will draw on information from national and international examples

Care Planning in Children and Young People's Nursing, First Edition.
Edited by Doris Corkin, Sonya Clarke, Lorna Liggett.
© 2012 Blackwell Publishing Ltd. Published 2012 by Blackwell Publishing Ltd.

when considering their contribution to care delivery. In addition, how these pathways can support the implementation of best practice guidelines and standardise care planning and delivery to children and their families will be included. In order to illustrate and appreciate the structure and support ICPs offer in delivering care to children and their families, an ICP for the management of bronchiolitis will be utilised in this chapter to outline how these documents can support care planning and delivery.

The origins of integrated care pathways

Integrated care pathways serve several purposes, including continuous quality improvement, reduction in variation of standards, minimising resource utilisation and education of healthcare staff (Kwan & Sanderwood 2005). Such reported activities have contributed to their development and utilisation in current healthcare practice. In attempting to identify the origins and use of these pathways it is therefore necessary to consider the strengths of these innovations and their contribution to the delivery of healthcare in the twenty-first century. Wakefield (2004) identified the origins of ICPs as being utilised in the USA and Australia from the 1980s, with their introduction in the UK in the 1990s. In responding to the reforms and modernisation of health services in the UK the need for an integrated approach to healthcare has been reinforced, whereby interprofessional, inter-organisational and user collaboration is seen as an essential component of best practice (Atwal & Caldwell 2002). This translates into putting children and their families at the centre of service planning and delivery alongside multidisciplinary teams. According to Whittle & Hewison (2007) and Middleton & Roberts (2000) this represents the vision for the modern NHS and the means of enhancing high-quality service delivery have been sought through ICPs.

Several authors identify reasons from a governance perspective for the introduction and development of ICPs in the UK; these include demonstrating evidence-based care through the utilisation of best practice guidelines, such as national service framework standards, developing benchmarking standards and thus addressing the clinical governance agenda (Allen *et al.* 2009; Campbell *et al.* 1998; Cunningham *et al.* 2008; MacLean *et al.* 2008; Wakefield 2004). Additional strengths of the ICP in care planning and delivery include reducing lengths of hospitalisation, facilitating decision making and supporting clinical judgement skills. These skills standardise and define the patient's programme of care and assess the impact on patient outcomes in terms of education and self-management (MacLean *et al.* 2008; Mirando *et al.* 2005; Whittle & Hewison 2007). Thus, ICPs have become part of contemporary healthcare practice in the UK.

What are integrated care pathways?

Within this chapter the term ICP is utilised; however, it is important to appreciate that within the literature several terms are used to identify these initiatives, including integrated case management, care map, clinical pathways, critical pathways and integrated care systems. The development and utilisation of these pathways are frequently individually unique to the unit or clinical environment in which they have been developed. They are created for specific purposes as creative solutions to issues in clinical practice, and are developed for managing the care of particular patient groups or situations. De Luc (2001) identifies the inclusion of all professionals involved in 'hands on' care in developing the

ICP relevant to the topic of interest, to develop and support the success of the initiative. Careful thought therefore needs to be given to their development and design if changes in practice are to be in the direction intended (Allen *et al.* 2009). Irrespective of their descriptive title it is important to consider what ICPs are.

Walsh (1998) identifies critical pathways as setting out plans of care to meet the needs of patients with the same medical problem, identifying goals to be achieved and defining outcomes against which progress can be measured, a view supported by Middleton & Roberts (2000). More contemporarily, ICPs are described as multidisciplinary care management tools which map chronologically, activities in healthcare systems which are to be achieved, whilst additionally having a quality improvement function (Allen 2009). Subsequently, having identified agreed goals and outcomes of care provision with other health professions involved in providing care to the individual, it is necessary to create a tool for recording and documenting these aspects which can be used by all involved in the delivery of care for the infant and family. Integrated care pathways have been developed to provide a framework for clinical and treatment decisions regarding care provision which incorporate and support the use of best evidence, by streamlining and standardising care for specific patient groups (NCNM 2006). Davis (2005) succinctly suggests ICPs as being crucial in delivering care which is safe, effective, patient-centred, timely, efficient and equitable in the modern NHS. Indeed, the use of ICPs can be perceived to address the following aspects of professional practice:

- Patient-centred care
- High quality and safe-care delivery
- Evidence base for care delivery utilised
- Timely delivery of care to meet needs of patient when required
- Efficiency through better management and use of services
- Equitable service for all patients

The pathway aims to identify significant factors and progression points along the patient's journey in relation to a particular disease process or access point to services.

Activity 7.1

Think about what benefits using an ICP would have for you individually as a professional in your current clinical environment.
Can you list what some of these might be?

What are the elements of an integrated care pathway?

The ICP will include several key aspects, which are initially based on the aim of tracing the expected journey of the infant through the illness. The patient's journey will have definitive start and end points and within the ICP will involve input from various health professionals who will contribute to care delivery and will aim to integrate evidence, clinical guideline information and recommendations (Mirando *et al.* 2005). This journey will be further refined considering what interventions are required, when these should be completed, by whom and in which setting (De Luc 2001). It is also important to identify and appreciate boundaries for the ICP, in order to ensure its effective utilisation in clinical practice, for example an infant who is admitted with a secondary pneumonia to the primary diagnosis of bronchiolitis may require consideration of possible variances in the ICP which may impact on expected care trajectories.

A variance is any deviation from the proposed standard of care listed in the pathway. It is the difference between the care stated within the time period and the actual event (Zander 2002). A variance from outcome is important at any time and should be addressed and documented and include possible reasons as to why the deviation has occurred. According to Zander (2002), variations from the pathway identify patients who are not progressing as expected and obviously allows for early and appropriate interventions to be instigated. Recording of variances assists professionals utilising personal autonomy to individualise care for the patient and their family (Atwal & Caldwell 2002). In addition, variances provide valuable information which may be collated and analysed (Hall, 2006), and as a result improvements for future practice may be identified.

The ICP, which contains the programme of care that has been developed for infants with bronchiolitis, will include areas to record holistic medical and nursing assessments of the patient in the initial stages of the journey. From a nursing perspective and in conjunction with the nursing process, these activities facilitate designing plans which meet the infant and family's individual needs, through the delivery of timely care and effective interventions. Additionally, areas of care particular to the individual infant's condition, investigations, communications, teaching and discharge plans are usually included in the document (see Appendix 2).

The ICP is aimed at providing a multiprofessional tool to detail and log the infant's journey through the illness or disease process, assisting professionals to create comprehensive documents which are developed by those involved in care delivery. The plan may also include criteria to help identify parameters of recovery or deterioration to assist the health professional in making timely decisions regarding management of the infant's condition. Timelines may be used within the pathway to monitor the patient's journey through the healthcare systems, with a multiprofessional focus. The inclusion of such information assists the professional practitioner to make timely clinical assessments and decisions based on the current condition of the infant and identify required interventions aimed at meeting the needs of the patient. As with many of the documents used in clinical practice these may vary in design from facility to facility and thus it is useful to provide an illustration of some of the elements of an ICP, to explore their content.

Activity 7.2

Think about an infant presenting with a possible diagnosis of bronchiolitis. What do you think would be key symptoms and indicators of severity of the disease process to observe?

List some of the symptoms and describe the altered physiology relevant to the symptoms identified.

Clinical scenario

If you consider the earlier identified example of bronchiolitis in a two-month-old infant, using an ICP will provide the children's nurse with guidance on presenting symptoms which will help to identify the likely diagnosis and the immediate care needs of the infant and family (see Appendix 2). Bronchiolitis is a seasonal, acute, infectious lower airway infection, usually caused by a virus affecting the bronchioles, and can cause acute respiratory distress including difficulty breathing, cough, irritability and even apnoea in young infants (Scottish Intercollegiate Guidelines Network (SIGN) 2006). As the most common lower respiratory tract infection in infants, bronchiolitis has several key features, including coryzal symptoms, snuffles, cough, wheeze, feeding difficulties, increasing respiratory rate, respiratory distress, pyrexia, tachycardia and fatigue (McDougall 2011; Peter & Fazakerley 2004). Nursing care management for infants with bronchiolitis is largely supportive, aimed at monitoring the infant's condition, relieving respiratory distress through use of prescribed therapies and ensuring adequate hydration and nutrition, and delivering effective infection control. Nevertheless, the children's nurse must be able to accurately determine the critical status of the infant and identify their immediate needs at the initial point of contact. The value of having clear criteria on which to base these clinical decisions is beneficial to all professionals and supports the provision of services in a timely manner. Incorporating guidelines and evidence such as that produced by SIGN (2006) assists the health professional to provide a high quality service which also meets the individual needs of the infant and family.

Signs of severe disease include:

- Respiratory rate >70/minute
- Oxygen saturation ≤94%
- Nasal flaring/grunting
- Severe intercostal recession
- Cyanosis/history of apnoea
- Lethargy
- Poor feeding <50% of feeding requirements

(SIGN 2006)

The ICP may also give the children's nurse information regarding possible interventions and guidance in relation to supportive care to the infant and family.

Subsequently, an example of a care pathway has been developed to illustrate some of the likely components of an ICP relating to the care of an infant with bronchiolitis. The ICP is used to record the patient's journey through their contact with professionals and the disease process. From a professional viewpoint, it allows practitioners to record and log details of care delivered, whilst also providing guidance on possible interventions required without repetition and duplication of information.

How do integrated care pathways contribute to evidence-based practice?

In developing ICPs an initial search of the literature which relates to the care pathway being created is undertaken. This will allow the development team to consider and integrate current clinical guidelines, information from recent studies and contemporary research in the area. The involvement of service users is also seen as key to ensuring the care pathway is responsive to patients' needs and also focuses the development of the initiative by keeping the patient at the centre of care delivery. Access to sample ICPs from other organisations may assist in considering the challenges and modifications of the developing ICP required and may prevent 'reinventing the wheel' processes. Additionally, review of sample ICPs may also facilitate focusing those involved in the initiative on key variances and ensure that best practice evidence is integrated into the process.

The development of ICPs is also strongly advocated and supported by Government both nationally and regionally within the UK, as it clearly supports multiprofessional working and partnerships which recognise the patient at the centre of service provision (DHSSPS 2004; DH 2004; OFMDFMNI 2006). The impetus of these government guidelines is to utilise the expertise of clinicians in delivering on modernising the health service in the UK to deliver high quality, evidence-based care within an efficient, finitely resourced service. With the developing partnerships amongst professionals in delivering care through ICPs, these interprofessional workings can cross traditional boundaries between health and social care settings, ensuring that the patient's journey is supported throughout.

As identified earlier in the chapter, ICPs also assists in achieving the clinical governance agenda through the delivery of evidence-based care which encompasses best practice guidelines and is subject to regular clinical audit and review (Middleton *et al.* 2001). Through this process of development, utilisation and evaluation of ICPs cognisance of contemporary research, clinical guidelines and current best practice, alongside review of clinical audit will be achieved. The ICP must be viewed as a dynamic and flexible tool which with regular review can incorporate changes occurring in clinical practice and which can adapt to meet the needs of patients for which the tool was designed.

Summary

In this chapter we have considered what an ICP is and how it contributes to the delivery of healthcare in the twenty-first century. ICPs have enjoyed the support of clinicians, academics and governmental policy in their development and growth in healthcare service delivery systems. The origins and use of ICPs have been explored, considering what they are and are not and what elements contribute to their structure and functionality. In developing such innovations an examination of how they require input from all professionals involved in the delivery of care is crucial to the success of such initiatives. This chapter has outlined major aspects of ICPs. However, it is by no means exhaustive and further independent study may assist in developing your appreciation of ICPs in contemporary healthcare services.

Acknowledgement

The authors would like to thank Dr Mike Smith, Consultant Paediatrician, for his generosity of time and commitment in commenting on and contributing to the content of this chapter.

References

Allen, D., Gillen, E. & Rixson, L. (2009) Systematic review of the effectiveness of integrated care pathways: what works, for whom, in which circumstances? *International Journal of Evidence Based Healthcare*, 7, 61–74.

Atwal, A. & Caldwell, K. (2002) Do multidisciplinary integrated care pathways improve interprofessional collaboration? *Scandiavian Journal of Caring Science*, **16**, 360–67.

Campbell, H., Hotchkiss, R., Bradshaw, N. & Porteous, M. (1998) Integrated care pathways. *British Medical Journal*, **316,** 133–7.

Cunningham, S., Logan, C., Lockerbie, L., Dunn, M.J.G., McMurray, A. & Prescott, R.J. (2008) Effect of an integrated care pathway on acute asthma/wheeze in children attending hospital: cluster randomised trial. *The Journal of Pediatrics*, **152**, 315–20.

Davis, N. (2005) *Integrated Care Pathways – a Guide to Good Practice*. Wales: National Leadership and Innovation Agency for Healthcare.

De Luc, K. (2001) *Developing Care Pathways: the Tool Kit*. Oxford: Radcliffe Medical Press.

Department of Health (2004) *National Service Framework for Children, Young People and Maternity Services: Executive Summary*. London: DH.

Department of Health, Social Services and Public Safety (DHSSPS) (2004) *A Healthier Future: a Twenty Year vision for Health and Wellbeing in Northern Ireland 2005–2025*. Belfast: DHSSPS.

Hall, J. (2006) Quality improvement. Chapter 2 in *Integrated Care Pathways in Mental Health*. London: Churchill Livingstone. Elsevier.

Kwan, J. & Sanderwood, P. (2005) In-hospital care pathways for stroke. An updated systematic review. *Stroke*, **36**, 1348–9.

MacLean, A., Fuller, R.M., Jaffrey, E.G., Hay, A.J. & Ho-Yen, D.O. (2008) Integrated care pathway for *Clostridium difficile* helps patient management. *British Journal of Infection Control*, **9**(6), 15–17.

McDougall, P.. (2011) Caring for bronchiolitic infants needing continuous positive airway pressure. *Paediatric Nursing*, **23**, 30–35.

Middleton, S. & Roberts, A. (2000) *Integrated Care Pathways: a Practical Approach to Implementation*. Oxford: Butterworth Heinemann.

Middleton, S., Barnett, J. & Reeves, D. (2001) What is an integrated care pathway? *Evidence-based Medicine*, **3**(3), 1–8.

Mirando, S., Davies, P.D. & Lipp, A. (2005) Introducing an integrated care pathway for the last days of life. *Palliative Medicine*, **19**, 33–9.

National Council for the Professional Development of Nursing and Midwifery (2006) *Improving the Patient Journey: Understanding Integrated Care Pathways*. Dublin: NCNM.

Office of the First Minister and Deputy First Minister (OFMOFM) (2006) *Our Children and Young People – Our Pledge, a Ten-year Strategy for Children and Young People in Northern Ireland 2006–2016*. Belfast: OFMDFM. www.allchildrenni.gov.uk (accessed 15 August 2010).

Peter, S. & Fazakerley, M. (2004) Clinical effectiveness of an integrated care pathway for infants with bronchiolitis. *Paediatric Nursing*, **16**(1), 30–35.

Scottish Intercollegiate Guidelines Network (SIGN) (2006) *Bronchiolitis in Children – a National Clinical Guideline*, 91. Edinburgh: SIGN.

Wakefield, L. (2004) An integrated care pathway for diabetic ketoacidosis. *Paediatric Nursing*, **16**(10), 27–30.

Walsh, M. (1998) *Models and Critical Pathways in Clinical Nursing – Conceptual Frameworks for Care Planning*. London: Baillière Tindall.

Whittle, C. & Hewison, A. (2007) Integrated care pathways: pathways to change in health care? *Journal of Health Organisation and Management*, **21**(3), 297–306.

Zander, K. (2002) Integrated care pathways: eleven international trends. *Journal of Integrated Care Pathway*, **6**, 101–107.

8

Interprofessional Assessment and Care Planning in Critical Care

Philomena Morrow

Introduction

A critically ill child is a child who is in a clinical state which may result in respiratory, cardiac, neurological, gastrointestinal, metabolic, renal and haematological complications. The immediate goal is prompt recognition and aggressive early treatment (Nadel & Kroll 2007) to prevent initial respiratory and circulatory insufficiency.

This requires rapid and systematic clinical assessment to detect physiological instability so that timely, prompt and effective resuscitation and stabilisation may occur before the onset of organ failure. To achieve the best possible outcomes and enhance patient safety requires interprofessional teamworking and collaboration, whereby formal decision making and care interventions are informed by the knowledge and skills within each of the professional roles.

This chapter will outline the approach required by the interprofessional team when involved in the assessment and subsequent care planning for a child with a critical illness. The case study relating to a child with meningococcal disease will illustrate each stage of the process within an ABCDE framework (Resuscitation Council (UK) 2007).

Case study

Martha, a two-year-old girl, has been admitted to hospital following emergency referral by her GP with a history of being unwell for the past 24 hours with high temperature, refusing to feed and vomiting. The GP reported that she had an increased heart rate and respiratory

Care Planning in Children and Young People's Nursing, First Edition.
Edited by Doris Corkin, Sonya Clarke, Lorna Liggett.
© 2012 Blackwell Publishing Ltd. Published 2012 by Blackwell Publishing Ltd.

rate and felt that she might be presenting with symptoms of meningococcal disease. The GP administered parenteral benzyl penicillin and secured intravenous access before Martha was transported to hospital by ambulance. Martha was accompanied by her mother who was extremely anxious about her daughter's condition. She was concerned that her child's hands and feet were very cold and remarked on her pale, mottled skin. Although Martha was constantly crying she was, according to her mother, becoming drowsy.

The history given by Martha's mother and the GP's initial diagnosis of meningococcal disease and subsequent administration of parenteral benzyl penicillin suggests that this child's condition is critical.

Meningococcal disease may present as septicaemia, as meningitis, or with a mixed picture and is caused by infection with *Neisseria meningitidis*, *Meningococcus*, *Streptococcus pneumoniae*, *Escherichia coli*, *Staphylococcus aureus* and *Haemophilus influenzae* type B (Hart & Thompson 2006). Despite the successful introduction of the conjugated meningococcal serogroup C vaccine in 1999, invasive meningococcal disease continues to cause substantial morbidity and mortality (Theilen *et al.* 2008).

The disease has an early non-specific stage, with signs such as fever, lethargy, irritability, nausea and poor feeding. Cold extremities and abnormal skin colour are associated with developing invasive meningococcal disease (Thompson *et al.* 2006), which progresses rapidly to clinical meningitis and/or septicaemia.

Clinical meningitis is characterised by fever, lethargy, vomiting, headache, photophobia, neck stiffness, and positive Kernig's sign and Brudzinski's sign. Petechiae or purpura may also be present. Meningococcal septicaemia is characterised by fever, petechiae, purpura and shock.

Martha's symptoms would suggest that she has progressed from the non-specific early stage of meningococcal disease and is rapidly developing disease patterns associated with clinical meningitis and/or meningococcal septicaemia.

Achieving the best possible outcomes for Martha as previously stated requires rapid and systematic clinical assessment to detect physiological instability so that timely, prompt and aggressive resuscitation and stabilisation will occur before the onset of organ failure. However, improving health outcomes for this child lies outside the scope of any single practitioner (Headrick *et al.* 1998). This assumption remains very evident in emergency care situations when the number of professionals involved and the importance of their ability to work collaboratively increases with the complexity of the child's condition. This highlights the need for developing interprofessional working models (DH 2005) whereby expertise in assessment, planning and treatment interventions are timely and promote stabilisation of the critically ill child. The expectation is that interprofessional team-based models of care will bring a range of professionals together to share different knowledge and experiences and will avoid gaps which are seen as factors which constitute an important risk for patient safety (Bion & Heffner 2004).

Interprofessional working

A powerful incentive for greater teamwork among professionals is created when there is respect and understanding of the role of each of the team members and recognition of the unique contribution of each individual in a critical care situation. In a well-practised team, each member knows in advance their role and regards the leader as the person who co-ordinates, directs the assessment, and consults with other members regarding problem identification and subsequent care or management planning. Therefore interprofessional working models require that the level of equality of esteem and power in formal decision making is balanced within the professional roles of doctor and nurse. Effective multidisciplinary teamworking is at the heart of providing high quality and safe care (DHSSPS 2007a).

The role of education in encouraging interprofessional working is crucial in promoting collaboration, teamworking and establishing roles and responsibilities (WHO 2010), particularly in a critical care situation. Education and competency-based training of interprofessional teams should include recognition of the acutely ill child, clinical assessment, appropriate interventions, and recognition of deterioration whereby senior assistance becomes necessary. Simulation as an educational strategy involves not only technological and computerised facilities, but includes important human interactions. High fidelity simulation using Simbaby provides opportunities for users at all levels, from novice to expert, to practice and develop skills with the knowledge that mistakes carry no penalties or fear of harm to patients or learners (Bradley 2006).

Using simulations within an interprofessional educational programme seeks to provide participants with a meaningful learning experience and has become increasingly recognised as having great potential in delivering elements of healthcare education (Bradley 2006). It integrates the cognitive, psychomotor and affective domains in a non-threatening and safe environment (Underberg 2003). Irrespective of a healthcare practitioner's chosen speciality, cognitive and psychomotor skills pertinent to assessing a patient's respiratory function, cardiovascular status and level of pain must be acquired (Rogers *et al.* 2001). Human patient simulators enable the replication of rarely witnessed critical events, ensuring all healthcare practitioners are exposed to the same standard of training. In addition, complex skills such as communication, critical thinking and decision making and teamworking thus receive attention.

Interprofessional development of protocols for the assessment and management of the sick child include physiological warning systems, whereby clinical parameters outside the normal ranges (see Table 8.1) indicating deterioration are subsequently detected and medical interventions can be implemented at an early stage.

The Glasgow Meningococcal Septicaemia Prognostic Scoring Tool is a scoring system which may determine the severity of the child's illness and subsequent deterioration (see Table 8.2).

Agreed assessment methods must consider the unpredictability of the timeframe, the multiple parameters that require observation and the swift spiral effect of deterioration in the sick child (Teasdale 2009). Prioritisation and effective action requires identification of one's own limitations and promptly identifying the most appropriate person within the multidisciplinary team to carry out an appropriate assessment and ensure that immediate action is taken (DHSSPS 2007a). This requires the utilisation of an effective communication strategy such as SBAR (Leonard *et al.* 2004). This is a situational briefing model which

Table 8.1 Normal ranges (Meningitis Research Foundation 2010).

Age	Respiratory rate	Heart rate	Systolic BP
<1	30–40	110–160	70–90
1–2	25–35	110–150	80–95
2–5	25–30	95–140	80–100
5–12	20–25	80–120	90–110
>12	15–20	60–100	100–120

Table 8.2   Glasgow meningococcal septicaemia prognostic scoring tool (Scottish Intercollegiate Guidelines Network 2008).

	Points
BP <75 mmHg systolic, age <4 y	3
<85 mmHg systolic, age >4 y	
Skin/rectal temperature difference >3°C	3
Modified coma scale score <8 or	3
Deterioration of > or =3 points in 1 hour	
Deterioration in hour before scoring	2
Absence of meningism	2
Extending purpuric rash or widespread ecchymoses	1
Base deficit (capillary or arterial) >8.0	1
Maximum score	15
1. Modified Glasgow scale	
(a) Eyes open:	
Spontaneously	4
To speech	3
To pain	2
None	1
(b) Best verbal response:	
Orientated	6
Words	4
Vocal sound	3
Cries	2
None	1
(c) Best motor response:	
Obeys commands	6
Localises to pain	4
Moves to pain	1
None	0
Add scores (a), (b), (c), to give result	
Score > or = to 8, or an escalating score is indicative of serious and rapidly progressing disease.	

Activity 8.1

With reference to the SBAR model, write down what you consider necessary to report regarding Martha's condition when communicating with the doctor.

helps ensure that important information is transmitted in a predictable structure, when summoning senior nursing and medical staff when support for the management of a child's deteriorating condition is vital.

SBAR stands for the following (Leonard *et al.* 2004):

- Situation – what is going on with the patient at present time?
- Background – circumstances leading up to situation or clinical background.
- Assessment – what do you think the problem is?
- Recommendation – what do you think should be done to correct problem?

Immediate assessment of the critically ill child

The hospital ward or emergency department will have been informed of Martha's anticipated arrival and this provides an opportunity for the nursing and medical team to prepare for immediate assessment and management of her clinical state in a systematic and organised way.

The hospital environment where the child is admitted to will have:

- Facilities to ensure adherence to infection control procedures
- Oxygen and suction with correct size of masks/catheters
- Emergency equipment available and an appropriately stocked resuscitation trolley with the necessary drugs and fluids

Fluid volumes, drug dosages and correct equipment size will depend on the weight of the child. Martha's mother may know what her weight is; if not then it may be worked out quickly to avoid delay in treatment interventions. Formula for estimating weight in kilograms is:

$$\text{Weight (kg)} = (\text{age} + 4) \times 2$$

✎ Activity 8.2

Based on the formula, work out Martha's estimated weight.

Assessment of the child will be rapid and sequential, with simultaneous management of life-threatening problems as they arise. Evaluation and systematic reassessment after each treatment intervention is essential. A combination of clinical features, laboratory results, ongoing monitoring and repeated assessment over time provide a foundation for predicting progress and informing care planning and treatment (SIGN 2008).

Martha's mother must be supported and encouraged to remain with her daughter and provided with information about her condition. Her concerns must be seriously considered and investigated.

ABCDE assessment framework

The use of the structured ABCDE approach promoted by the Resuscitation Council (UK) (2007) is a framework that helps to ensure that potentially life-threatening problems are identified and dealt with in order of priority.

Assessment of airway

The aim is to assess if the airway is patent or if there are signs of obstruction as indicated by difficulty in breathing, increased respiratory effort and noisy breathing, for example stridor, wheeze, coughing or grunting. Silence may be a sign of complete obstruction.

Box 8.1

Problem identification

Potential problem for obstruction due to intense muscle contraction associated with the release of tumour necrosis factor and other inflammatory mediators. Secretions such as vomitus may further impede the airway.

A progressive developing hypoxic state will result in apnoea.

Goal: to maintain patency of the airway to ensure adequate respiratory ventilation to prevent hypoxia, vital organ failure and cardiorespiratory arrest.

Care interventions with rationale

- Observe Martha for signs of airway obstruction – if obstruction is evident place child in supine position.
- Open the airway by performing a jaw thrust or chin lift manoeuvre and head tilt – check for possible airway obstruction.
- Clear excessive secretions, vomitus or other secretions using appropriate size and type of suction catheter, maintaining suction pressure as low as possible and taking care to prevent adverse effects such as hypoxia.
- If Martha's airway becomes compromised insert correctly sized airway adjunct, for example Guedeal airway to open a channel between the base of the tongue and posterior pharyngeal wall (Resuscitation Council (UK) 2007).
- If airway patency cannot be maintained tracheal intubation will be required to be carried out by the anaesthetist in a controlled and safe environment.

Assessment is based on the following observations:

- Detect airway obstruction – look at the child's chest/abdomen for signs of respiratory movement.
- Listen to breathing sounds and feel for air movement at the child's face and mouth.
- Assess child's responsiveness and ability to talk, cry or cough.
- Unless contraindicated, assess for possible cause of airway obstruction by looking in the mouth for gastric contents or mucous.

Martha is crying at the time of initial assessment which indicates patency of airway.

Assessment of breathing and ventilation

The aim in assessing breathing and ventilation is to determine whether there is adequate gas exchange to provide sufficient oxygen for Martha's tissue requirements and prevent her from developing respiratory acidosis.

Assessment is based on observation of:

- The work of breathing, as it may be compromised due to pulmonary oedema resulting from capillary leakage.

- Body position and visual movements of chest and abdomen and breathing pattern.
- Use of accessory muscles.
- Evidence of minimal movement of chest wall.
- Sternal supraclavicular substernal or intercostal recession.
- Presence of nasal flaring.
- Respiratory rate fast, slow or normal – see Table 8.1 for normal respiratory rate values according to age. Tachypnoea is the first indication of respiratory insufficiency.
- Evidence of central cyanosis indicates severe hypoxia and is a pre-terminal state.
- Air movement if audible on auscultation.
- Arterial oxygen saturation, although this may be unreliable when a child has poor peripheral circulation. A saturation of <90% in room air or <95% in supplemental oxygen indicates respiratory failure.

Box 8.2

Problem identification

Martha is presenting with signs of increasing hypoxia as indicated by increased respiratory rate and effort.

   She has the potential to become fatigued if hypoxia state persists, with progression to respiratory failure and bradypnoea.

   Goal: to immediately ensure effective delivery of oxygen through a patent airway to maintain O_2 saturations above 95% and prevent metabolic acidosis, cellular damage and cell death from hypoxia.

Care interventions with rationale

- Apply high flow oxygen 10–15 litres through a rebreathable oxygen facemask to ensure Martha receives adequate oxygenation to allow normal metabolism of cells.
- Attach pulse oximetry to assess oxygen saturations which aim to be maintained above 92–95%.
- A reading below 92% for Martha with 100% mask oxygen could be an indication that she requires assisted ventilation.
- Respiratory rate, heart rate and oxygen saturations should be monitored relative to the child's condition and accurately documented.
- Reference to early warning scoring system to ascertain clinical deterioration.
- Support respiratory effort by nursing Martha, who is distressed, in upright position unless her clinical state contraindicates this position.
- Keep communicating with the multidisciplinary team informing them of Martha's condition.
- If breathing is absent or if Martha is hypoventilating, i.e. with slow respiratory rate or weak respiratory effort, she should be supported with oxygen by valve mask device and an airway adjunct needs to be inserted. Effective bag-mask ventilation remains the cornerstone of providing effective emergency ventilation (Nadkarni & Berg 2009).
- If Martha is exhausted and needs ongoing respiratory support or cardiorespiratory arrest is imminent tracheal intubation will be necessary.

Assessment of circulation

The aim is to assess adequate cardiovascular function to maintain oxygenation and tissue perfusion.

Assessment is based on observation of the following:

* Hypovolaemia, due to increased vascular permeability causing water and plasma proteins to leak out of capillaries as indicated by:
* Skin colour for pallor or mottling.
* Cold hands and feet due to vasoconstriction, which reduces blood flow to the skin, which in turn increases capillary refill time.
* Respiratory function, as previously indicated for increased respiratory rate.
* Pulse rate for indication of tachycardia or bradycardia.
* Pulse quality reflects the adequacy of peripheral perfusion. A weak central pulse may indicate decompensated shock and a peripheral pulse that is difficult to find, weak or irregular suggests poor peripheral perfusion and maybe a sign of shock.
* Blood pressure – see Table 8.1 for ranges across the age span. Low recording is an indication of decompensated shock.

Assessment of disability

Review care planning (see Chapter 16), for reference to detailed disability assessment to identify Martha's neurological status, which may be deranged as a result of respiratory failure, cardiovascular failure and her neurological condition, meningitis. Meningitis causes severe inflammation of the meninges and capillary leak, which gives rise to fluid and electrolyte imbalance. This causes fluid shift and predisposes the child to developing cerebral oedema, thus raising intracranial pressure. Inadequate oxygen perfusion of the brain as a result of shock causes altered levels of consciousness. Hypoglycaemia and high body temperature may cause seizure activity.

Assessment is rapid and is determined by:

* The APVU score (Resuscitation Council (UK) 2007).
* Ongoing monitoring using the Glasgow Coma Scale.
* Appropriate pain assessment tools:
  — A alert
  — P response to stimuli
  — V response to voice
  — U unresponsive
  — Glasgow Coma Scale
  — Pain Assessment
  — Kernig's and Brudzinski's signs as indicated previously are positive in child with meningococcal meningitis
  — Neck stiffness and photophobia may be evident

Glasgow Meningococcal Septicaemic Prognostic Scoring Tool (see Table 8.2) will determine the severity of Martha's condition.

Box 8.3

Problem identification

Martha is presenting with signs of compensated shock as indicated by tachycardia and tachypnoea. Her cold hands and feet and skin colour represent changes in peripheral circulation and are the early symptoms of sepsis (Thompson *et al.* 2006).

Potential problem of progressing to decompensated shock which will be evident if Martha presents with bradycardia and lowered blood pressure and increased capillary refill time.

Goal: to immediately enhance circulatory function to provide adequate delivery of O_2 and nutrients to meet the metabolic demands of tissues.

Care interventions with rationale

- Monitor the heart rate, pulse quality and skin temperature, oxygen saturations and blood pressure. Compare findings on Paediatric Early Warning Score Chart or Glasgow Meningococcal Septicaemia Prognostic Scoring Tool, see Table 8.2 and report to medical team.
- Assist in obtaining additional vascular access and blood samples if possible.
- Monitor capillary refill, which is normally less than two seconds. If >2 seconds then assist in administering immediate fluid resuscitation of 20 ml fluid/kg of either crystalloid as normal saline or colloid such as human plasma protein, administered usually as a bolus injection to restore circulating volume, blood pressure and tissue perfusion.
- Continue to monitor heart rate, blood pressure, peripheral perfusion and oxygen saturations throughout fluid resuscitation and report.
- Maintain accurate record of fluid input and output.
- Follow prescription for required fluid maintenance – see Table 8.3. However, it may be necessary to restrict fluids so recheck prescription and discuss with the doctor if concerned.
- Check blood glucose as increased cellular activity increases the metabolic demands for glucose. Hypoglycaemia may cause seizures.
- After each treatment intervention reassessment of Martha's status is necessary to ascertain response or identify further deterioration.
- Call senior medical staff and additional nursing support if concerned.
- If the pulse rate falls below 60 and there are no or minimal signs of life commence cardiopulmonary resuscitation.

Intraosseous puncture may be necessary to deliver fluids and emergency drugs such as inotropic support, which may be administered to increase contractility of the heart and cardiac output. Child needs to be transferred to paediatric intensive care (NICE 2007).

Table 8.3 Fluid maintenance requirements (DHSSPS 2007b).

Body weight	Daily fluid requirement ml/kg	Hourly fluid requirement ml/kg
First 10 kg	100	4
Second 10 kg	50	2
Subsequent kg	20	1

Box 8.4

Problem identification

Martha is presenting with signs of early neurological impairment as she is irritable but becoming drowsy and is vomiting.

Goal: to recognise early signs of neurological disturbance, i.e. raised intracranial pressure, so that treatment interventions aimed at preventing complications of hypoxia and hypoperfusion may be commenced.

Care interventions with rationale

* Maintain oxygenation to ensure adequate oxygen perfusion to Martha's brain.
* Monitor blood glucose levels to ensure they are maintained within normal limits to prevent seizure activity.
* Monitor temperature and administer antipyretic drugs as prescribed to prevent seizure activity (NICE 2007).
* Assess neurological status using the APVU scoring system and Glasgow Coma Scale to detect signs of raised intracranial pressure.
* Immediately summon medical assistance if there are signs of raised intracranial pressure – if Martha becomes drowsy, pupils are abnormal, pulse rate decreases or presents with seizures.
* Assist in preparation and checking of drugs for administration. Initial antibiotic treatment will commence before definitive microbiological diagnosis. This is crucial for optimising the outcome of bacterial meningitis (Holub *et al.* 2007).
* Prepare child and family for lumbar puncture if considered necessary by the doctor to obtain sample of cerebral spinal fluid for diagnostic purposes to determine causative organisms and sensitivities to antibiotic treatments.

Exposure

To carry out an assessment of the body for signs of bruising, rashes or other skin abnormalities the child will need to be exposed for a brief period of time. Rashes will require further assessment to determine if it is non-blanching as this may be an indication of septicaemia. Rash may develop in minutes or initially present as a blanching, maculopapular rash. A generalised petechial rash, or a purpuric rash in any location, in an ill child is strongly suggestive of meningococcal septicaemia (Theilen *et al.* 2008).

Those who have been exposed to prolonged contact in a household setting with a child with meningococcal disease during the seven days before the onset of illness should be offered chemoprophylaxis. Chemoprophylaxis should be offered to healthcare workers who have been directly exposed to droplet or respiratory secretions during the acute illness phase, prior to completion of 24 hours of antibiotic (SIGN 2008).

Debriefing

Debriefing after Martha's clinical status has been stabilised is an important reflective process for individuals involved and for the team. The debriefing process is a feedback method that is applied to the actual situation whereby the team evaluates what they did well collectively, what were the challenges and what could be done differently next time. This creates opportunities for shared learning across disciplines as well as identifying the need for improvement in practices, which ultimately contributes to promoting safe effective care for the critically ill child.

Summary

Achieving the best possible outcomes for a critically ill child requires rapid and systematic clinical assessment to detect physiological instability so that timely, prompt and aggressive resuscitation and stabilisation will occur before the onset of organ failure. In emergency care situations there is a need for interprofessional working models (DH 2005), whereby expertise in assessment, planning and treatment interventions are timely and promote stabilisation of the critically ill child. The use of the structured ABCDE approach (Resuscitation Council (UK) 2007) as a framework will help ensure that potentially life-threatening problems are identified and dealt with in order of priority. Debriefing after a critical care event will enable professionals to reflect on their practice and identify strategies which may improve future assessment and care management of the critically ill child.

References

Bion, J.F. & Heffner, J.E. (2004) Challenges in the care of the acutely ill. *Lancet*, **363**(9413), 970–7.

Bradley, P. (2006) The history of simulation in medical education and possible future directions. *Medical Education*, **40**, 254–62.

Department of Health (2005) *Creating a Patient-led NHS*. Department of Health. London: Stationery Office.

Department of Health and Social Services and Public Safety (DHSSPS) (2007a). *Promotion of Safe, High Quality Health and Social Care in Undergraduate Curricula*. London: Stationery Office.

Department of Health and Social Services and Public Safety (DHSSPS) (2007b). *Paediatric Parenteral Fluid Therapy (1month–16 years). Initial Management Guidelines*. London: The Stationery Office.

Hart, L. & Thompson, A. (2006) Meningococcal disease and its management in children. *British Medical Journal*, **333**, 685–90.

Headrick, L.A., Wilcock, P.M. & Batalden, P.B. (1998) Interprofessional working and continuing medical education. *British Medical Journal*, **316**(7133), 1–9.

Holub, M., Beran, O., Dzupova, O., *et al.* (2007) Cortisol levels in cerebrospinal fluid correlate with severity and bacterial origin of meningitis. *Critical Care*, **11**(2), 1–9. http://ccforum.com/content/11/2/R41 (accessed 26 April 2011).

Leonard, M., Graham, S. & Bonacum, D. (2004) The human factor: the critical importance of effective teamwork and communication in providing safe effective care. *Quality and Safety in Health Care*, **13**, 85–90.

Meningitis Research Foundation (2010) Algorithm, 5th edn. *Early Management of Meningococcal Disease in Children*. Meningitis Research Foundation. www.meningitis.org (accessed 26 April 2011).

Nadel, S. & Kroll, J.S. (2007) Diagnosis and management of meningococcal disease: the need for centralised care. Federation of European Microbiological Societies. *Microbiological Review*, **31**, 71–83.

Nadkarni, V.M. & Berg, R.A. (2009) Pediatric cardiopulmonary resuscitation. In: Wheeler *et al.* (eds). *Resuscitation and Stabilization of the Critically Ill Child*. London: Springer-Verlag.

National Institute Clinical Excellence (NICE) (2007) *Feverish Illness in Children. Assessment and Initial Management in Children Younger than 5 Years.* London: NICE.

Resuscitation Council (UK) (2007) *Paediatric Immediate Life Support,* 1st edn. London: Resuscitation Council (UK).

Rogers, P.L., Jacob, H., Rashwan, A.S. & Pnsky, M.R. (2001) Quantifying learning in medical students during a critical care medicine elective: a comparison of three evaluation instruments. *Critical Care Medicine,* **29**(6), 1268–73.

Scottish Intercollegiate Guidelines Network (SIGN) (2008) *Management of Invasive Meningococcal Disease in Children and Young People. A National Clinical Guideline.* Scotland: NHS.

Teasdale, D. (2009) Chapter 2. In: Dixon, M., Crawford, D., Teasdale, D. & Murphy, J. (eds). *Nursing the Highly Dependent Child or Infant.* London: Wiley- Blackwell.

Theilen, U., Wilson, l., Wilson, G., Beattie, J, O., Qureshi, S. & Simpson, D. (2008) Management of invasive meningococcal disease in children and young people: summary of SIGN guidelines. *British Medical Journal,* **336**, 1367–70.

Thompson, M.J., Ninis, N., Perera, R., Mayon-White, R., Phillips, C., Bailey, L. & Harnden, A. (2006) Clinical recognition of meningococcal disease in children and adolescents. *Lancet,* **367**, 397–403.

Underberg, K.E. (2003) Experiential learning and simulation in health care education. *Surgical Services Management,* **9**(4), 31–6.

World Health Organisation (WHO) (2010) *Framework for Action on Interprofessional Education and Collaborative Practice.* Geneva: Department of Human Resources for Health, WHO.

9

Practice Education Facilitator, Mentor and Student – Supporting the Planning of Care

Michael Davidson and Nuala Devlin

Introduction

In 2006 (revised 2008) the Nursing and Midwifery Council (NMC) published *Standards to Support Learning and Assessment in Practice* (NMC 2006; 2008), which reflected the response to two previous consultations on the standards themselves and on fitness to practice at the point of registration (NMC 2005; UKCC 1999). These standards were published to ensure the protection of the public by implementing systems that guarantee competency of nursing and midwifery students at the point of registration or recording a qualification with the NMC. These standards define and describe the knowledge and skills nurses need to apply in practice when supporting and assessing students undertaking NMC approved programmes that lead to registration or a recordable qualification. Although there are many interpretations to the term mentor, with regard to pre-registration nursing the NMC states that a mentor:

'Is a registrant who, following successful completion of an NMC approved mentor preparation programme – or comparable preparation that has been accredited by an AEI (Approved Educational Institution) as meeting the NMC mentor requirements – has achieved the knowledge, skills and competence required to meet the defined outcomes.'

(NMC 2008, p19)

Care Planning in Children and Young People's Nursing, First Edition.
Edited by Doris Corkin, Sonya Clarke, Lorna Liggett.
© 2012 Blackwell Publishing Ltd. Published 2012 by Blackwell Publishing Ltd.

Role of mentors

Mentors have a key role in supporting students in practice (Aston & Hallam 2011). Elcock & Sookhoo (2007) suggests that the quality of mentorship in pre-registration nursing education is highly variable and at times may be a cause for concern, particularly since mentors are the people assessing students' fitness for practice at the point of registration. One response to these concerns and the publication of the standards has been the implementation of new roles, with a remit to facilitate and thus enhance practice learning.

In response to this standard, different parts of the UK have established infrastructures to support teachers, such as link lecturers, mentors and nursing students in practice settings (Cardwell & Corkin 2007; Ness *et al.* 2010). There appears to have been variable approaches, with Scotland (http://www.nes.scot.nhs.uk/nursing/) (NES 2006), Northern Ireland and the Republic of Ireland (Department of Health & Children 2001) taking a committed, strategic and integrated approach to the development of these roles, providing education and support for mentors in practice. However, in England and Wales there appears to be a more varied regional approach to the development of these roles, with a range of titles and responsibilities which are subject to local education policy and variable funding commitment (Mallik & McGowan 2007). From an international perspective there does appear to be some recognition of the need for the preparation and support for mentors. However, difficulties with the actual definition of mentorship in relation to nursing makes it difficult to identify what roles and mechanisms are in place to develop and support nurses in a more global context (Fulton *et al.* 2007).

Within the Belfast Health and Social Care Trust and across Northern Ireland, practice education coordinators were appointed to manage teams of practice education facilitators, whose role is to support mentors/teachers in practice, as well as supporting learning within the practice environment and providing practice education leadership across the organisation. Implementation of robust evaluation processes to ensure the quality of placement experiences and maximise learning and development opportunities are also part of their remit in ensuring improvements in patient safety. Funding for these roles came from the Department of Health, Social Services and Public Safety for Northern Ireland.

Throughout the UK and Republic of Ireland there are a wide variety of roles and responsibilities to support education and mentoring. In practice, however, within the context of Northern Ireland there was an expectation that the practice education facilitators would be registered nurses on Part 1 of the NMC register. These roles were appointed at band 7 with an expectation that the individuals appointed to these roles would have experience at band 6 or above, having previously worked with students in a mentorship or practice teacher role. Although desirable it was not essential to have a recognised teaching qualification, but this is encouraged as part of the ongoing professional development within the role.

Practice education facilitator role

The main focus of the practice education facilitator role is one of collaboration and partnership, working within the practice setting and liaising with higher education institutions, placing an emphasis on the support of mentors in the assessing and supervising of nursing students in practice. These roles have a wide remit to enhance the quality of the practice learning experience and positively contribute to the development of a well-educated and practice-competent future nursing/midwifery workforce. More specifically the role entails:

- Mentorship support
- Support of learning in practice
- Ensuring the quality of the practice learning environment
- Communication links between the practice setting and higher education institution (HEI)
- Involvement in updating mentors and the process of development from mentor to sign-off mentor status
- Supporting mentors and students where there are concerns about a student's performance in practice and assisting with the documentation of this, for example creating action plans
- Auditing practice placements in liaison with the HEIs and clinical areas
- Working with clinical placement managers to manage the local register of available mentors, ensuring that staff are updated and the records are accurate
- Advising mentors where a student has disclosed a support need
- Developing newsletters, maintaining the local register of mentors and devising teaching materials
- Contributing to the teaching on the mentorship preparation programme (MPP) in partnership with the HEIs

It is important to recognise that mentors support students and help to facilitate their learning by identifying objectives, planning programmes of learning and negotiating action plans. Assessment and the provision of timely and appropriate feedback are vital to the role and any challenging issues are discussed and managed. The importance of the mentor role is acknowledged with the introduction of the practice education facilitator role to support the mentors who, in turn, support the students in achieving the NMC outcomes of their nursing programme.

The NMC (2006; 2008) stipulated the duration and the academic level of the mentorship preparation programme (MPP). A mentorship preparation programme must be:

- At a minimum academic level of HEI level
- A minimum of ten days, of which at least five days are protected learning time
- Include learning in both academic and practice settings
- Include relevant work-based learning, for example experience in mentoring a student under the supervision of a qualified mentor, and have the opportunity to critically reflect on such an experience
- Normally be completed within three months

As part of this programme within Northern Ireland, developed regionally (five NHS trusts) in conjunction with Queen's University Belfast, the Open University and the University of Ulster, trainee mentors are expected to complete a portfolio providing evidence of their ability to support and assess student nurses in practice. Content of this portfolio includes activities to develop the trainee mentors' skills in assessing student nurses in practice, such as the development of a four-week plan of working with a student and the experience and learning which will take place as a result of this plan; consideration of learning styles and how this may impact on the students' ability to learn in practice; the student journey and the importance of reflection. This mentorship programme within Northern Ireland also has a regionally agreed quality assurance process ensuring standards for mentor preparation are met.

As a facilitator of learning the practice education facilitator needs to possess some very specific skills which seem to reflect what Nash and Scammell (2010) describe as essential in pre-registration mentorship. These include: knowledge of learning theory, including adult learning; practice-based teaching and assessment; integration of theory and practice; and a knowledge and insight of the curriculum, as well as developed communication and relationship skills (ENB & DH 2001; Nash & Scammell 2010). The importance of these factors in mentorship is supported through research by Spouse (2001), who suggested that the most important factor in influencing professional development within the practice setting is the quality of the mentorship. Previous research (Burns & Patterson 2005; Carlisle *et al.* 2009) has indicated that the quality and effectiveness of mentorship within the clinical setting influences the students' ability to learn and to adjust to the demands within the clinical setting. There is also evidence to suggest that negative experiences with mentors and on clinical placements contribute to the overall attrition rate of students on pre-registration nursing programmes (Scott 2005; Urwin *et al.* 2010). There is also a wider context of issues affecting the quality of mentorship which inevitably impacts on the student. These issues concern nursing staff shortages, competing demands of clinical and teaching work that the mentor has to 'juggle' with on a daily basis, lack of preparedness of mentors and lack of motivation of some mentors to carry out the role effectively (Elcock & Sookhoo 2007). The impact of role modelling has been identified as significant within mentoring (Donaldson & Carter 2005; Murray & Main 2005); it is recognised that it is more than just imitating behaviour and that it can actually lead to behaviour change in an individual who has observed the behaviour of another. Nursing students, anecdotally and from research, indicate that they want good role models to both observe and practice skills and behaviours such as care planning (Donaldson & Carter 2005; Sharp & Maddison 2008). However, the importance of role modelling needs to be made explicit in mentorship and this is part of the role of the practice education facilitator to ensure that the mentor in practice is well supported and developed to gain all the skills above in order to be able to function effectively as a mentor.

In order to enter the NMC register nurses must achieve the standards of proficiency in the practice of their specific field of nursing – in this case children's nursing. One of these standards is to: 'formulate and document a plan of nursing care, where possible in partnership with patients, clients, their carers and family and friends, within a framework of informed consent' (NMC 2004, p5).

To exemplify the role of the practice education facilitator in supporting the mentor working with student nurses in the practice setting the following case study will explore the key points relating to the development of skills in care planning. The case study is taken from the perspective of a student not performing to the required standard of practice.

Case study

Jane is a registered children's nurse working in a busy medical ward within the regional children's hospital. She has just finished the Mentorship Preparation Programme (MPP), with the Health and Social Care Trust in partnership with Queen's University Belfast. Jane is the mentor for a second-year student nurse, Kelly, and has been working closely with her on a number of care planning issues which had been identified as a core clinical skill and is concerned that she is failing the placement. Having undertaken the MPP Jane has become more self-aware and has identified that the student appears to be lacking in motivation and her performance appears to be declining. Jane has advised the student to contact her link lecturer and Jane contacted the practice education facilitator (PEF) for her area in order to discuss and explore the issues of concern with Kelly's performance. Jane is aware of the need to reflect on the situation in order to learn from it as this is an ongoing process and a means of new learning and understanding (Gibbs 1988).

Initially Jane felt the student was failing the placement, as she appeared disinterested, lacked motivation and rarely asked questions regarding the care of patients on the ward. Through discussion and critical reflection with the PEF several key points were raised and Jane reflected on one particular episode when the student was being supervised as she gave advice to an 11-year-old girl who had been recently diagnosed with diabetes. Jane reflected that what she had observed throughout was that the student ignored the patient and spoke directly to her parents. As a result, the student was unable to perform care planning safely and effectively as clearly identified in the student's ongoing record of achievement (clinical portfolio). Specifically, the student was unable to:

- Set realistic goals in partnership with the child and family
- Identify the child's preference regarding care and respect choices within the limits of professional practice
- Apply the philosophy of family-centred care
- Demonstrate ability in formulating and documenting care interventions relevant to child's needs
- Document adequately in the care plan

During this reflection with the PEF, Jane acknowledged that it was possible that the student did not have any insight into diabetes, thus ignoring the patient and that this could impact on the student's ability to plan care for the patient. The mentor was able to relate to the specific domains as outlined in the NMC standards to support learning and assessment in practice (NMC 2008). In order for the student to progress, an action plan would need to be agreed between Jane and Kelly. Jane would have to discuss issues of poor care planning with the student, recognising that the discussion may be challenging but drawing on her experience through the MPP and the development of the portfolio and problem-based learning. Jane felt confident that she could provide the student with support and guidance. The development of the portfolio was crucial in giving focus and working specifically within the domains of:

- Establishing effective working relationships
- Facilitation of learning
- Evaluation of learning
- Creating an environment for learning

The completion of the MPP has given Jane greater confidence in being able to give students constructive feedback and Jane was also aware of the difference in learning styles and the importance of being flexible and responsive and of creating a good learning environment. Through considerable discussion with the student Jane ascertained that the student had been reluctant to engage with the patient as her theory on the subject was limited and she was afraid of looking 'stupid in front of the child'. The student also stated that she was worried about her level of knowledge and understanding and was reluctant to ask questions not because she was disinterested, but rather because she felt she should know this. Subsequently, the student agreed to evaluate which areas she specifically needed to focus on within this placement. Furthermore, an action plan was constructed to help the student meet the specific issues raised and a facilitation contract was devised:

- The mentor agreed to have one-to-one teaching sessions with the student regarding the treatment of common conditions on the ward.
- The mentor agreed to supervise and guide the student in relation to care planning.
- The student agreed to revise the common conditions on the ward as instructed by the mentor.
- The mentor agreed to give the student constructive feedback in a timely fashion.
- Both student and mentor agreed to meet on a weekly basis to evaluate the ongoing needs of the student.

Through this mode of facilitation the needs of both the mentor and student were acknowledged and therefore progress was achieved. The PEF continued to monitor the situation with Jane to ensure as a mentor she felt adequately supported.

Through critical reflection the practitioner is able to analyse events more clearly and recognise that it is an essential element of learning (Sharp & Maddison 2008). Although, it may be a gradual process and is ongoing from previous experiences it should not be seen as a checklist. The ability to plan care for individuals is a fundamental requisite of the role of the registered nurse. However, like many skills, it is something that must be taught and it should not be assumed that the individual has the ability to carry out the task without focused instruction.

The ability to identify underperforming students and manage the situation properly requires skill and knowledge acquisition (Duffy 2003). Through the support of the practice education team ultimately the mentor is supported and encouraged to develop a culture of learning where nursing staff act as role models, and articulate their practice and decision making while sharing knowledge (Benner *et al.* 1996). Indeed, timely intervention can often mean that mentors are able to support 'failing' students with sensitivity and confidence, which can lead to the student achieving a satisfactory outcome of learning objectives (Carlisle *et al.* 2009). The role of the mentor within the clinical setting is of vital importance for the experience of the student, where practice-based assessment is complex and it is difficult to manage objectively (Carr 2004). It is imperative that the mentor is adequately prepared and supported so that they have the necessary skills needed to support students. The development of the trainee mentor portfolio is based around the eight domains of learning as stipulated by the NMC (2008). These eight domains are: establishing effective relationships; facilitation of learning; assessment and accountability; evaluation of learning; creating an environment of learning; context of practice; evidence-based practice and leadership. This portfolio is designed to help the trainee mentor integrate theory into practice. It provides an organised and systematic way of documenting all the practical and learning activities which demonstrate that they have met the competencies for the mentor programme, as described in the NMC *Standards to Support Learning and Assessment in Practice* (NMC 2008). In practice-based disciplines portfolios are increasingly seen as a useful apparatus in the assessment of practice competencies (Jasper & Fulton 2005). If used properly a portfolio could not just encourage reflection of practice but also inspire new learning (Wade & Yarbrough 1996).

Indeed, the practice education facilitator actively encourages the mentor to reflect and critically analyse the situations and under the domain of 'Facilitation of learning' it is stated that mentors: 'support students in critically reflecting upon their learning experiences in order to enhance future learning' (NMC 2008, p51).

Critical analysis is often something that is feared as it invokes feelings of disapproval (Sharpe & Maddison 2008). However, this crucial skill of self-awareness and critical thinking is embraced by the practice education team and it plays an integral role in the development of the mentor and how they can support students in their area. In the above case study both mentor and student were able to resolve pertinent issues affecting the performance of the student by critically discussing the incident, gaining insight and developing an action plan which met the needs of all parties.

Summary

The authors have attempted to inform future practice development. Evidence suggests that the role of the practice education facilitator is appreciated and valued as a resource by both mentors and stakeholders (Carlisle *et al.* 2009). Their availability to support mentors experiencing challenges managing a 'failing' student means that mentors feel more equipped to deal with the situation confidently and effectively. In addition, they are able to manage the student in a sensitive and professional manner. This is exemplified in the case study by Jane's sensitive and supportive management of Kelly, the student nurse.

References

Aston, L. & Hallam, P. (2011) *Successful Mentoring in Nursing*. Exeter: Learning Matters.

Benner, P., Tanner, C. & Chesla, C. (1996) *Expertise in Nursing Practice: Caring, Clinical Judgment and Ethics*. New York: Springer.

Burns, I. & Patterson, I.M. (2005) Clinical practice and placement support: supporting learning and practice. *Nurse Education in Practice*, **5**(1), 3–9.

Cardwell, P. & Corkin, D. (2007) Mentorship: the art and science. *Paediatric Nursing*, **19**(4), 31–2.

Carlisle, C., Calman, L. & Ibbotson, T. (2009) Practice-based learning: the role of practice education facilitators in supporting mentors. *Nurse Education Today*, doi: 10.1016/jnedt2009.02.018

Carr, S.J. (2004) Assessing clinical competency in medical senior house officers: how and why should we do it? *Postgraduate Medical Journal*, **80**(940), 63–6.

Department of Health and Children (2001) *National Evaluation of the Role of the Clinical Placement Co-ordinator*. Dublin: Department of Health and Children.

Donaldson, J.H. & Carter, D. (2005) The value of role modelling: perceptions of undergraduate and diploma (adult) nursing students. *Nurse Education in Practice*, **5**, 353–9.

Duffy, K. (2003) *Failing Students: a Qualitative Study of Factors that Influence the Decisions Regarding Assessment of Students' Competence in Practice*. Nmc-uk.org (accessed 9 June 2010).

Elcock, K. & Sookhoo, D. (2007) Evaluating a new role to support mentors in practice. *Nursing Times*, **103**(49), 30–31.

English National Board for Nursing, Midwifery and Health Visiting, Department of Health (2001) *Placements in Focus: Guidance for Education in Practice for Healthcare Professions*. London: ENB/DH.

Fulton, J., Bohler, A., Storm, Hansen., *et al.* (2007) Mentorship: an international perspective. *Nurse Education in Practice*, **7**(6), 399–406.

Gibbs, G. (1988) *Learning by Doing: A Guide to Teaching and Learning Methods.* London: FEU.

Jasper, M. & Fulton, J. (2005) Marking criteria for assessing practice-based portfolios at masters' level. *Nurse Education Today*, **25**, 377–89.

Mallik, M. & McGowan, B. (2007) Issues in practice-based learning in nursing in the United Kingdom and the Republic of Ireland: results from a multi-professional scoping exercise. *Nurse Education Today*, **27**(1), 52–9.

Murray, C.J. & Main, A. (2005) Role modelling as a teaching method for mentors. *Nursing Times*, **101**(26), 30.

Nash, S. & Scammell, J. (2010) Skills to ensure success in mentoring and other workplace learning approaches. *Nursing Times.net* www.nursingtimes.net/nursing-practice-clinical-research/students/skills-to-ensure-success-in-mentoring-and-other-workplace-learning-approaches/5010479.article?referrer=RSS (accessed 2 July 2010).

Ness, V., Duffy, K., McCallum, J. & Price, L. (2010) Supporting and mentoring nursing students in practice. *Nursing Standard*, **25**(1), 41–6.

NHS Education Scotland (2006) www.nes.scot.nhs.uk/nursing/

Nursing and Midwifery Council (2004) *Standards of Proficiency for Pre-registration Nursing Education.* London: NMC.

Nursing and Midwifery Council (2005) *Consultation on Fitness for Practice at the Point of Registration.* London: NMC.

Nursing and Midwifery Council (2006) *Standards to Support Learning and Assessment in Practice: NMC Standards for Mentors, Practice Teachers and Teachers.* NMC, London. www.nmc-uk.org/aFrameDisplay.aspx?DocumentID=1914 (accessed 8 June 2010).

Nursing and Midwifery Council (2008) *Standards to Support Learning and Assessment in Practice: NMC Standards for Mentors, Practice Teachers and Teachers.* NMC, London. www.nmc-uk.org/Documents/Standards/ nmcStandards toSupportLearningAndAssessmentInPractice.pdf (accessed 8 June 2010).

Scott, H. (2005) Report claims that a third of student nurses don't qualify. *British Journal of Nursing*, **14**(4), 189.

Sharp, P. & Maddison, C. (2008) An exploration of the student and mentor journey into reflective practice. Chapter 4. In: Bulman, C. & Schutz, S. (eds), *Reflective Practice in Nursing*, 4th edn. Oxford: Blackwell Publishing.

Spouse, J. (2001) Bridging theory and practice in the supervisory relationship: a sociocultural perspective. *Journal of Advanced Nursing*, **33**(4), 512–22.

United Kingdom Central Council for Nursing, Midwifery and Health Visiting (UKCC) (1999) *Fitness for Practice, The UKCC Commission for Nursing and Midwifery Education.* London: UKCC.

Urwin, S., Stanley, R., Jones, M., Gallagher, A., Wainwright, P. & Perkins, A. (2010) Understanding student nurse attrition: learning from the literature. *Nurse Education Today*, **30**(2), 202–207.

Wade, R.C. & Yarbrough, D.B. (1996) Portfolios: a tool for reflective thinking in teacher education? *Teaching & Teacher Education*, **12**(1), 63–79.

10

Holistic Care – Family Partnership in Practice
Erica Brown

Introduction

Lifestyles are changing dramatically throughout the Western world (Smart & Neale 1999). In the past attention has largely focused on the traditional model of a nuclear family and neglected diversity in family composition. Although family structures vary, many people would agree that the central purpose of the family is to create and nurture a common culture that encourages the wellbeing of the people concerned, providing physical and emotional support (Bjornberg & Buck-Wiklund 1990).

Family members are interdependent. Therefore, anything that affects one member will affect the family as a whole. There is extensive literature concerning the way in which parents are first told about their child's illness. Diagnosis may well be a watershed between two different lifestyles – the pre-diagnostic life with normal ups and downs and post-diagnostic life, where parents feel that their future is unknown and everything is at the mercy of their child's illness. The situation may render them confused and in a state of extreme anxiety (Davis 1993).

One of the first dilemmas of having a child with a serious or life-limiting illness is the shattering experience of how to cope with something which was unexpected and how to accept, as a parent, what is unacceptable (Cooper 1999). Several authors write about the isolation which parents face as they struggle to come to terms with their shock (Carpenter

Care Planning in Children and Young People's Nursing, First Edition.
Edited by Doris Corkin, Sonya Clarke, Lorna Liggett.
© 2012 Blackwell Publishing Ltd. Published 2012 by Blackwell Publishing Ltd.

1997; Hornby 1998). The task of coping is a process in which parents find themselves constantly adjusting to the new demands that their child's illness makes. Murgatroyd and Woolfe (1993) refer to this process as 'recurrent crises'.

Family-centred care

Family-centred care was implemented in major teaching hospitals from the late 1970s, and in 1988, Casey introduced a family-centred nursing model. Together with other models developed from the Casey (1988) principles, existing nursing models were revised and the family's need to be involved in the care of their child was taken into account. Built upon the principles of partnership and negotiation, these models encourage family members to participate in assessment, planning and delivery of care.

Many practitioners consider family-centred care to be a cornerstone of paediatric practice, yet there is no single definition of family-centred care in existence (Shields *et al.* 2006). One definition is 'negotiation between health professionals and the family, which results in shared decision-making about what the child's care will be and who will provide it' (Corbett & Twycross 2006). Others interpret the concept as a list of elements of care. Thus, whilst family-centred care considers the wider needs of the child and family, in practice this may be at a relatively superficial level, depending on the depth of the assessment and the interpretation and communication of the information received from individual families.

Assessment will also depend on a definition of 'family' and who the child considers as core members of their 'family?' For some children, their grandparents may be the main carers, for others their parent's partner may be a crucial support and influence, even though they are not related. The situation may be further complicated by former partner's relatives, step-siblings, foster carers, home care teams, etc.

Family-centred care is grounded in the participation and involvement of the family but there is much evidence to suggest that this is not always a reality and in many cases mere lip service is paid to the process. It is well recognised that experienced nursing staff are generally confident in enabling decision-making, but negotiation of care and the assessment of need may be affected by the expectations of both staff and parents, issues of control and the lack or quality of information (Corbett & Twycross 2006). Family-centred care may also be less successful where family involvement in care is influenced by resource issues such as staff shortages or poor facilities.

All families need to achieve a balance between stability and change, but roles and relationships may need to alter to accommodate developments in the physical, social or emotional life of family members (Down & Simons 2006). This means that the assessment of care must be constantly revisited.

Families adapting to their child's illness

Within each of the phases of illness experienced by the child, the family will have to develop strategies for adjusting and coping. These will differ throughout the trajectory of the illness, but they may include:

• Recognising the symptoms, pain and physical changes
• Adjusting to medical intervention, treatment and in some cases to palliative care

- Developing strategies to manage stress
- Communicating effectively with professional people and carers
- Maintaining the family identity
- Preserving relationships with partners and friends
- Expressing emotions and fears

A number of frameworks explore the adaptation process (Brown 2007; Hornby 1999). Families vary in the ways in which they deal with the stress. Factors that influence family adjustment include:

- The demands of the illness, including onset, progression, severity of symptoms and symptom visibility
- The impact of the illness on everyday living
- The personality of the child and family and their ways of communicating with each other

Traditionally, there has existed a tension between the coping strategies adopted by parents and those preferred by professionals. Parents need to be encouraged and empowered to develop the coping strategies which are best for them. The challenge to professionals is in helping parents to develop those tactics which will enable the strategies to work (Goldman 2002).

Professionals who work with parents after their child's diagnosis should not assume that because a family has been coping for some time they are no longer in need of constant support. The coping strategies which families learn and the skills they acquire need to be acknowledged. All parents will need:

- Continued support in adjusting to their emotional and psychological reactions
- Assistance in seeking professional support
- Support in recouping their physical strengths
- Assistance in ensuring resources to meet their needs
- Adequate information at each stage of the child's illness

The care of sick children is multidisciplinary, requiring a range of services and skills. In order to provide flexible comprehensive support to all members of a child's family, services must be co-ordinated so that the wide range of agencies across health, social and voluntary sectors are able to make a valid contribution. This requires effective networking, co-operation and commitment to collaborative partnerships in practice.

Hain (2002) says that the early assumption that all aspects of care of children were the paediatrician's domain has, in more recent times, given way to appreciation of the skills of other members of a multidisciplinary team.

Models of care are different. Some children with life-limiting illnesses are cared for in the community, some in children's hospices and some in hospital. Wherever the care setting, the overall aim is to meet the needs of the child and their family and to maintain the equilibrium of life as far as possible. Seamless care follows the child from one environment to another and recognises the skills and expertise of the multiprofessional team. Goldman and Schuller (2006) believe that the problems faced by children and young people are dependent on many variables. Recently there has been a commitment by many agencies to work collaboratively with families and with each other. For example, ACT has campaigned for many years about the need for services to be co-ordinated around the individual needs of each family, taking account of their views and recognising the central role and expertise that parents have in the care of their children.

In 2005, Al Aynsley Green, the Children's Commissioner for England, acknowledged that top level managers and those charged with governance and strategic decision- making, have in the past failed sick children by perceiving them as 'small adults needing small beds'. Aynsley Green expressed a commitment towards extending and developing the historical success and efficacy of social reformers such as Barnardo, Rowntree and Dickens. He believes that the role of children's commissioner must support a transformation of children's services.

Families are often overwhelmed by the number of professionals involved with them. The DfES (2005) document, *Professional Guidance for Children with Additional Needs*, recommends that parents and carers should have one practitioner who acts as a single point of contact for them and supports them in making informed choices about the care they need; who ensures they receive appropriate help at the right time, delivered by skilled and appropriate practitioners; who makes sure that professional duplication and inconsistency are avoided. Such a person can make a real difference to the quality of experience families enjoy, especially if the paediatrician remains involved in caring for the child and works alongside a range of service providers.

Each family's needs are individual and may change over a period of time. Therefore, a wide range of services will be required in order to provide flexible care that complements each family's own skills and the contribution of primary care teams.

Empowering parents

Since the early 1980s, a tremendous amount has been written about working with parents who have a child with a disability. Authors such as Carpenter (1997), Brown (2007) and Hornby (1998), have described the importance of working collaboratively in practice. However, it was not until 1999, that Hornby developed a theoretical model that recognised the collaborative relationship between parents and professionals. Although Hornby's model was originally designed for educational settings, Brown (2007) suggests that with some adaptations the Hornby model is relevant to professionals working with families who have a sick child.

The diamond in Figure 10.1 represents parental needs and the contributions that parents are able to make to their child's care. The model also demonstrates how some parents will need greater guidance, whilst others are able to make extensive contributions. For example, all parents need professionals who are able to communicate with them and some may need individual counselling.

Information about their child

All parents have a wealth of knowledge about their child. Indeed, they *are* the experts about their child's behaviour, likes and dislikes and daily care, including medical care. Professionals need to work with parents in order to be able to tap into this knowledge. They will also need to possess excellent communication and listening skills in order to enter into meaningful conversations with families.

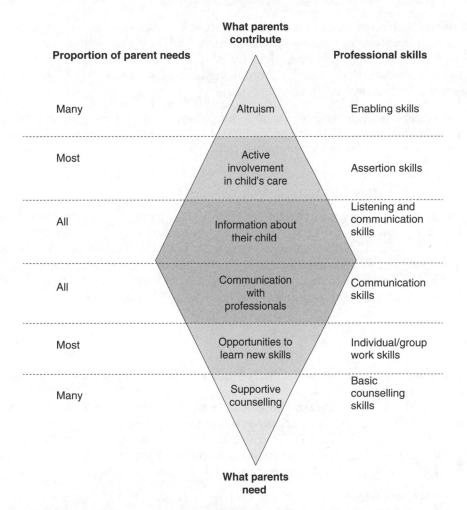

Figure 10.1 Meeting parents needs – the supportive role of professionals (based on Hornby 1999). Source: Brown (2007). Reproduced with kind permission.

Involving parents in their child's care

Many parents develop complex skills in their child's care, including medical procedures, symptom control and pain management. Professionals are often astounded by the expertise of parents. They need to encourage and empower parents to make decisions on behalf of, or with, their child, whilst also being available to give advice and support when it is needed. A flexible working partnership involves listening to parents' needs and helping them to be assertive, in order to communicate their ideas, needs and concerns, so that they are able to gain the best care for their child. Professionals also need to be assertive with colleagues from within and outside their own service in order to act as advocates for families.

Altruism

Many families with a sick child seem to possess the capacity to reach out and to support other parents, taking comfort from shared experience. At Acorns children's hospices this is lived out in practice in groups such as men's groups, Asian mothers' groups, grandparent groups and user involvement groups. Other parents, both bereaved and non-bereaved, speak at professional conferences and open days, or write in journals and newsletters. It should be recognised, however, that parents should never be exploited but enabled by professionals to make the contribution that is right for them:

> 'I felt less isolated when I was able to chat to other mums. The common ground we shared was nothing to do with where we lived or what kind of employment we were in. At a basic level it was about having a very poorly child.' (anonymous)

Opportunities to learn new skills

Most parents welcome opportunities to learn new skills in caring for their child. Sometimes parents prefer to develop new capacities through attending groups, but more often skills are acquired through modelling care and medical procedures carried out by professionals. Whatever the setting, in addition to learning, parents will benefit from being able to share their own ideas and to raise their concerns, a process that can be facilitated by professionals who have developed teaching and group-work skills.

Summary

Resource allocation in the future is likely to be determined by efficacy and also on cost effectiveness, with the result that where efficacy is lacking funds will not be provided. The care of sick children and their families is at a critical stage in its evolution. Amongst the challenges will be the necessity for rigorous assessment of the quality of everyday practice matched to the needs of individual family members so that services are worthy of being deemed to be excellent and the relationship between professionals and families truly demonstrates collaborative partnership in practice.

References

Aynsley Green, A. (2005) Interview, 29 June 29, *Children Now*.

Bjornberg, U. & Buck-Wiklund, M. (1990) *The Organisation of Everyday Family Life in the Family and the Neighbourhood*. Goteborg: Daidalos.

Brown, E. (2007) *Supporting the Child and the Family in Paediatric Palliative Care*. London: Jessica Kingsley.

Carpenter, B. (ed.) (1997) *Families in Context: Emerging Trends in Family Support and Early Intervention*. London: David Fulton.

Casey, A. (1988) A partnership with the child and family. *Senior Nursing*, **8**(4), 8–9.

Cooper, C. (1999) *Continuing Care of Sick Children – Examining the Impact of Chronic Illness*. Salisbury: Quay Books.

Corbett, J. & Twycross, A. (2006) Negotiation of care by children's nurses – lessons from research. *Journal of Palliative Nursing*, **18**(8), 34–7.

Davis, H. (1993) *Counselling Parents of Children with Chronic Illness or Disability*. Leicester: BPS Books.

Department for Education and Skills (DfES) (2005) *Professional Guidance for Children with Additional Needs*. London: DfES.

Down, G. & Simons, J. (2006) Communication. In: Hain, R., Goldman, A. & Liben, S. (eds) *The Oxford Textbook of Palliative Care for Children*. Oxford: Oxford University Press.

Goldman, A. (ed.) (2002) *Care of the Dying Child*, 2nd edn. Oxford: Oxford University Press.

Goldman, A. & Schuller, I. (2006) Models of curative and palliative care relationships. In: Cooper, J (ed.) *Occupational Therapy in Oncology and Palliative Care*. London: John Wiley.

Hain, R. (2002) The view from a bridge. *European Journal of Palliative Care*, 9(2), 75–7.

Hornby, G. (1998) *Counselling in Child Disability*. London: Chapman and Hall.

Hornby, G. (1999) *Working with Parents of Children with Special Needs*. London: Cassell.

Murgatroyde, S. & Wolfe, R. (1993) *Coping with Crisis: Understanding and Helping People in Need*. Birmingham: Open University.

Shields, L., Pratt, J. & Hunter, J. (2006) Family-centred care: a review of qualitative studies. *Journal of Clinical Nursing*, **15**, 1317–23.

Smart, C. & Neale, B. (1999) *Family Fragments?* Cambridge: Policy Press.

11

From Hospital to Home – Parents' Reflective Account

Ian and Nicola Markwell

Introduction

Ryan was born on Christmas Day 2000, after a fast journey down the motorway to the maternity hospital. He was born 15 weeks premature, weighed in at 1 pound 11 ounces (762 g) and was delivered by Caesarean section. Since the time that Nicola had realised that she was having contractions at home, things all happened so quickly that we did not have time to think of names. When we were shown into the neonatal unit to see him for the first time, we were introduced to him as Joseph, but by that time we had already decided on Ryan as a name and quickly got it corrected. Ryan was not actually due until April 2001, and as we sat and watched him in the incubator over that Christmas period, it was hard to comprehend what would be in front of us over the coming months and years.

Medical history – the first nine months

As Ryan was born at 25 weeks, he was ventilated for 60 days and developed chronic lung disease (see Figure 1.1). His early weeks in hospital were very difficult, as he lost weight, was given phototherapy for jaundice and was tube fed. Over these weeks, the aim of the medical and nursing staff was to reduce Ryan's dependence on ventilation and they made steady progress towards this goal.

Care Planning in Children and Young People's Nursing, First Edition.
Edited by Doris Corkin, Sonya Clarke, Lorna Liggett.

Nevertheless, it soon became apparent that Ryan would be difficult to extubate. On one occasion we had a difficult situation, when Ryan extubated himself and the medical staff found it difficult to re-intubate him.

After this episode, it was concluded that he had sub-glottic stenosis, and therefore the best way to reduce his dependence on the ventilator would be for him to have a tracheostomy. This was successfully completed on the 21 February 2001, and within a matter of days Ryan's dependence on the ventilator had stopped, although he remained on low flow oxygen for the remainder of his time in hospital.

Gradually, Ryan started to gain weight and improve to the point that the medical staff started to talk about discharging him, but this was on the assumption that we would take him home attached to an oxygen cylinder which was connected to his tracheostomy tube. Although this was initially a very daunting prospect, the medical staff, nurses and technicians prepared us well for what was involved in handling the oxygen cylinders and managing Ryan's care, whilst on oxygen. We therefore started to prepare to bring him home, and he was finally discharged from hospital in May 2001.

Unfortunately, this was not the end of the medical problems as within a week of discharge, we were back in intensive care due to Ryan aspirating on his food and milk and a significant reduction in his lung function to the point that he stopped breathing at home. It was a long week in intensive care, but fortunately Ryan made a full recovery and was discharged again, after a revision of his medication. Over the next period of months, Ryan was in and out of hospital on a regular basis, only remaining at home for 1–2 weeks at a time. We seemed to be going round in a vicious circle. Ryan had a gastro-oesophageal reflux and he was aspirating milk into his lungs which were already badly damaged, causing severe chest infections, which required hospitalisation. To try and treat this, the medical options were thickened milk and food, to try and prevent the reflux and other medication to try and empty the contents of his stomach quickly.

Eventually, it was concluded that the best solution would be to conduct a fundoplication, which is a surgical procedure where the top of the stomach is tightened to prevent the stomach contents from refluxing back and entering the windpipe. This was completed in September 2001, and it was soon clear that the issue with the reflux had been solved. The cycle of hospital visits was broken for now.

Planning care

From September 2001, Ryan's care was primarily managed at home. He had a tracheostomy tube, which needed changing weekly and required regular suction. In order to maintain Ryan's breathing he required low-flow oxygen via a cylinder 24 hours a day and he also received nebulisers four times a day. His feeds were thickened with carobel and he was given domperidone medication daily to help prevent the reflux (despite the fundoplication).

In order for us to care properly for Ryan at home we had to transform his bedroom and other parts of the house into what looked like a small 'medical' centre. The essential equipment and facilities which we needed were:

- Two full size oxygen cylinders (one upstairs and one downstairs)
- One small handheld oxygen cylinder for use in the car or when on trips out
- Two suction machines (one portable and one electric)

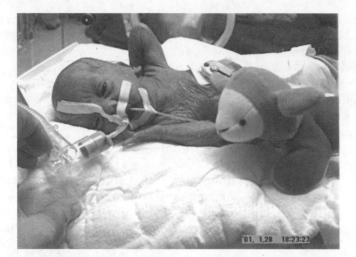

Figure 11.1   Ryan in neonatal unit.

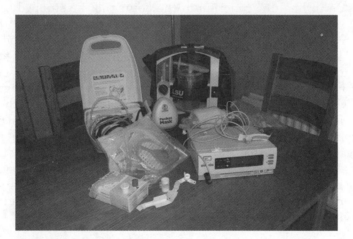

Figure 11.2   Ryan's equipment at home.

- Nebuliser medication and equipment (Figure 11.2)
- Tracheostomy tubes and humidifiers
- Oxygen saturation monitor (Figure 11.2)

The treatment of Ryan's medical issues changed as he became older:

- His dependence on bottled oxygen: gradually over the first three months, we were able to slowly reduce the level of oxygen which Ryan required, whilst still maintaining his oxygen saturation levels. It got to the stage where we could remove the bottled oxygen and from that point forward he only required oxygen when suffering reduced lung performance due to chest infections.
- The presence of the tracheostomy tube: this was the most obvious sign of Ryan's medical problems. From a medical perspective this was a source of chest infections, it required

regular suction, led to difficulties in Ryan learning to talk and, as he became older, it led to an element of social awkwardness.
- He was very susceptible to chest infections, and from time to time he required hospitalisation and treatment with intravenous antibiotics.
- The presence of his fundoplication meant that he could not vomit, and on one occasion, when he had a serious gastro-intestinal infection, this led to emergency treatment in hospital, as he could not get rid of the infection.

As Ryan began to be regularly assessed through the community nursing system, a number of other medical or developmental issues emerged:

- Ryan was diagnosed as having reduced hearing due to the presence of glue ear, and had vents put in to correct this. He was quite susceptible to ear infections because of the issues with his ears.
- Ryan was assessed as being developmentally delayed and therefore required additional assistance, although he was able to enter mainstream school.
- Ryan was slow to begin to learn to talk because of the presence of his tracheostomy tube, as the air bypassed his mouth and nose. He began to learn to talk, by dropping his chin over the entrance to his tube, thereby forcing the air through his mouth and nose and in this way could talk. Despite this mechanism, which Ryan developed himself, he could not make some specific word sounds and could not speak for long periods without pausing to take a breath.

Each of these issues tended to be dealt with by a different group of people, either community or hospital based, and it was one of our main frustrations, particularly in the early days of Ryan's care at home, that there did not seem to be one person charged with Ryan's overall care.

Hospital to home

With Ryan's medical history and treatment, we have spent a significant portion of time in hospitals. Particularly over the first nine months of Ryan's life, we seemed to spend half of our lives in hospital. This meant that we came to know quite a few of the medical staff fairly well. As Mum, Nicola, was qualified in adult nursing, she seemed to slip easily into the ward routine, particularly those wards where Ryan was cared for over longer periods of time.

Ryan's hospital notes seemed to grow and grow, and with each new visit to hospital we found that when Ryan was admitted to a new ward in the hospital we always ended up repeating Ryan's life story to a new doctor or nurse. At home we had become very used to handling Ryan's various medical needs, such as tracheostomy care, suction and nebulisers, and at times seemed to be more aware of how to treat him than some of the hospital staff. This usually led to them backing off slightly from providing 'front-line' care in those aspects and allowing us to take the lead in those areas. This usually worked well for both parties, as the hospital staff could then concentrate on treating Ryan's condition, which had led to that particular hospital admission.

Although on the whole the medical staff were very good, it is also true to say that the hospital visits allowed us to come into contact with other non-medical people, who were able to give us additional advice which led to our care of Ryan in the home becoming that little bit easier. Hospital technicians quite often had little hints and tips on how to operate or use some of the equipment which was necessary to have in the home. This allowed us to resolve some of the problems, which gave us sleepless nights from time to time, such as a poor signal on an oxygen monitor. During hospital visits, we also met other parents who were trying to cope with a similar set of circumstances to ours, and it was always quite therapeutic to compare notes with each other. This was particularly true of the treatment of children with a tracheostomy, where the medical staff rely on other more experienced parents to provide guidance to those who are faced with managing a child with a tracheostomy. This was a service which we have felt the benefits of, having participated as experienced tracheostomy carers ourselves.

Living with Ryan and his tracheostomy

Ryan had his tracheostomy tube inserted in February 2001, and up until July 2008 there were three unsuccessful attempts to remove Ryan's tracheostomy tube in Northern Ireland. On each occasion, Ryan encountered difficulties breathing without the tracheostomy tube for more than 48 hours and so the tracheostomy tube was reinserted. This meant that we became used to dealing with a child with a tracheostomy, even though Nicola would have admitted that this was one of the tasks which she hated most whilst she was doing her nurse training. The main issues with tracheostomy care were:

- The tracheostomy tube required replacement with a new tube on a weekly basis.
- Ryan had difficulty coughing up mucus and therefore required suction at home. This needed to be more frequent when Ryan had a cold or chest infection.
- We had to be careful with his clothing and mindful of the activities which Ryan could do, to ensure that the tracheostomy tube was never covered and that he did not participate in activities which could have led to materials entering his tube, for example swimming or playing in the sand pit. Anything which had the potential to block Ryan's tube would essentially have blocked his airway and therefore would have been a serious risk to his health.

We both received training on tracheostomy care from the medical and nursing staff, but once we were in the home environment and became used to doing the various tasks routinely, we realised that the training that we had been given was not necessarily the most practical, and was really derived from textbooks. One very simple example of this was the emphasis, which some staff in the hospital placed on linen tracheostomy tapes, which could be tied around Ryan's neck and which were supplied as standard with each tracheostomy tube. However, over time we learnt that Velcro tapes were available, and although we were aware of the potential safety risks (can easily open), Velcro was in fact a more practical and comfortable solution to keeping Ryan's tracheostomy tube in place.

The various aspects of tracheostomy care also needed to be emphasised to the staff at the local school, prior to Ryan becoming a pupil, and this was backed up by training for Ryan's teachers in how to deal with him should a difficulty be encountered at school, and this training was delivered by Mum, Nicola. It is fair to say that the school staff willingly participated in the training, and this gave us great comfort in ensuring that Ryan was in safe hands whilst at school.

As indicated above, the path to removing Ryan's tracheostomy tube was not a smooth one, and led to intense frustration on our part, as the only surgeon based in Northern Ireland who could perform these types of operations retired, and it was not obvious if (or when) a replacement would take up the post. This meant that there was minimal medical assistance locally, and after several years of frustration with the lack of progress, we eventually wrote to our MP to bring the matter to his attention. Thanks to his intervention, and with the help of senior consultants in Northern Ireland, we managed to get a referral to a children's hospital in England.

We journeyed over to England to attend our first appointment with a feeling of trepidation over what might be in front of us, but were met with a very experienced and highly competent team, dealing with children with tracheostomies. The medical team in England took ownership of Ryan's care, in terms of his tracheostomy tube and history of sub-glottic stenosis, and within a matter of months an operation was successfully performed to surgically correct his condition and remove his tracheostomy tube. To summarise our experience, after an initial assessment appointment, we arrived in England on a Monday and when leaving the children's hospital the following Monday, Ryan was discharged without his tracheostomy tube and no ill effects. After one year at home that is still the case.

Parents as carers

As Ryan has developed and grown, and his medical conditions have steadily improved, the role which we have played as parents has gradually changed from one of full-time carers to a normal parent-child relationship. In the early days, when Ryan was hospitalised, our life was made up of daily visits to the neonatal unit to visit Ryan, and this was despite having to care for his two older sisters, aged three and five years at the time. Upon reflection, it was difficult to sit beside him in the incubator, particularly when we were not allowed to hold him, and when he gripped your hand through the incubator glove port it was a whole different experience.

After his discharge from hospital, we became Ryan's main carers, with Mum, Nicola, giving up her career to devote 100% of her time to Ryan and the girls. The first few months of his time at home were very stressful, as we had a lot of medical equipment in the home and had to carry an oxygen cylinder *everywhere* that we went, including trips to the shops, to visit family and friends and on holidays. Over this time, there were very regular spells of hospitalisation, and several ambulance or fast car journeys, as on occasions we found that his condition deteriorated very quickly. On the whole these hospital spells brought some respite to our lives, as it was not necessary for one of us to stay in hospital with Ryan and we were able to recharge the batteries.

In our experience, the caring situation resulted in varying degrees of depersonalisation brought about by:

- Lack of sleep
- Loss of privacy and personal space
- Loss of freedom of choice in personal and family matters
- Loss of leisure activities, including holidays, and social isolation

Although a lot could be said about any of the problems listed above, perhaps the most difficult to cope with was the combination of disturbed sleep and inadequate sleep. This was particularly applicable for us in the early days when Ryan was discharged from hospital, or on occasions when he was unwell at home. It is not surprising that there is a sense of unreality about the world which we live in when we are acting as the primary carers.

The fear and stress of caring does not arise solely from the physical act of caring. Relationships can become strained and this can lead to the possible breakdown of marriage due to the loss of time spent together by husband and wife. One person may have to give up their job to become the primary carer at home and this can also bring an additional financial burden on the family budget.

However, the caring role can also arise due to the complex nature of the support systems which exist in the community, i.e. it may become difficult to determine who to turn to for assistance in the various agencies. In our case, this took quite some time to organise, as the community children's nursing service had just been established. After unsuccessfully trying several avenues, it was finally with the help of our MP, that we were able to have a children's nurse to stay in our home and care for Ryan overnight.

This was still only for one day over several weeks, and although it did give us the required respite for a short period, we soon came to the conclusion that it was not worth the hassle of sorting out the house and medication, organising the girls and having someone else in our home, for just a few hours' respite. There was a sense that we had lost ownership of our home, the professional carer could go home after her shift, while we had to return to our role as primary carers as soon as the children's nurse left the house.

As Ryan became older, the trips to hospital became less frequent, but when he was admitted this proved to be quite challenging as the management of the rest of the family placed additional stresses on us as parents. For each of these stays in hospital, one of the parents had to stay, and in these periods we went through a cycle where the parent staying in hospital lived in an unreal situation of boredom and quick bites of something to eat as Ryan was having treatment. Ryan himself grew to dislike these trips to hospital and hated being left alone.

Siblings and extended family

To fully understand the impact that Ryan's medical conditions and treatment have had on his sisters, you need to consider it from their perspective. They woke up on Christmas Day in 2000 to find that their mum gone and to be told that they had a new baby brother. Although they were both very excited at that time, this excitement soon changed as our new pattern of living emerged. They did not actually get to visit their new baby brother until 17 March 2001, and spent parts of every weekend from then to September 2001, either in hospital visiting him, or with relatives as we visited him. The girls were quite accepting of Ryan's tracheostomy and the various medicines which we had to dose him with, and they treated him like any other little brother.

When Ryan's problems with reflux were resolved in September 2001, everyone was relieved that we could settle into some semblance of a normal family life, albeit interrupted occasionally by Ryan's follow-up visits to hospital. When this happened the girls could have become quite annoyed and afraid for him, but generally when they were allowed to see him in hospital and they could see that he was improving, they were quite accepting of the reality of the situation.

Until Ryan's premature birth, the girls had enjoyed a relatively normal family life and although this was occasionally seriously disrupted, as we went through the ups and downs of Ryan's hospitalisation and treatment, the girls never displayed any resentment towards him; their reaction has rather been to be very protective of him, and display a relatively mature concern for his wellbeing.

Our son Ryan

Within a matter of days of Ryan's premature birth, it was apparent that he was a determined character, as he moved around the incubator as much as he could and extubated himself a couple of times, much to the consternation of the medical staff. Our view has consistently been that it is this element of his character which has helped him get over the various medical hurdles that he has had to overcome.

When Ryan was at home, he was a very quiet baby due to the presence of the tracheostomy and he never really cried, as the air escaped through his tracheostomy, rather than going through his mouth and nose. He never really crawled, but developed a way of moving around the floor on his side, which he became quite good at.

As Ryan grew up, he developed quite well socially and mixes well with his own age group and with other children and adults, and he is a very happy little boy, despite his medical history.

Furthermore, Ryan's reaction to his intermittent stays in hospital over the years has been what you might expect from a child, in that he did not like to be left alone, and when he had started to recover he was keen to get home. One of the most traumatic times for Ryan, in recent years, was when he was preparing to go to England to have his tracheostomy removed. The entire family was concerned as to how successful the operation would be, and the emotions were running very high in the days before the trip, to such an extent that Ryan himself became more aware of the significance of this operation. Fortunately the operation was successful and it has seen Ryan take another step forward in terms of improving his speech and reducing his dependence on nebulisers. Ultimately the medical staff believe that it will help his chronic lung disease in the longer term.

Ryan's education

One of the key challenges which we have faced as Ryan has developed and grown has been the question as to whether he could be placed in mainstream schooling, given his medical and developmental needs. Fortunately, we already had a relationship with the local primary school as both of our other children attended the school and Mum, Nicola, was involved in the parent teacher association. This did assist us in the long run, but nevertheless we had to go through the necessary red tape to finally achieve a place for Ryan. The first steps towards school were through a visit by the educational psychologist to the playgroup which Ryan attended, to conduct an assessment of him. This led to the requirement to have a statutory assessment of Ryan's educational needs carried out by the local Education and Library Board. This resulted in a recommendation that Ryan could attend mainstream schooling with the presence of a classroom assistant for a few hours each day, but the extent of red tape involved was such that we only finally got this recommendation in October, with the school year commencing in September. It was thanks to the good relationship with the school that they permitted Ryan to attend from September.

Each year the validity of the statement was reviewed and an assessment made. We also faced an additional challenge when Ryan's tracheostomy was removed, as this was the primary medical need on which the statement was based and therefore we had to go through the whole process all over again to be reassessed from a developmental perspective. Fortunately this also resulted in support being continued and that is where we are today.

Giving something back

We have been quite fortunate that we have had an opportunity to give something back to the nursing profession in that the community children's nursing sister, who assisted us in the early days at home, took up an educational post in Queen's University Belfast. Since then Nicola has been invited into the School of Nursing and Midwifery to present Ryan's journey to pre-registration second-year child branch nursing students. This yearly classroom tutorial is based on the 'lived experience' which we have had and does not rely on any reference to textbooks, thus giving the nursing students an insight into what it is really like to be the primary carer of a child with life-threatening needs in the community setting. Planning care for Ryan's complex healthcare needs initially brought a major upheaval into the lives of the whole family and this has lead to a long-standing relationship with the main healthcare professionals. We are very pleased to be able to give something back to our healthcare system which has provided us with so much practical training over the years and supported the planning of care for our precious son.

This unique journey with our son Ryan has taught us as parents to think outside the box, to explore all possible avenues and to ensure we are fully informed, using specialist input where needed. Home was recognised as the best place to care for Ryan and he was only admitted to hospital if the care he required could not be provided within his home, despite the fact that, as you may appreciate, this proved to be extremely challenging at times for everyone involved. Nevertheless, we his parents and the whole family have ultimately been rewarded for our perseverance.

Section 2

Care Planning – Pain Management

12

Managing a Neonate in an Intensive Care Unit
Clare Morfoot and Susanne Simmons

Scenario

Molly is a 32-week gestation preterm infant born by normal vaginal delivery, following spontaneous rupture of membranes. Her Apgar score (Pinheiro 2009) was 7 at one minute and 10 at five minutes. Following delivery, Molly had shallow, irregular respirations with a heart rate less than 100 beats per minute. She was dusky in colour, but had good tone and some movement of her limbs. Molly received five inflation breaths which improved her heart rate. However, as her respiratory effort remained poor continuous positive airway pressure (CPAP) was commenced for transfer to the neonatal unit.

On admission to the unit, Molly weighed 1.4 kg and was placed into a closed incubator. Bubble CPAP was applied and an orogastric tube sited. Over the next few days, Molly's respiratory function improved and CPAP pressures were weaned until it was discontinued on day three. During these first three days of life, Molly required a number of painful invasive diagnostic procedures: 15 heel pricks for newborn blood spot screening, blood gases and glucose screening; 5 venepunctures and 12 cannulations (including unsuccessful attempts). Subsequently, Molly continued to receive invasive diagnostic procedures although their frequency reduced during Molly's admission.

Care Planning in Children and Young People's Nursing, First Edition.
Edited by Doris Corkin, Sonya Clarke, Lorna Liggett.
© 2012 Blackwell Publishing Ltd. Published 2012 by Blackwell Publishing Ltd.

Questions

1. Assessment: how would you assess whether Molly is in pain?
2. Planning: how would you prepare Molly and her family for painful invasive diagnostic procedures?
3. Implementation: what pain management strategies might you use to support Molly during painful invasive diagnostic procedures?
4. Evaluation: what might be the consequences of not managing Molly's pain effectively?

This chapter will focus on the non-pharmacological management of pain in the neonate. Although the scenario is based on a premature infant, the principles of care outlined in the chapter are also relevant to the term neonate and infant. Therefore, this theory can be applied to practice in any child healthcare setting, as well as the neonatal unit. Pharmacological pain measures will not be addressed as these are covered in other relevant chapters.

Answers to questions

Activity of living: communication.

Question 1. Assessment: how would you assess whether Molly is in pain?

Although historically, neonates were regarded as incapable of experiencing and interpreting noxious stimuli, it is now known that neonates do possess the neurological capacity to perceive pain from twenty weeks' gestation (Anand & Hickey 1987; Simons & Tibboel 2006). Additionally, it is now believed that premature infants may be hypersensitive to noxious stimuli and something that would not normally produce pain feels painful (Ballweg 2007). This is thought to be due to the immaturity of descending inhibitory pathways, larger pain perception areas in the spinal cord and more concentrated pain receptors lying closer to the skin.

Most definitions of pain recognise the subjective, emotional and sensory nature of the pain experience. However, as they include an emotional component, these definitions may not accurately reflect the neonatal pain experience. It is also important to acknowledge that neonatal pain may encompass stress, distress (Mathew & Mathew 2003) and discomfort and it may be difficult to differentiate between these. Therefore, the management strategies which are used to alleviate distress, stress, discomfort and pain may overlap.

At 32 weeks' gestation, Molly is capable of feeling pain and, therefore, the healthcare professional must observe Molly for specific pain indicators, in order to accurately assess her pain. Pain indicators in neonates (see Table 12.1) include behavioural, physiological and chemical changes (Ballweg 2007; Labonia 2007).

The available neonatal pain assessment tools normally include observations of behavioural responses and physiological parameters, as chemical indicators may only be demonstrated by further painful, invasive, diagnostic procedures. A few examples of commonly cited and validated neonatal pain assessment tools include:

1. *Premature Infant Pain Profile (PIPP)*. This uses seven behavioural and physiological indicators, each attracting a score of 0–3, depending on the infant's gestational age. It

Table 12.1 Examples of neonatal pain indicators.

Behavioural responses	Physiological parameters	Chemical changes
Facial expression, for example cupped tongue, brow bulge, naso-labial furrow, open mouth, eye squeeze	↑↓ heart rate	↑ stress hormone production
Cry (may be silent if intubated)	↑↓ respiratory rate	↑ blood glucose
Body movement, for example splayed digits, arching, hand swiping, clenching of fists and toes, limb withdrawal, rigidity, flaccidity	↑↓ oxygen saturations	↓ insulin
Changes in sleep/wake cycle, for example hyper-alert or lethargic, irritability	↑↓ blood pressure	

can be used on preterm and term infants and has been validated for acute procedural pain (Stevens *et al.* 1996).

2. *Neonatal Infant Pain Score (NIPS)*. This uses six behavioural and physiological indicators, each attracting a score of 0–1 (except for cry, which scores 0–2), with a maximum score of seven. It is currently used for both preterm and term infants and has been validated for acute procedural pain (Lawrence *et al.* 1993).

3. *CRIES (Crying, Requires oxygen, Increased vital signs, Expression, Sleepless)*. This uses five behavioural and physiological indicators, each attracting a score of 0–2 and is a neonatal post-operative pain assessment tool (Krechel & Bildner 1995).

It is important to remember that the sick, preterm, sedated, paralysed or ventilated neonate may not be capable of demonstrating the anticipated behavioural responses to pain. For example, an extremely premature neonate will have insufficient glucose reserves and may lack the energy to cry or move their body (as outlined in Table 12.1). Although this makes neonatal pain assessment challenging, a tool enables the health professional to demonstrate objectivity in assessing neonatal pain. Research undertaken by BLISS (2005) informed the publication of *The BLISS Baby Charter*, incorporating seven core values for neonatal care. Key findings from this report highlighted that a pain scale is only used by about 20% of neonatal units in the UK and that less than 60% of units regularly use analgesia for pain relief. It could be argued that without effective pain assessment, appropriate pain management strategies may not be implemented.

Question 2. Planning: how would you prepare Molly and her family for painful invasive diagnostic procedures?

Preparing Molly

The *in utero* environment facilitates normal neurodevelopment through appropriate and controlled stimuli which meet the needs of the gestational stage of the infant. In contrast, the premature infant on a neonatal unit is exposed to noise, light and excessive noxious handling at a time when they would normally still be developing *in utero*. A recent Cochrane Review (Symington & Pinelli 2006) highlighted the benefits of implementing developmental care strategies, such as reducing noise, light and handling, in order to reduce the inappropriate level and pattern of stimulation that these infants are constantly exposed to. Failure to minimise the impact of the neonatal environment can jeopardise normal development.

Table 12.2 Examples of behavioural cues.

Avoidance behaviour	Approach behaviour
Sneezing	Hands together, clasping
Hiccoughing	Grasping
Yawning	Moving hand to face
Grimacing	Hand to mouth
Tongue thrust	Smooth movements
Limp or stiff posture	Orientation to voice or sound
Sudden or jerky movement	Softly, flexed posture
Tremulousness	Relaxed, open face
Finger splay	Mouth pursing to make 'ooh' face
Arms extended/outward facing palms ('high guard' hands)	Sucking
Crying	Smooth state change, for example sleep to wake
Looking away	Snuggling

Infant behaviour corresponds to the stage of maturity of the central nervous system. Assessment of behavioural cues (Table 12.2) will allow the healthcare professional to interpret how the infant is coping with the stressors of the environment (Als & Butler 2008; Warren & Bond 2010). For example, Molly may display avoidance behaviours such as splayed digits and side swiping during attempts at venepuncture. If avoidance behaviours are demonstrated, the environment should be modified and if appropriate, procedures should be delayed. During procedures, pain management strategies must be employed.

The timing of procedures should be individually assessed and planned to ensure that Molly is allowed periods of rest to promote growth and development. Procedures should coincide with other caregiving activities whenever possible. Invasive procedures are best timed away from Molly's feed times to avoid vomiting and the risk of aspiration.

Preparing Molly's family

It is known that having a premature infant on a neonatal unit can be extremely stressful for the family. The concept of family-centred care concerns the parents' relationship with their infant, their participation in their infant's care and any decisions that are made about their infant (Reid & Freer 2010). It represents a holistic approach to care, which enables and empowers families to be equal partners with the healthcare professional (Smith *et al.* 2002), thereby minimising the detrimental effects of being separated from their infant.

During this time, parents will be vulnerable and may not be able to absorb the large amount of information given by healthcare professionals (Reid *et al.* 2007). It is therefore important to use clear, consistent explanations, which should be repeated as often as necessary. Medical jargon and abbreviations should be avoided. The reason for the procedure should be given, along with the risks and benefits. Verbal information should be supported by written resources and all information should be available in the parents' first language. The fifth core value of the *BLISS Baby Charter* identifies the information and support needed by parents to help them care for their baby and achieve the best quality of life possible (BLISS 2005). As with all interventions, parental consent should be ascertained prior to the procedure (Alderson 2006).

Molly's parents may wish to be involved in supporting her during the procedure. However, some parents may choose not to stay and this decision should be respected (Lee 2004). Although Molly's parents may choose to be present for one procedure, it should not be assumed that they wish to be present for each intervention. Similarly, explanations regarding procedures should be repeated each time.

Preparation of the practitioner

It is imperative that the practitioner undertaking the procedure is the most appropriate person for the job. Consideration should be given to the practitioner's time availability and level of competence. The healthcare professional should ensure that two people are available throughout the procedure: one to support Molly and one to undertake the procedure.

In addition, the equipment should be collected and easily accessible. The immediate environment should be prepared, with consideration for health and safety. This may include using a height adjustable incubator for Molly and ensuring a functioning, mobile light source is available.

Aseptic, non-touch techniques should be employed at every stage of the procedure, which includes effective handwashing, use of alcohol hand rub and appropriate personal protective equipment, for example aprons and gloves (Aziz 2009). The number of attempts for venepuncture and cannulation should be limited (normally no more than three attempts) and if unsuccessful, Molly should be allowed to recover and a more senior practitioner asked to undertake the procedure.

Question 3. Implementation: what pain management strategies might you use to support Molly during painful invasive diagnostic procedures?

There are several appropriate, non-pharmacological pain management strategies which can help Molly prepare for, cope with and recover from painful or stressful procedures. Some strategies lead to the endogenous release of natural endorphins to relieve pain, while others modify the pain response through distraction (Cignacco *et al.* 2007).

Comfort holding and positive touch

Positive touch provides an essential contrast to the negative effects of noxious handling by healthcare professionals (Bond 2002). This aspect of developmental care consists of firm but gentle holding, responding to individual behavioural cues. Parents are the best placed and most appropriate providers of positive touch and their involvement can promote empowerment and participation in care (Warren 2002).

Touch may be used as a gentle disturbance, prior to a procedure, which will allow Molly the opportunity to prepare for what is going to happen next (Halimaa 2003). The healthcare professional should place both hands on Molly to promote her awareness of the imminent procedure. The strategy of comfort holding (also known as containment holding or facilitated tucking) can then be used to support Molly during the painful and stressful intervention (Bond 2002). However, it might also be used as a means to maintain security and calm Molly at other times. Comfort holding can be described as the still holding of an infant in a flexed, midline position. One hand may be placed on the infant's head, while the other hand maintains the flexion of the lower body/legs (Figure 12.1). Comfort holding has been described as an effective, non-pharmacological, pain relieving intervention for acute pain (Huang *et al.* 2004; Ward-Larson *et al.* 2004). Involving and supporting Molly's parents to provide this comfort measure may also empower parental participation in care.

Swaddling and positioning

Swaddling or wrapping the infant may provide some pain relieving effects (Huang *et al.* 2004; Prasopkittikun & Tilokskulchai 2003). However, use of this strategy may restrict

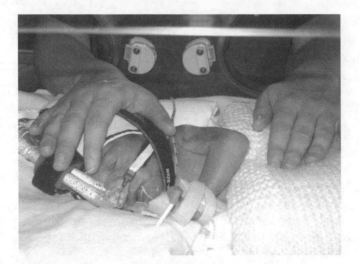

Figure 12.1   Comfort holding.

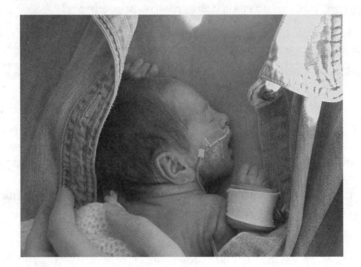

Figure 12.2   Kangaroo care.

physical access to the infant for the procedure. The prone position may provide a means of pain relief, although the evidence for this is inconclusive (Cignacco *et al.* 2007). Nonetheless, the prone position is known to improve cardiovascular, respiratory and gastrointestinal function in the compromised neonate. The provision of boundaries (rolled blankets, nests and positioning aids) to contain Molly's limbs is also known to promote self-calming and forms an important part of developmental care (Warren 2002).

Kangaroo care

Kangaroo care or skin-to-skin contact describes the contact between the prone, naked neonate and their parent's bare chest (Curran *et al.* 2008) (Figure 12.2). Maternal contact during kangaroo care has been shown to decrease the physiological and behavioural pain responses and facilitate quicker recovery time for even very preterm neonates undergoing painful procedures (Castral *et al.* 2008; Johnston *et al.* 2008). This endogenous beneficial effect of skin-to-skin contact is known to be more rapid and powerful, however, in older preterm neonates (Johnston *et al.* 2008).

Reduction of auditory and visual environmental stressors

The reduction of noise and light serves to minimise the impact of the constant environmental onslaught within the neonatal unit, thereby promoting homeostasis and calm for the infant. The use of individual spotlights and covering Molly's eyes, during the procedures, for example, may help to limit the number of stressful stimulants for the infant. This approach may also benefit Molly's parents and healthcare professionals (Hamilton *et al.* 2008).

Conversely, the use of music or voice as a method of distraction and soothing has also been explored. However, the optimum gestational age, length of exposure and volume in relation to this therapy still requires clarification (Standley 2002).

Non-nutritive sucking

Non-nutritive sucking refers to the promotion of sucking behaviour without nutrition (Cignacco *et al.* 2007). The use of non-nutritive sucking during invasive painful procedures could help to produce a calming effect in Molly, since it reduces pain behaviours and increases attentiveness (Bellieni *et al.* 2001; Corbo *et al.* 2000). Although pacifier use is traditionally thought to interfere with breastfeeding (WHO 1998), recent research suggests that it is not detrimental to breastfeeding outcomes (O'Connor *et al.* 2009). In view of the controversy regarding the effects of pacifier use on breastfeeding, it is vital that local guidelines are followed.

The administration of oral sucrose to reduce pain responses in neonates during procedures, such as heel pricks and venepuncture has recently received much debate (Leslie & Marlow, 2006; Stevens *et al.* 2009). The effect is enhanced when used in conjunction with non-nutritive sucking (Bellieni *et al.* 2001). Harrison *et al.* (2009) suggest that there is no reduction in the effectiveness of oral sucrose when repeated doses are given during painful procedures throughout the infant's hospital stay. Breastfeeding or breast milk is also associated with a reduction in pain responses (Shah *et al.* 2009).

Question 4. Evaluation: what might be the consequences of not managing Molly's pain effectively?

The pain experienced by Molly, during her time in the neonatal unit, could have long-lasting deleterious consequences. This early exposure to pain and stress can produce neurodevelopmental, behavioural, cognitive, motor, emotional and social effects (Grunau 1998). It is important to acknowledge that Molly will not only have pain responses that are immediate (seconds to minutes), but also those that are persistent (days to weeks) and prolonged (outlasting her hospital stay) (Fitzgerald & Beggs 2001). For example, some children are known to become increasingly sensitised or preoccupied with pain later, while other sequelae include: deficits in learning; poor motor performance; behavioural problems; attention deficits; impulsivity and poor adaptive behaviour.

References

Alderson, P. (2006) Parents' consent to neonatal decisions about feeding and discharge. *Journal of Neonatal Nursing*, **12**(1), 6–13.

Als, H. & Butler, S. (2008) Newborn individualized developmental care and assessment program (NIDCAP): changing the future for infants and families in intensive and special care nurseries. *Early Childhood Services*, **2**(1), 1–20.

Anand, K.J.S. & Hickey, P.R. (1987) Pain and its effects in the human neonate and fetus. *The New England Journal of Medicine*, **317**, 21.

Aziz, A.M. (2009) Variations in aseptic non-touch technique and implications for infection control. *British Journal of Nursing*, **18**(1), 26–31.

Ballweg, D. (2007) Neonatal and pediatric pain management: standards and application. *Pediatrics and Child Health*, **17**(1), 61–6.

Bellieni, C.V., Buonocore, G., Nenci, A., Franci, N., Cordelli, D.M. & Bagnoli, F. (2001) Sensorial saturation: an effective analgesic tool for heel-prick in preterm infants. *Biology of the Neonate*, **80**, 15–18.

BLISS (2005) *Special Care for Sick Babies: Choice or Chance*. London: BLISS – the Premature Baby Charity.

Bond, C. (2002) Positive Touch and massage in the neonatal unit: British approach. *Seminars in Neonatology*, **7**, 477–86.

Castral, T.C., Warnock, F., Leite, A.M., Haas, V.J. & Scochi, C.G.S. (2008) The effects of skin to skin contact during acute pain in preterm newborns. *European Journal of Pain*, **12**, 464–71.

Cignacco, E., Hamers, J.P.H., Stoffel, L., *et al.* (2007) The efficacy of non-pharmacological interventions in the management of procedural pain in preterm and term neonates. A systematic literature review. *European Journal of Pain*, **11**, 139–52.

Corbo, M.G., Mansi, G., Stagni, A., *et al.* (2000) Non-nutritive sucking during heelstick procedures decreases behavioural distress in the newborn infant. *Biology of the Neonate*, **77**(3), 162–7.

Curran, R.L., Genesoni, L., Ceballos, A.H. & Tallandini, M.A. (2008) A kangaroo mother care research study: a work in progress. *Infant*, **4**(5), 163–5.

Fitzgerald, M. & Beggs, S. (2001) The neurobiology of pain: developmental aspects. *Neuroscientist*, **7**, 246–57.

Grunau, R.E. (1998) Long term effects of pain. *Clinical and Research Forums*, **20**(4), 19–29.

Halimaa, S.-L. (2003) Pain management in nursing procedures on premature babies. *Journal of Advanced Nursing*, **42**(6), 587–97.

Hamilton, K., Moore, R. & Naylor, H. (2008) Developmental care: the carer's perspective. *Infant*, **4**(6), 190–95.

Harrison, D., Loughnan, P., Manias, E., Gordon, I. & Johnston, L. (2009) Repeated doses of sucrose in infants continue to reduce procedural pain during prolonged hospitalizations. *Nursing Research*, **58**(6), 427–34.

Huang, C., Tung, W., Kuo, L. & Chang, Y. (2004) Comparison of pain responses of premature infants to the heelstick between containment and swaddling. *Journal of Nursing Research*, **12**(1), 31–9.

Johnston, C.C., Filion, F., Campbell-Yeo, M., *et al.* (2008) Kangaroo mother care diminishes pain from heel lance in very preterm neonates: a crossover trial. *BMC Pediatrics*, **8**(13), 1–9.

Krechel, S.W. & Bildner, J. (1995) CRIES: a new neonatal postoperative pain measurement score: initial testing and reliability. *Paediatric Anaesthesia*, **5**, 53–61.

Labonia, M. (2007) Pain management for children: the OPBG experience – newborn pain. *Paediatrics and Child Health*, **17**, S71–4.

Lawrence, J., Alcock, D., McGrath, P., Kay, J., MacMurray, S.B. & Dulberg, C. (1993) The development of a tool to assess neonatal pain. *Neonatal Network*, **12**(6), 59–66.

Lee, P. (2004) Family involvement: are we asking too much? *Paediatric Nursing*, **16**(10), 37–41.

Leslie, A. & Marlow, N. (2006) Non-pharmacological pain relief. *Seminars in Fetal and Neonatal Medicine*, **11**, 246–50.

Mathew, P.J. & Mathew, J.L. (2003) Assessment and management of pain in infants. *Postgraduate Medical Journal*, **79**, 438–43.

O'Connor, N.R., Tanabe, K.O., Siadaty, M.S. & Hauck, F.R. (2009) Pacifiers and breastfeeding: a systematic review. *Archives of Pediatrics and Adolescent Medicine*, **163**(4), 378–82.

Pinheiro, J.M.B. (2009) The Apgar cycle: a new view of a familiar scoring system. *Archives of Disease in Childhood Fetal and Neonatal Edition*, **94**, F70–72.

Prasopkittikun, T. & Tilokskulchai, F. (2003) Management of pain from heel stick in neonates. *Journal of Perinatal and Neonatal Nursing*, **17**(4), 304–312.

Reid, T., Bramwell, R., Booth, N. & Weindling, M. (2007) Perceptions of parent-staff communication in neonatal intensive care: the findings from a rating scale. *Journal of Neonatal Nursing*, **13**(2), 64–74.

Reid, T. & Freer, Y. (2010) Developmentally focused nursing care. In: Boxwell, G. (ed.) *Neonatal Intensive Care Nursing*, 2nd edn. London: Routledge.

Shah, P.S., Aliwalas, L.L & Shah, V.S. (2009) Breastfeeding or breast milk for procedural pain in neonates (review). *The Cochrane Library Issue* 2.

Simons, S.H.P. & Tibboel, D. (2006) Pain perception, development and maturation. *Seminars in Fetal and Neonatal Medicine*, **11**, 227–31.

Smith, L., Coleman, V. & Bradshaw, M. (2002) *Family Centred Care: Concept, Theory and Practice*. Basingstoke: Palgrave.

Standley, J.M. (2002) A meta-analysis of the efficacy of music therapy for premature infants. *Journal of Pediatric Nursing*, **17**(2), 107–13.

Stevens, B.R.N., Johnston, C., Petryshen, P. & Taddio, A. (1996) Premature infant pain profile: development and initial validation. *The Clinical Journal of Pain*, **12**(1), 13–22.

Stevens, B., Yamada, J. & Ohlsson, A. (2009) Sucrose for analgesia in newborn infants undergoing painful procedures (review). *The Cochrane Library* Issue 2.

Symington, A. & Pinelli, J. (2006) Developmental care for promoting development and preventing morbidity in preterm infants. *The Cochrane Database of Systematic Reviews* Issue 2.

Ward-Larson, C., Horn, R. & Gosnell, F. (2004) The efficacy of facilitated tucking for relieving procedural pain of endotracheal suctioning in very low birthweight infants. *American Journal of Maternal/Child Nursing*, **29**, 151–6.

Warren, I. (2002) Facilitating infant adaptation: the nursery environment. *Seminars in Neonatology*, **7**, 459–67.

Warren, I. & Bond, C. (2010) *A Guide to Infant Development in the Newborn Nursery*, 5th edn. London: Winnicott Baby Unit.

World Health Organization (WHO, 1998) *Evidence for the Ten Steps to Successful Breastfeeding*. Geneva: World Health Organisation, Division of Child Health and Development.

13

Epidural Analgesia

Michelle Bennett and Sharon Douglass

Scenario

John is a 15-year-old boy who was diagnosed with Crohn's disease three years ago. Conservative management is no longer effective; therefore he has been admitted electively for a right hemi-colectomy; the aim being to improve John's quality of life.

A hemi-colectomy can be performed either as a laparoscopic or an open procedure. It involves the tying of the right colic artery, ileocolic artery and also, if needed, the right branch of the middle colic artery (Thomas 2001). John is having an open procedure, which involves interruption of all tissue and muscle layers. In addition, previous frequent acute exacerbations of his Crohn's disease have resulted in thickening of the intestinal wall with swelling and scar tissue. Crohn's also causes ulcers (fistulas) that tunnel through the affected area into the surrounding tissues. Therefore this surgery may involve significant handling of the bowel and surrounding organs. As a result, this procedure is potentially very painful and will require *multi-modal and advanced analgesic techniques.*

It is essential to take into consideration any child's underlying condition when planning postoperative pain management. In John's case non-steroidal anti-inflammatory drugs (NSAIDs) such as ibuprofen and diclofenac are contra-indicated as one of the side effects is gastric irritation, which is already a symptom of Crohn's disease. Therefore suitable analgesia includes paracetamol, opiates and local anaesthetics.

The route of administration must also be considered and in the immediate postoperative period, the oral route would not be appropriate for the following reasons: being nil by mouth, presence of a paralytic ileus, nasogastric tube on free drainage, nausea and vomiting.

Also, Crohn's is known to have a negative impact on absorption in the body. After major surgery such as a hemi-colectomy the Association of Paediatric Anaesthetists of Great Britain and Ireland (APAGBI 2008) recommend use of intravenous paracetamol alongside an advanced analgesic technique such as an epidural infusion and/or an intravenous opiate patient controlled analgesia (PCA) infusion. When the anaesthetist visits John and his family pre-operatively they discuss the options and decide on an epidural infusion.

Care Planning in Children and Young People's Nursing, First Edition.
Edited by Doris Corkin, Sonya Clarke, Lorna Liggett.
© 2012 Blackwell Publishing Ltd. Published 2012 by Blackwell Publishing Ltd.

Activity 13.1

Recommended reading:

Association of Paediatric Anaesthetists of Great Britain and Ireland (2008) *Good Practice in Postoperative and Procedural Pain.* http://www.apagbi.org.uk

Twycross, A., Dowden, S., Bruce, E. & Blackwell, L.B. (2009) *Managing Pain in Children: A Clinical Guide.*

*Especially guidelines regarding pain assessment, management and pharmacology.

Questions

1. What is epidural analgesia?
2. Reflecting upon the nursing process and a model of care, how would the children's nurse prepare this young person, John, and his family for having an epidural infusion?
3. What general aspects of nursing management would you need to address when considering epidural analgesia for John?
4. Discuss the postoperative nursing care John will require whilst an epidural infusion is in progress.

Answers to questions

Question 1. What is epidural analgesia?

Epidural analgesia is the administration of local anaesthetic drugs with or without other analgesic medications into the epidural space via a fine bore catheter. The local anaesthetic reversibly blocks the transmission of peripheral nerve impulses by inhibiting the entry of sodium ions into the nerve cells, preventing depolarisation and the nerve transmission being passed on from cell to cell (Stannard & Booth 2004).

A continuous epidural infusion of a local anaesthetic in combination with low dose opiate reversibly blocks pain transmission along the pain pathway and offers unique benefits in the relief of acute and peri-operative pain. Used to its full potential, it offers children pain-free post-surgical recovery and is associated with a reduction in postoperative and post-trauma morbidity, particularly in the high-risk patient (e.g. children with respiratory disease, poor lung function and complex disability).

Epidural analgesia can provide excellent effective, long-lasting pain relief both intra-operatively and postoperatively, blunting the stress response to surgery and reducing the need for other analgesic medications (Morton 1998; Twycross *et al.* 2009). High quality analgesia with minimal sedation allows better lung expansion and improves the patient's ability to cough and clear secretions. In older patients there is a decrease in the risk of deep vein thrombosis. The reduced quantity of opiate drugs used in combination with the local anaesthetic decreases the degree of ileus after abdominal surgery and may also decrease or abolish the incidence of nausea and vomiting, which are recognised side effects of opiates (Twycross *et al.* 2009).

Activity of living: maintaining a safe environment.

Question 2. Reflecting upon the nursing process and a model of care, how would the children's nurse prepare this young person, John, and his family for having an epidural infusion?

Assess: ensure that both John and his parents/carers have an appropriate level of knowledge and understanding regarding epidural analgesia. This is essential to ensure that they can make an informed decision when approached for consent.

Plan: the children's nurse must ensure that John and his parents are given appropriate pre-operative preparation at ward level. This will involve explaining the physical and psychological impact of the surgery, postoperative recovery and observations, and interventions associated with the analgesic technique used. All planned care should adopt an appropriate model of nursing, for example the Roper-Logan-Tierney Model (Holland *et al.* 2008, with Casey 1988).

Implement/pre-operative interventions

- Pre-operative assessment – achieved through attending a pre-admission clinic (if available).
- Verbal information should be supported with written information leaflets, which the family may take home to read and digest the information at a later time. These can also be used to prepare John further pre-operatively.
- Discuss with John and his family the importance of regular pain assessment, demonstrate available pain assessment tools, negotiate on the most appropriate and offer a demonstration on its use. The 0–10 Visual Analogue Scale would be appropriate for a 15-year-old young person, where 0 is 'no pain' and 10 is the 'most imaginable pain' (RCN 2009).
- Discuss potential pain management options:
  — Patient controlled analgesia (PCA)
  — Continuous epidural infusion (Clarke 2003)
  — Intravenous paracetamol (Clarke and Richardson 2007) and step-down medication

Wherever possible demonstrate the use of the equipment which will deliver the analgesic technique. First, this enables recognition postoperatively, which reduces levels of anxiety, but more importantly it allows the nurse to assess whether the correct level of understanding and manual dexterity is present to ensure effective delivery of analgesia is achievable.

N.B. Although epidural analgesia is the advanced technique chosen, John and his family still need to be prepared for patient controlled analgesia which may be used in conjunction with or to replace the epidural infusion.

Evaluate all nursing interventions and documentation.

Question 3. What general aspects of nursing management would you need to address when considering epidural analgesia for John?

Pre-requisites

These pre-requisites should be met before discussion and the informed consent of John/carer obtained.

1. Patient suitability – establish whether any contraindications are present:
   (a) Local skin infection
   (b) Systemic infection
   (c) Coagulation disorders
   (d) Known allergy to local anaesthetics
   (e) Patient/parent refusal
   (f) Spinal deformities
   (g) Neurological disease
   (h) Raised intracranial pressure
   (i) Extreme obesity
   (j) Certain cardiac conditions

2. Patient safety – establish the following:
   (a) Bed availability – in line with local trust guidelines (e.g. either on PICU, HDU or on a ward where John can be closely observed).
   (b) The workload of the ward allows the child to be observed closely.
   (c) Minimum trained staff numbers in line with local trust guidelines.
   (d) Minimum of one epidural trained nurse per shift. This must be a nurse who has completed the appropriate theoretical and practical training and has been assessed competent in line with local trust guidelines.
   (e) Intravenous access must be available at all times.

Activity 13.2

Reflect upon ward policy and procedures regarding safety issues.

Activity of living: maintaining a safe environment (Holland *et al*. 2008)

Question 4. Discuss the postoperative nursing care John will require whilst an epidural infusion is in progress.

See Table 13.1.

See Appendix 3 RCN Recommendations and good practice points or go to: www.rcn.org.uk/childrenspainguidelines.

Table 13.1 Proposed answer plan.

Action	Rationale
Assess and plan post operative interventions	
1. John should be identified and prepared for the technique pre-operatively by the anaesthetist, pain nurse and child's nurse.	To ensure that John/carer understands the technique and experienced staff are available to care for John postoperatively.
2. John/parent/carer should be given the epidural information sheet.	To ensure that John/carer understands and is able to absorb the information and ask questions at their own pace.
3. Epidural infusion pump and yellow tubing should be sent to theatre with John. Ensure previous rates on the machine are zeroed.	To ensure a pump is available prior to operation.

continued

Table 13.1   (*Continued*)

Action	Rationale
Implement, document and evaluate all nursing interventions – this is a continuous cycle	
4. On collecting John from theatre recovery ensure that: (a) The machine is working. Place 'Epidural drugs in use' sign on the machine and ensure the giving set is labelled with yellow epidural stickers. (b) The rate of the infusion complies with the prescribed regime. (c) The drug complies with the prescription. (d) Both the recovery nurse and the ward nurse record the readings on the infusion pump and ensure pump is locked. (e) The catheter site is secure with a transparent dressing. (f) Venous access is available and patent.	To ensure continuity of the analgesia. To ensure all staff are aware that an epidural infusion is in progress. To ensure the prescription, infusion rate and solution are the same as the prescription to prevent errors. To comply with the National Patient Safety Agency Alert (2007). See also http://www.apagbi.org.uk. To prevent the catheter from falling out and ensure the site can be observed at all times. To facilitate resuscitative measures if severe side effects occur.
5. One hourly observations of the following must be recorded throughout the duration of the infusion and after removal of the epidural catheter until normal sensation returns to the site of the anaesthetised area: (a) Continuous oxygen saturation monitoring. (b) Record respiratory rate, heart rate, sedation score, pain score and oxygen saturation level every 15 minutes in recovery until condition stabilises, then half hourly for two hours and hourly thereafter. (c) Blood pressure, sensory level and motor block must be recorded hourly for the first four hours then every four hours thereafter. If these observations remain within limits written on the prescription sheet. (d) Recording of blood pressure, sensory level and motor block must revert back to hourly or more frequent in the following circumstances: (i) The sensory block is higher than prescribed. (ii) John becomes hypotensive. (iii) A change has been made to the infusion rate. (iv) The motor block score is 3. (v) The pain score is 3 (severe). (vi) The sedation score is 3.	To ensure John is receiving adequate pain control. To ensure that the block is working and the level is not above that prescribed by the anaesthetist. To monitor side effects. To monitor for potential complications: 1. Excessive sedation 2. Respiratory depression 3. Hypotension 4. Nausea and vomiting 5. Itching 6. Urinary retention 7. Altered lower limb function To ensure that the drug has been adequately eliminated from the body. John's motor function and level of motor block is assessed by using the Bromage scale: Score 0 (none) – full flexion of the knees Score 1 (partial) – just able to move knees Score 2 (almost complete) – able to move feet only Score 3 (complete) – unable to move knees or feet (Department of Anaesthesia and Pain Management, RCH, Melbourne 2007, cited in Twycross *et al.* 2009).
6. Side effects of the infusion should be noted in John's records and the anaesthetist informed.	To ensure that staff are aware of adverse reactions to the drug for future reference. To ensure that John receives appropriate analgesia. To counteract any adverse effects promptly.

Table 13.1 (*Continued*)

Action	Rationale
7. Administer concurrent analgesia as prescribed. If opiates are already being infused in the epidural, no other opiates or central nervous system depressants should be given whilst the infusion is in progress.	To ensure that John receives regular, combined analgesia.
8. Read and record the amount of infusion hourly.	To facilitate an accurate record of the analgesia given to John.
9. A clear dressing will be used over the catheter insertion site and the site should be checked at least once each shift.	To ensure connections are secure. To observe for leakage or infection (Lin & Greco 2005; Seth *et al.* 2004).
10. Nurse John in a comfortable position and check skin integrity and pressure areas at least once per shift. If appropriate depending on the postoperative instructions regarding mobilising. John may be helped to sit in a chair by the bed with the support of two nurses when his motor score is 0–1.	To reduce the risk of pressure sores developing due to immobility, poor skin integrity or altered lower limb function. Low concentration solutions of levobupivicaine produce complete sensory blockade and are associated with a very low incidence of motor block.
11. Monitor urinary output and ensure that children/young people with lumbar epidurals are catheterised in theatre.	To ensure that John does not have urinary retention.
12. If the epidural infusion contains an opiate, monitor for side effects such as pruritis and nausea and vomiting (APAGBI 2009). Ensure the appropriate medication is prescribed and administered.	To counteract any side effects promptly.
13. The anaesthetist or nurse with appropriate competencies is responsible for the removal of the epidural catheter and the completion of the audit sheet on the prescription protocol.	To monitor the state of the catheter on removal (Lin & Greco 2005; Seth *et al.* 2004).

References

Association of Paediatric Anaesthetists of Great Britain and Ireland (2008) *Good Practice in Postoperative and Procedural Pain.* www.apagbi.org.uk

Association of Paediatric Anaesthetists of Great Britain and Ireland (2009) *Guidelines on the Prevention of Post-operative Vomiting in Children.* www.apagbi.org.uk

Casey, A. (1988) A partnership with child and family. *Senior Nurse*, 8(4), 8–9.

Clarke, S.E. (2003) Postoperative pain in children: a retrospective audit of continuous epidural analgesia in a paediatric orthopaedic ward. *Journal of Orthopaedic Nursing*, 7(1), 4–9.

Clarke, S.E. & Richardson, O. (2007) Using intravenous paracetamol in children following surgery: a literature review. *Journal of Children's and Young People's Nursing*, 1(6), 273–80.

Holland, K., Jenkins, J., Soloman, J. & Whittam, S. (2008) *Applying the Roper Logan Tierney Model in practice*, 2nd edn. Edinburgh: Churchill Livingstone.

Lin, C. & Greco, C. (2005) Epidural abscess following epidural analgesia in pediatric patients. *Pediatric Anesthesia*, **15**, 767–70.

Morton, N.S. (1998) *Acute Paediatric Pain Management. A Practical Guide.* London: W.B. Saunders.

National Patient Safety Agency (2007) *Patient Safety Alert: Safer Practice with Epidural Injections and Infusions.* www.npsa.nhs.uk

Royal College of Nursing (2009) *The Recognition and Assessment of Acute Pain in Children: Clinical Practice Guidelines*. London: RCN. www.rcn.org.uk/childrenspainguideline (see Appendix 3 in this volume).

Seth, N., MacQueen, S. & Howard, R.F. (2004) Clinical signs of infection during continuous postoperative epidural analgesia in children: the value of catheter tip culture. *Pediatric Anesthesia*, **14**, 996–1000.

Stannard, C. & Booth, S. (2004) *Pain*, 2nd edn. London: Churchill Livingstone.

Thomas, M.G. (2001) *Guide to Colorectal Surgery*. Portsmouth: Bishops Printers Limited.

Twycross, A., Dowden, S., Bruce, E. & Blackwell, L.B. (2009) *Managing Pain in Children: A Clinical Guide*. Chichester: Wiley-Blackwell.

Section 3

Care of Children and Young Persons with Special Needs

14

Young Person with a History of Epilepsy
Alan Forster

Scenario

Robert is a highly motivated, mature 17-year-old who is studying for his AS levels. Last year, he achieved excellent grades at GCSE, and intends studying mechanical engineering at university next year. He plays rugby, enjoys Adventure Scouting, is currently undertaking the Duke of Edinburgh Gold award and also learning to drive.

Robert has an unremarkable medical history, though six months ago he was admitted to hospital for a second time with severe concussion following injury in a rugby match when the scrum collapsed. Recently, he has been feeling very tired at times and having tingling and slight twitching in his right arm and hand, but put it down to leaning on his arm while studying. He had not mentioned this to his parents.

One evening, unusually after some coaxing by his friends, Robert went to the local snooker club. After missing several easy shots which he blamed on pins and needles in his right hand and a sore arm, Robert suddenly fell to the ground, his body stiffened and then started shaking uncontrollably. His concerned friends quickly responded by calling for an ambulance, but by the time it arrived Robert was sitting up, but was obviously disorientated. So his friends told the paramedics what had happened and they transported him immediately to hospital, while his friends then rang his parents.

Care Planning in Children and Young People's Nursing, First Edition.
Edited by Doris Corkin, Sonya Clarke, Lorna Liggett.
© 2012 Blackwell Publishing Ltd. Published 2012 by Blackwell Publishing Ltd.

On arrival at the A&E department his worried parents were immediately taken to see Robert. While being examined, his body suddenly stiffened again and began to shake violently. His now distraught parents were ushered out of the cubicle by a nurse as the doctor dealt with the situation.

While waiting, Robert's friends explained to them what had happened earlier. Eventually, the doctor came and spoke to them all. She explained that Robert had what appeared to be an epileptic seizure but he was now resting comfortably and she was admitting him to the neurological unit for further specialist investigations.

The epilepsies

In the UK and in adolescents, epilepsy is named as the most common chronic disabling neurological condition (Mitchell *et al.* 2008; Stokes *et al.* 2004). It is a complex spectrum of disorders (Fisher *et al.* 2005) found worldwide, regardless of sex, age, class or race, which can manifest itself in up to 50 different types (Joint Epilepsy Council (JEC) 2008). The main characteristic is recurrent, unprovoked seizures (Glasper & Richardson 2010), due to the presence of excess electrical activity in the brain, which causes a temporary disruption in the normal nerve impulses passing between brain cells (Epilepsy Research UK 2010). Hauser and Banerjee (2008) further add that the recurrent seizures are separated by more than 24 hours. In some cases, it is possible for one person to have several types of seizure.

Activity 14.1

Refer to books and the following websites to select a definition which best describes epilepsy for you:
www.epilepsy.org.uk/info/whatisepilepsy.html
www.epilepsyresearch.org.uk/about_epilepsy/ERUK_introduction_what_is_epilepsy.htm
www.jointepilepsysycouncil.org.uk/About-Epilepsy.html

Epilepsy affects approximately 1:242 children and young people under the age of 18 years in the UK (JEC 2005), although people who have other neurological problems, for example a learning disability, show a higher incidence (Whittaker 2004). It is most commonly diagnosed during the first year, after a child has had two or more unprovoked seizures (Camfield & Camfield 2006). Though normally diagnosed in childhood, it can affect people of any age as a result of brain injury or infection, for example (Ricci & Kyle 2009).

The causes of epilepsy fall into three categories (National Society for Epilepsy (NSE) 2010a; Wolraich *et al.* 2008):

• Idiopathic epilepsy: has no apparent cause, but a genetic defect is thought to be involved. It is known that epilepsy can be inherited. In some cases single or combinations of two or more genes can be involved, and environmental factors cannot be underestimated.

- Symptomatic epilepsy: has a definite cause, for example meningitis, birth trauma, anoxia or congenital abnormalities, for example hydrocephalus.
- Cryptogenic epilepsy: has a likely cause, but for which nothing definite can be found.

According to Scheffer *et al.* (2007) there is growing evidence of the role of genes in symptomatic and cryptogenic epilepsies. Gene defects do not lead directly to epilepsy, but can affect the excitability of the brain, making it more susceptible to seizures. Each of us is born with a genetically inherited seizure threshold. Those with low thresholds are more susceptible to having a seizure when exposed to certain circumstances or *triggers*, for example sleep deprivation. Conversely, those with higher thresholds are less likely to have a seizure in similar circumstances. According to the NSE (2009a) anyone has the potential to have a seizure given the right circumstances, or a strong enough stimulus (Whittaker 2004).

Seizures are a clinical manifestation or symptom of epilepsy associated with a disturbance of the electrical activity in the brain; however, not all seizures are due to epilepsy. They may also be associated with other non-epilepsy conditions, such as CNS infections, hypoglycaemia, syncope, hyponatraemia and hypoxia, which can disturb the neuronal environment. Whilst the seizures may have much in common, they differ in their cause, which must be investigated when making an accurate diagnosis.

To understand how epilepsy occurs, you need to know about the electrical activity in the brain and how it is produced.

Questions

1. Explain what is meant by the resting membrane potential of a neuron.
2. Explain how an action potential is generated in a neuron.
3. As a friend and witness to Robert's first seizure, what could you tell the doctor that might help with a diagnosis?
4. Apart from the example given earlier, list six triggers that may cause a susceptible person to have a seizure.
5. Distinguish between pre-ictal, ictal, post-ictal, and inter-ictal phases.

Answers to questions

Question 1. Explain what is meant by the resting membrane potential of a neuron.

The resting membrane potential is a measure of the electrical difference between the inside (intracellular) and outside of the cell (extracellular). Depending on the neuron, it can vary from approximately −40 to −70 mV when measured using a voltmeter (see Figure 14.1).

The electrical difference is due to separation of the ionic composition of the intracellular and extracellular fluids giving rise to a relative excess of positive charges, mainly Na^+ outside, and negative charges, mainly phosphates (PO_4^{3-}) and proteins inside the cell close to the cell membrane (see Figure 14.2). At this point, the cell membrane is described as being *polarised*.

The separation of charges is maintained by the lipid bi-layer construction which 'controls' the diffusion of the various ions. At rest the membrane is only slightly permeable to Na^+

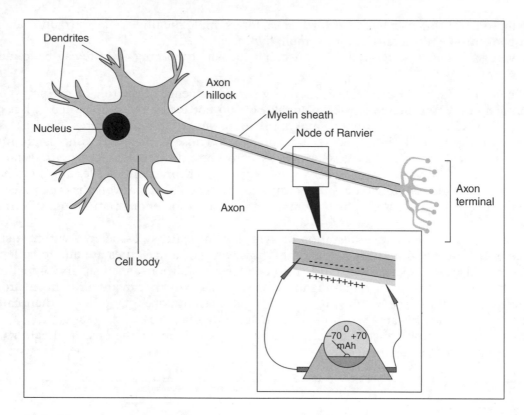

Figure 14.1   Measurement of a neuron.

entering, and impermeable to the large intracellular, negatively charged proteins which remain inside the cell. However, K^+ is much more permeable than Na^+, and Cl^- is relatively freely permeable. The higher membrane permeability of K^+ to Na^+ allows more K^+ to 'leak' out of the cell down its concentration gradient than Na^+ can enter. The net result is more positive ions diffuse out of the cell than enter, causing the inside of the cell to have a negative charge. The sodium-potassium ATPase pump prevents equal concentrations of sodium (Na^+) and potassium (K^+) occurring inside and outside the cell, thus maintaining their concentration gradients.

Question 2. Explain how an action potential is generated in a neuron.

Neurons (and muscles) are able to communicate with each other because they have excitable membranes capable of generating and propagating action potentials. In neurons, action potentials are transmitted from the cell body down the axon, and are often referred to as *nerve impulses*.

Figure 14.3 represents the electrical activity in a neuron when in a resting (polarised) state (area 'A') and the subsequent generation of an action potential following stimulation. For descriptive purposes, it can be divided into three phases:

- Depolarisation phase (areas 'B' and 'C')
- Repolarisation phase (area 'D')
- Hyperpolarisation (area 'E')

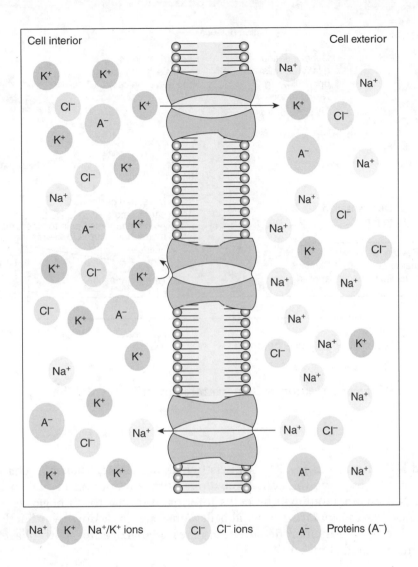

Na⁺   K⁺   Na⁺/K⁺ ions   Cl⁻   Cl⁻ ions   A⁻   Proteins (A⁻)

Figure 14.2   Polarisation of a cell.

Depolarisation phase

Stimulation of the neuron causes changes in the permeability of the membrane by opening and closing specific voltage-gated membrane channels for Na^+ and K^+. As Na^+ moves in, the membrane potential becomes more positive (moving from $-70\,mV$ towards $-55\,mV$).

The firing of an action potential is described as an *'all-or-none'* event. This is dependent on a crucial point called *threshold* (approx $-55\,mV$) being reached. If depolarisation to threshold does not occur, then the action potential does not occur. At threshold, further $Na+$ channels open until eventually they all open. The resulting rapid influx of Na^+ causes the cell's interior to become positively charged. As the membrane potential passes $0\,mV$, a change in the influx of Na^+ is triggered as Na^+ channels begin to close, and the intracellular environment resists the influx of Na^+, causing the action potential to cease rising

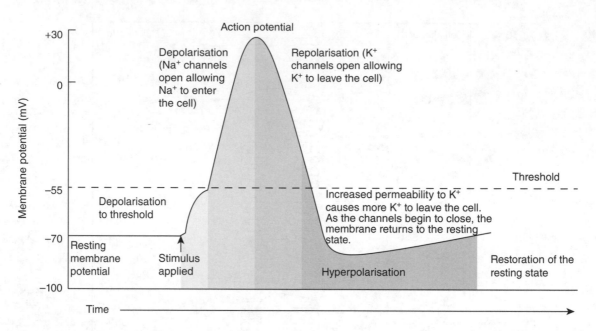

Figure 14.3   Electrical activity in a neuron.

beyond +30 mV. Depolarisation is demonstrated by an upward deflection from the resting potential.

Repolarisation phase

Threshold also stimulates the K⁺ channels (which are slower than Na⁺ channels) to open, thus allowing K⁺ to leave the cell. This, along with a reduction of Na⁺ influx due to the closing of Na⁺ channels allows the cell's interior to return to its negative state (−70 mV). This is referred to as *repolarisation* and is demonstrated by a downward deflection. During this phase, the resting membrane potential is restored. Together, both phases last approximately 1 millisecond (1 msec).

Hyperpolarisation

Because the K⁺ channels respond more slowly, K⁺ permeability lasts longer than required to re-establish resting potential. This results in excess K⁺ efflux causing a hyperpolarisation, seen as an 'undershoot' on the graph. Redistribution of ions via the ATPase pump re-establishes ionic concentration on both sides of the membrane, at which point the membrane potential returns to its resting state.

Seizures

The NSE (2010b) classifies seizures into two main groups. This classification was carried out by the International League against Epilepsy (ILAE 1981), based on the manifestation of seizure activity and is currently under review, with new recommendations having been made (Berg *et al.* 2010). Until they are adopted, we will consider the two main categories currently described.

Box 14.1   Types of partial seizure

	Manifestations
Simple partial seizure	Occurs without loss of consciousness or awareness. The person may experience sensory or motor symptoms such as:

- Tingling or numbness in a limb
- Limpness, stiffening or twitching in a limb
- Déjà vu (feelings that events have happened before) or jamais vu (events that never happened before)
- Sensory abnormalities affecting vision, hearing, taste and smell

Complex partial seizure   This seizure is accompanied by altered consciousness, which may be displayed as unusual behaviour such as:

- Pulling and plucking at clothing
- Repetitive vocal sounds
- Turning of head and eyes
- Lip smacking, chewing or swallowing
- Not responding to verbal commands
- Being unaware of surroundings or preceding events

Complex partial seizures account for 20% of all seizures experienced by people with epilepsy.

Partial seizures

Partial seizures (focal or localised seizures), affect a small area of the cerebral cortex, for example a single lobe. Consciousness is not usually lost, but can be altered, as typically the motor or sensory areas are affected (Glasper & Richardson 2010); thus the symptoms can vary depending on which part of the brain is involved. There are two types of partial seizure as shown in Box 14.1.

In some people, a partial seizure can extend as the electrical activity spreads to involve both cerebral hemispheres. Such seizures are referred to as *partial seizures, secondarily generalized* resulting in loss of consciousness.

Generalised seizures

Generalised seizures involve both hemispheres of the cerebral cortex and are characterised by bilateral synchronous electrical discharges from the onset. Consciousness is usually lost. The main types are described in Box 14.2.

Classification of seizures by type alone in many instances ignores other important clinical manifestations, such as age of onset, triggers, genetics, EEG readings or presence of a learning disability. Taking all these into consideration can define a particular epilepsy syndrome, for example West syndrome, Lennox-Gastaut syndrome, Angelman syndrome, Rett syndrome and Ohtahara syndrome, which can present during childhood.

In the hours or days preceding a seizure (*prodromal period*) some people may experience mood or behavioural changes manifesting as insomnia, anxiety, depression or aggression. These are harbingers of a forthcoming seizure, but are not part of it (Panayiotopolus 2010).

Box 14.2   Generalised seizures

Type of generalised seizure	Manifestations
Absence seizures	Mainly affects children. Can occur several times a day – child abruptly stops activity. Causes a loss of awareness of surroundings for up to 20 seconds. Child may appear to stare vacantly into space, sometimes mistaken for day-dreaming. There may be fluttering of eyes or lip-smacking. Child's school performance may be affected.
Myoclonic seizures	Causes sudden twitching of the limbs or trunk. Sometimes the whole body can be involved. Usually last less than a second. Consciousness is not usually lost; however, if the legs are involved, the person may fall to the ground.
Clonic seizures	May be similar twitching as in myoclonic jerks. Can continue for several minutes. Consciousness may be lost.
Atonic seizures	Sudden loss of muscle tone causing the body to go limp. The person suddenly collapses to the ground.
Tonic seizure	Muscles suddenly stiffen causing the person to lose balance and fall to the ground. Can occur during sleep
Tonic-clonic seizure	The seizure passes through two stages: **Tonic stage** • Loss of consciousness, usually without warning. • Sudden generalised muscle contraction causing the body to stiffen and fall to the ground, the person may also cry out. • Teeth are clenched. • Pallor, with cyanosis due to apnoea. • Pupil dilation and eye rolling. • This stage lasts approximately 10–30 seconds. **Clonic stage** • Twitching or jerking of the arms, legs and head due to alternating contraction and relaxation of muscles. These gradually reduce in frequency. • There can be frothing from the mouth as a result of excess salivation, which sometimes is bloodstained if the patient has bitten his tongue or cheek. • Hyperventilation can occur. • Sweating and increased pulse. • Incontinence can occur. • This stage can last approximately 30–60 seconds. The seizure normally lasts up to three minutes, after which consciousness returns but the person may sleep afterwards. The patient usually has no recollection of the seizure but may complain of headache or muscle soreness afterwards. This type of seizure accounts for approximately 60% of all seizures experienced by people with epilepsy.

They should not be confused with *auras*, which occur minutes to seconds before a seizure and are considered part of the seizure. Auras differ in individuals but manifest themselves in symptoms similar to a simple partial seizure which becomes secondarily generalised (David 2009). Normally it is not possible to prevent the seizure from occurring; however, it is possible in some cases to act on the warning signs.

Establishing a correct diagnosis is important to ensure appropriate treatment. To achieve that, accurate history taking is important; additionally, a number of investigative procedures will be performed to confirm the diagnosis and rule out other possible causes.

Question 3. As a friend and witness to Robert's first seizure, what could you tell the doctor that might help with a diagnosis?

Obtaining an accurate history of events is important in achieving an accurate diagnosis. In epilepsy, this is often given by parents, carers or witnesses to the events, as the patient is often unaware of what happened, though they may be able to assist with events during the prodromal period, or after the seizure event.

As a friend who was with him at the time, and from your knowledge of him you might be able to provide some of the following information.

From your friendship:

- You know that he 'works hard and plays hard'.
- You may know about his rugby injury and subsequent hospitalisation.
- He may have confided in you about his tiredness and tingling and twitching in his arm.

Immediately before the event (prodromal period or aura?):

- He was complaining of being very tired that evening.
- He had to be coaxed to come out.
- He complained of pins and needles in his right hand and a sore arm.
- He missed a lot of easy shots.

During the event (ictal period):

- He suddenly fell to the ground, his body stiffened and began shaking.
- Location and time of seizure.
- Were there any injuries?
- Was consciousness lost?
- How long did the body stiffening last?
- How long did the shaking last?
- Did he bite his tongue?
- Was he incontinent?
- Did his colour change?
- How long did the seizure last?

After the event (post-ictal period):

- Did he sleep – if so, for how long?
- Was he confused/disorientated afterwards?

Any information, no matter how apparently insignificant, can help in determining an accurate diagnosis.

Question 4. List six triggers that may cause a susceptible person to have a seizure.

- *Fatigue* – late nights, over-exertion, insomnia.
- *Stress* – school, studying, work, peers, etc.
- *Medication* – missing or over medicating with anti-epileptic drugs (AED) or other prescription or non-prescribed medication. Some prescribed medications, for example anti-depressants, can lower the seizure threshold, while aspirin can enhance phenytoin (BNF 2010).
- *Alcohol* – binging or intoxication, especially if taking some AEDs.
- *Drug abuse* – recreational drugs can have both direct and indirect effects (e.g. cocaine can cause seizures). Some drugs can cause sleep deprivation or cause the person to forget to take AED.
- *Infection* – in some susceptible children a raised temperature can induce a seizure (not to be confused with a febrile convulsion).
- *Hormone changes* – particularly in females in relation to their menstrual cycle.
- *Environmental stimulants* – in those with rare reflex epilepsy certain individual stimulants can cause a seizure, for example flickering lights, noise, music, reading or tone of voice. Photosensitive epilepsy is the most common form. Reflex epilepsy affects 4–7% of people with epilepsy (Panayiotopoulos 2010).
- *Some people may have no apparent triggers or differ from those listed.*

Question 5. Distinguish between pre-ictal, ictal, post-ictal, and inter-ictal phases.

Pre-ictal phase refers to the period immediately before a seizure, which may include an aura.

Ictal phase refers to the seizure itself and the events which occur during it.

Post-ictal phase refers to the recovery period following the seizure when the person may be confused or sleepy. This phase generally lasts longer than the ictal phase.

Inter-ictal phase refers to the period of time between seizures after the patient has recovered from the post-ictal phase.

A diagnosis of epilepsy was eventually confirmed, based on Robert's presenting history and results from the diagnostic procedures, and he and his parents were informed of the diagnosis.

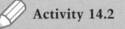 **Activity 14.2**

Consider five evaluation/diagnostic tools (e.g. electroencephalograph) that could be used to confirm Robert's condition, including an appropriate rationale for their use. Please refer to Appendix 4.

During his stay in hospital Robert's care was planned based on the initial assessment data completed on admission. It involved the setting of priorities, establishing goals, determining nursing interventions and documenting care plans. The main objectives in managing his care were to include preventing injury during a seizure, preventing or reducing seizure activity by the administration of suitable anti-epileptic drugs (AEDs), and providing information and support to the patient and their family.

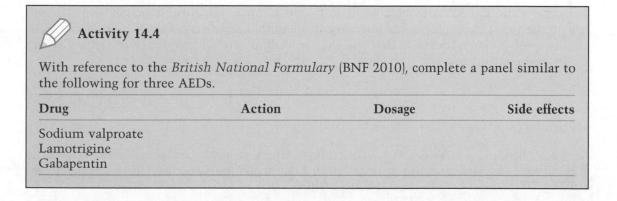

Activity 14.3

With reference to the activities of living, *'maintaining a safe environment' and 'working & playing'* (Roper *et al.* 2004), complete the nursing care plan below to meet the needs of Robert and his family. Please refer to Appendix 5.

A/L	Nursing Assessment	Nursing Problem	Goal/ objective	Nursing interventions	Rationale
Maintaining a safe environment	Robert has had several seizures				
	Robert is a newly diagnosed patient with epilepsy				
	Robert and his family know little about epilepsy				
Working & Playing	Robert and his family know little about epilepsy				

In order to reduce the likelihood of seizure and the risk of complications, patients are usually commenced on anti-epileptic drugs (AEDs) in the first instance. There is a wide variety of such medications available today, and treatment strategies are based on individual requirements.

Activity 14.4

With reference to the *British National Formulary* (BNF 2010), complete a panel similar to the following for three AEDs.

Drug	Action	Dosage	Side effects
Sodium valproate			
Lamotrigine			
Gabapentin			

Robert and his family are eager to find out more about epilepsy.

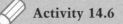

Activity 14.5

Considering Robert's lifestyle, with reference to *The Epilepsies: Diagnosis and Management of the Epilepsies in Children and Young People in Primary and Secondary Care* (NICE 2004), ascertain what *specific* information Robert and his family might require to help them live with this condition. See also:

www.epilepsyontario.org/client/EO/EOWeb.nsf/web/Wellness+&+Quality+of+Life+(kit) and www.epilepsysociety.org.uk/AboutEpilepsy/Epilepsyandyou/Youngpeople-1

People with epilepsy have a 2–3 times higher mortality rate than the general population (Nashef & Langan 2003). Although seizures are generally self-limiting, one major seizure event which can put a patient's life at risk is a state called status epilepticus. This is a medical emergency requiring prompt treatment to prevent a fatality. Another cause of fatality is sudden unexpected death in epilepsy (SUDEP). Although rare, there is a suggestion that young adult males may be more at risk of SUDEP (NSE 2009b).

Activity 14.6

Refer to *The Diagnosis and Management of the Epilepsies in Adults and Children in Primary and Secondary Care* (Stokes *et al.* 2004) found at www.nice.org.uk/nicemedia/ live/10954/29533/29533.pdf and obtain a definition of status epilepticus and SUDEP.

For some children, AEDs alone are not sufficient to reduce seizure frequency and, depending on the type of epilepsy, some have to consider other adjunctive techniques (NICE 2004) to gain control. Such therapies that you may read about include surgery, ketogenic diet and vagus nerve stimulation.

References

Berg, A.T., Berkoric, S.F., Brodie, M.S., *et al.* (2010) Revised terminology and concepts for organization of seizures and epilepsies: report of the ILAE Commission on Classification and Terminology, 2005–2009. Special Report. *Epilepsia*, **51**(4), 676–85.

Camfield, P.R. & Camfield, C.S. (2006) Pediatric epilepsy: an overview, Chapter 40. In: Swaiman, K., Ashwal, S. & Ferriero, D. (eds). *Pediatric Neurology Principles and Practice*, 4th edn. Philadelphia, Mosby Elsevier.

Commission on Classification and Terminology of the ILAE (1981) Proposal for revised clinical and electroencephalographic classification of epileptic seizures. *Epilepsia*, **22**, 489–501.

David, R.B. (2009) *Clinical Pediatric Neurology*, 3rd edn. New York: Desmos Medical Publishing.

Epilepsy Research UK. *What is Epilepsy?* www.epilepsyresearch.org.uk/about_epilepsy/ERUK_introduction_what_is_epilepsy.htm (accessed 11 June 2010).

Fisher, R.S., van Emde Boas, W., Blume, W., *et al.* (2005) Epileptic seizures and epilepsy: definitions proposed by the International League Against Epilepsy (ILAE) and the International Bureau for Epilepsy (IBE). *Epilepsia*, **46**(4), 470–72.

Glasper, A. & Richardson, J. (2010) *A Textbook of Children's and Young People's Nursing*. Edinburgh: Churchill Livingstone, Elsevier.

Hauser, W.A. & Banerjee, P.N. (2008) Epidemioloy of epilepsy in children, Chapter 9. In: Pellock, J.M., Dodson, W.E. & Bourgeois, B.F.D. (eds). *Pedriatric Epilepsy: Diagnosis and Therapy*, 3rd edn. New York: Demos Medical Publishing.

Joint Epilepsy Council (2005) *Epilepsy Prevalence, Incidence and Other Statistics*. Leeds: Joint Epilepsy Council of the UK & Ireland.

Joint Epilepsy Council (2008) *About Epilepsy*. www.jointepilepsycouncil.org.uk/About-Epilepsy.html (accessed 10 June 2010).

Joint Formulary Committee (2010) *British National Formulary*, 59th edn. London: British Medical Association and Royal Pharmaceutical Society of Great Britain.

Mitchell, W.G. Partikian, A. & Neinstein, L.S. (2008) Epilepsy, Chapter 21. In: Neinstein, L.S. (ed.) *Adolescent Health Care: a Practical Guide*, 5th edn. Philadelphia: Lippincott, Williams & Wilkins.

Nashef, L. & Langan, Y. (2003) Sudden unexpected death in epilepsy (SUDEP). Review Article. *Advances in Clinical Neurosciences and Rehabilitation (ACNR)*, **2**(6), 6–8.

National Institute for Clinical Excellence (2004) *The Epilepsies. The Diagnosis and Management of the Epilepsies in Adults and Children in Primary and Secondary Care*. London: NICE.

National Society for Epilepsy (2009a) *Epilepsy. An Introduction to Epilepsy – What is it?* Chalfont St Peter: National Society for Epilepsy.

National Society for Epilepsy (2009b) *Sudden Unexplained Death in Epilepsy (SUDEP)* (online) (updated 30 July 2009). www.epilepsy.org.uk/info/sudep.html (accessed 10 June 2010).

National Society for Epilepsy (2010a) *Epilepsy: an Introduction to Epileptic Seizures*. Chalfont St Peter: National Society for Epilepsy.

National Society for Epilepsy (2010b) *Causes of Epilepsy?* www.epilepsysociety.org.uk/AboutEpilepsy/Whatisepilepsy/Causesofepilepsy (accessed 10 June 2010).

Panayiotopoulos, C.P. (2010) *A Clinical Guide to Epileptic Syndromes and Their Treatment*, 2nd edn. London: Springer.

Ricci, S.S. & Kyle, T. (2009) *Maternity and Pediatric Nursing*. Philadelphia: Lippincott Williams & Wilkins.

Roper. N., Logan. W.W. & Tierney, A.J. (2004) *The Roper, Logan and Tierney Model of Nursing: Based on Activities of Living*. Philadelphia: Churchill Livingstone Elsevier.

Scheffer, I, E., Dibbens, L., Berkovic, S.F. & Mulley. J.C. (2007) What is the role of genetics in epilepsy? In: Sisodiya, S., Cross, J.H., Blümcke, I., *et al.* Genetics of Epilepsy: Epilepsy Research Foundation Workshop Report. *Epileptic Discord*, 9(2), 194–236.

Stokes, T. Shaw, E.J. Juarez-Garcia, A. Camosso-Stefinovic, J. & Baker, R. (2004) *Clinical Guidelines and Evidence Review for the Epilepsies: diagnosis and management in adults and children in primary and secondary care*. www.nice.org.uk/nicemedia/live/10954/29533/29533.pdf (accessed 10 June 2010).

Whittaker, N. (2004) Epilepsy. In: Whittaker, N. *Disorders and Interventions*. New York: Palgrave Macmillan.

Wolraich, M.L. Dworkin, P.H. Drotar, D.D. & Perrin, E.C. (2008) *Developmental-behavioral Pediatrics: Evidence and Practice*. Philadelphia: Mosby Inc.

Websites for further reading

www.epilepsysociety.org.uk/AboutEpilepsy/Livingwithepilepsy/Epilepsyandleisure
www.epilepsysociety.org.uk/AboutEpilepsy/Livingwithepilepsy/Epilepsyandsafety
www.epilepsysociety.org.uk/AboutEpilepsy/Whatisepilepsy/Seizures#d
www.epilepsy.org.uk/info/driving
www.yourepilepsy.org.uk/indcx.html
www.epilepsy.org.uk/info/parents.html
www.epilepsy.org.uk/info/ketogenic.html
www.epilepsy.org.uk/info/vagal.html

15

Nut Allergy – Anaphylaxis Management
Diane Gow

Scenario

Katie is a four-year-old child who lives with her parents in a five-bedroom house in a semi-rural location. She has a three-year-old brother and her mother is 25 weeks pregnant, expecting her third child. Katie was diagnosed with atopic eczema at the age of one month, and asthma at the age of two years.

Whilst attending a family wedding reception, Katie becomes distressed. Her eyes have swollen, and she says her 'tummy aches', and subsequently she vomits. Katie's concerned parents notice she appears to have a nettlerash on her face. Her parents take her home, and she gradually starts to feel better.

The next day her parents contact their GP, who arranges for Katie to be referred to a specialist allergy clinic to be tested for suspected nut allergy. There is a four-month waiting period.

 Questions

1. How prevalent is nut allergy in children?
2. Explain the current approaches to diagnosing nut allergy.
3. Discuss the current approaches to management of nut allergy at home/school.
4. What is anaphylaxis?
5. Describe the emergency treatment of anaphylaxis.

Care Planning in Children and Young People's Nursing, First Edition.
Edited by Doris Corkin, Sonya Clarke, Lorna Liggett.
© 2012 Blackwell Publishing Ltd. Published 2012 by Blackwell Publishing Ltd.

Answers to questions

Question 1. How prevalent is nut allergy in children?

Foods have been known to cause adverse reactions in susceptible individuals for almost 2000 years. Both Hippocrates and Galen reported allergic reactions to milk. One of the earliest references to food allergy is found in the often quoted aphorism:

'One man's meat is another man's poison'

Lucretious, BC 55, cited by Fox (1999)

Although nut allergy is a relatively new condition the prevalence has tripled amongst children since the mid-1990s. The House of Commons Health Committee (2004) placed the figure as high as 1 in 50 children being affected. This has been accompanied by a dramatic 700% increase in the rate of hospital admissions for anaphylactic reactions between 1990 and 2004 (Gupta *et al.* 2006), described by Hourihane *et al.* (1996) as an apparent epidemic, which is increasing exponentially with each generation. The age of onset is decreasing, with children often being diagnosed in the first year of life.

Possible causes

The reason for the dramatic increase in this allergic disease remains unclear, although it is thought to be influenced by increased exposure to widespread use of peanuts in food manufacture. The hygiene hypothesis also asserts that too hygienic an environment may set the stage for allergic disease later in life as immunity is not being challenged in affluent homes. The emergence of nut allergy also appears to relate directly to the increase in prevalence of allergic asthma and eczema, in predominantly westernised populations.

Whilst there have been some encouraging developments in desensitisation programmes, at present nut allergy is likely to be lifelong, with only 10% of children developing a tolerance to the allergen.

Allergy to peanuts and other types of nuts and seeds is the most serious form of food allergy, characterised by more severe symptoms than other food allergies, wherein sensitivity is often extreme, with minute amounts of the allergen being capable of triggering a rapid and severe type 1 allergic response. The course of anaphylaxis is by nature rapidly progressive, and failure to recognise the severity of these reactions and to administer adrenaline promptly, significantly increases the risk of a fatal outcome.

Question 2. Explain the current approaches to diagnosing nut allergy.

Diagnosis is based on clinical history, along with skin prick test, or quantisation of allergen-specific immunoglobulin E (IgE), and oral food challenges, when indicated in a specialist allergy clinic.

IgE specific blood tests – venepuncture

Assess: as the children's nurse caring for the needs of the child and family whilst undergoing these tests in an allergy clinic, what approaches would you consider appropriate to help the child cope with the anticipated skin prick test and venepuncture?

How would you support the family in terms of the anxiety whilst undergoing these procedures and awaiting confirmation of diagnosis in the clinic?

Please visit allergy UK website below for more detailed information on how skin prick testing is performed. This includes a ten-minute demonstration video:

http://www.allergyuk.org/allergy_skintest.aspx

Plan/implement:

- Give family information in advance of procedure.
- Explore with the family any previous experience the child has had of injections or venepuncture. This can provide valuable information for planning the procedure.
- Work in conjunction with a play specialist where possible. For younger children, consider providing a teddy or medical kit for the child to 'practise' with, to gain some familiarity and element of control.
- Provide choices – would they prefer to sit on the parent's lap, be sitting up, use the right or left hand, choose their sticking plaster.
- Ensure provision of adequate pain relief – local anesthetic cream or ethyl chloride spray.
- Encourage child to have had a good fluid intake – if they are well hydrated this promotes easier venous access.
- Ensure child keeps warm – to promote vasodilatation and easier venous access.
- Consider using age appropriate distraction during the procedure – read from a book, sing a favorite song, count backwards or blow bubbles.
- Comfort and praise child.

Supporting parents: this is an uncertain and anxious time. Give parents information on an ongoing basis and provide opportunities for clarification. Receiving the diagnosis for some parents can be like a bombshell and has the potential for profound changes in family life.

The technique involves using either a needle or lancet to puncture the epidermis through an extract of a food by specifically trained staff. The test site is examined after 10–20 minutes. A local weal and flare response indicates the presence of food specific IgE antibody. The preferred site is either along the inner forearm or on the child's back.

Question 3. Discuss the current approaches to management of nut allergy at home/school.

Once the diagnosis is confirmed, the only current management approach is strict avoidance of all nuts and nut products. This may appear relatively straightforward, but as Collins (2000) suggests, avoidance is easier to advocate than to undertake. There is the potential risk of inadvertent cross contamination in food manufacture, children sharing food, etc. The literature is replete with accidental exposure to the very allergen they are trying to avoid (Sampson *et al.* 2003).

Adults responsible for the care of children are therefore advised to diligently read food labels. This level of constant vigilance creates the conditions for living under the threat of inadvertent exposure and consequent severe reaction.

In addition, parents and other adult carers need to be taught how to recognise the signs of anaphylaxis, and to administer adrenaline (epinephrine) via auto injector (i.e. Epipen®, Anapen®) when necessary and to be able to give basic life support/CPR (Rescuscitation Council 2008).

The groups of adult carers who will need to be advised on Katie's nut allergy management will include her parents, nursery/school staff and other family members. A management plan will be required for Katie's school/nursery.

Specific guidance for managing medicines in schools, nurseries and similar settings can be found via www.allergyinschools.org.uk and www.medicalconditionsatschool.org.uk.

Question 4. What is anaphylaxis?

Anaphylaxis is a severe, life-threatening, generalised or systemic hypersensitivity reaction. There is an exaggerated response to an allergen, characterised by rapidly developing, life-threatening airway and/or breathing and/or circulation problems usually associated with skin and mucosal changes.

When the specific allergen has been ingested it can react in widespread areas of the body with basophiles of the blood and the mast cells located immediately outside the small blood vessels, giving rise to a widespread allergic reaction throughout the vascular system and in closely associated tissues.

The large quantities of histamine released into the circulation causes widespread peripheral vasodilatation as well as increased permeability of the capillaries and marked loss of plasma from the circulation. This leads to potentially catastrophic circulatory shock within minutes, unless treated with epinephrine to oppose the effects of histamine.

Also released from the cells are leukotrienes, which cause spasm of the smooth muscle of the bronchioles, giving rise to asthma-like symptoms.

Urticaria results from antigen entering specific skin areas causing local reactions. Locally released histamines causes:

1. Local vasodilatation, inducing an immediate red flare.
2. Increased local permeability of capillaries that leads to swelling of the skin, known as hives.

Angioedema is deep swelling around the eyes, lips and sometimes the mouth and throat.

Activity 15.1

Whilst at school Katie says the back of her throat is tickling, and her voice is becoming hoarse. She says she feels poorly, is frightened, wheezy and is losing consciousness. Katie has some swelling around the lips.

You are called to help. What are your priorities in this situation, and how would you assess Katie?

Your priority is to recognise that she is seriously unwell, and that this is potentially an anaphylactic reaction. Call for help. Treat the greatest threat to life first. Initial treatment should not be delayed by the lack of complete history or definite diagnosis.

Recognition of an anaphylactic reaction

The Resuscitation Council Guidelines (2008) state that anaphylaxis is likely when all of the following three criteria are met:

*   Sudden onset and rapid progression of symptoms.
*   Life threatening **A**irway and/or **B**reathing and/or **C**irculation problems.
*   Skin and/or mucosal changes (flushing, urticaria, angioedema).

Please note, generalised urticaria, angiodema, rhinitis, gastro-intestinal symptoms (e.g. vomiting, abdominal pain) would not be described as an anaphylactic reaction, because the life-threatening features, such as airway problem, respiratory difficulty and hypotension are not present.

The emergency treatment for suspected anaphylaxis should be based on general life support principles using ABCDE approach (Resuscitation Council 2008).

A Airway problems:

- Airway swelling, tongue, throat, patient feels their throat is closing up
- Hoarse voice
- Stridor – indicating upper airway obstruction

B Breathing problems:

- Shortness of breath
- Wheeze
- Becoming tired
- Confusion (caused by hypoxia)
- Cyanosis (late sign)
- Respiratory arrest

C Circulation problems:

Signs of shock – pale, clammy the child will look and feel unwell:

- Increased pulse rate – tachycardia
- Low blood pressure – feeling faint, dizzy, collapse – DO NOT STAND CHILD UP
- Decreased level of consciousness
- Cardiac arrest

D Disability problems:

There may be altered neurological status due to decreased brain perfusion; there may be confusion, agitation and loss of consciousness and the child is usually anxious, panicky, and can experience an 'impending sense of doom'.

E Exposure:

- Skin and/or mucosal changes often the first feature (present in over 80% of anaphylactic reactions)
- Can be subtle or dramatic
- May be erythema – a patchy, or generalised, red rash
- Urticaria (also called hives, nettlerash, weals or welts anywhere on the body)
- Angioedema – swelling of deep tissues, for example eyelids, lips sometimes mouth and throat

Differential diagnosis – life-threatening conditions

- Asthma (particularly in children)
- Septic shock (hypotension with petechial/purpuric rash)

Differential diagnosis – non-life-threatening

- Vasovagal episode
- Panic attack
- Breath-holding episode
- Idiopathic, non-allergic urticaria or angioedema

NB: SEEK HELP EARLY IF THERE ARE ANY DOUBTS ABOUT THE DIAGNOSIS

Question 5. Describe the emergency treatment of anaphylaxis.

- Act immediately.
- Call for an ambulance.
- Do not make child vomit following ingestion.
- Loosen tight clothing, take a history from anyone present.
- Locate Epipen®/Anapen® and be prepared to administer.

Patient positioning

All patients should be placed in a comfortable position, taking into account the following:

- Patients with airway and breathing problems may prefer to sit up as this will make breathing easier.
- Lying flat with legs raised is helpful for patients with low blood pressure. If feeling faint DO NOT stand them up – this can induce cardiac arrest.
- If breathing and unconscious they should be placed on their side in recovery position.

Administration of Epipen®/Anapen®

Adrenaline (epinephrine) is the most important drug for the treatment of an anaphylactic reaction. It works by:

- Constricting the small blood vessels, causing a rise in blood pressure
- Relaxing smooth muscle in the lungs, improving breathing by dilating bronchial airways
- Stimulates the heart contractility
- Reverses peripheral vasodilatation, reducing oedema/swelling around the face and lips
- Suppresses histamine and leukotriene release, reducing the severity of the IgE mediated allergic reaction

The intramuscular (IM) route is used by most healthcare providers; IV can only be administered by specialists, such as intensivists or anaesthetists.

Adrenaline is administered into the muscle via a pre-loaded syringe (such as Epipen® or Anapen®), which provides a single dose of epinephrine.

Using an adrenaline autoinjector Epipen®/Anapen® (Figure 15.1)

The injection is administered intramuscularly into the middle of the outer/front thigh. It can be given through clothing.

- Remove the injector from the packaging.
- Remove the safety cap (grey coloured if Epipen®, black with red if Anapen®).

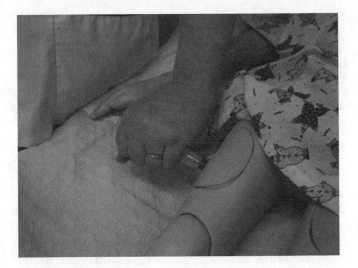

Figure 15.1   Adrenaline autoinjector.

- Hold the injector firmly in your fist, 10 cm away from outer thigh, with the black tip at right angles to the thigh.
- Epipen®: press hard (there should be a click).
  Anapen®: press the trigger at the top.
- Hold in place for ten seconds.
- Remove the pen and massage the area for ten seconds.
- Stay with the child and be prepared to administer basic life support.
- Check H/R, R/R and if no improvement occurs be prepared to give a second dose after five minutes.
- The child will need to be transferred to hospital via ambulance.

These are the current recommended dosages for intramuscular adrenaline supplied by Resuscitation Council 2008:

Adult or child over 12 yrs	500 micrograms IM (0.5 ml)
Child 6–12 yrs	300 micrograms IM (0.3 ml)
Child 6 months–6 years	150 micrograms IM (0.15 ml)
Child less than 6 months	150 micrograms IM (0.5 ml)

For video demonstrations of this please visit www.epipen.co.uk and www.anapen.co.uk

After use

The needle remains exposed and will need to be carefully disposed of. Be alert to the potential for needlestick injury to the finger. Adrenaline has a potent peripheral vasoconstrictive action, and accidental injection may cause acute ischemia of the end arteries of a distal digit.

Activity 15.2

As a children's nurse working in an acute hospital, if you come across a child outside hospital having an anaphylactic reaction, are you allowed to use their adrenaline auto-injector to give them IM adrenaline?

There is no legal problem in any person administering adrenaline that is either prescribed for a specific person or in administering adrenaline to an unknown person in such a lifesaving situation (though there are specific exemptions in the Medicines Act). However, the nurse involved must work within the Nursing & Midwifery Council (NMC) standards, and must therefore be competent in being able to recognise the anaphylactic reaction and administer adrenaline using an auto-injector. Furthermore, it would be sensible for trusts/employers to ensure that such a provision is included in their first aid or anaphylaxis guidelines (Resuscitation Council 2008).

References

Collins, L. (2000) *Caring for Your Child with Severe Food Allergies*. Chichester: John Wiley and Sons.

Fox. D, & Gaughan, M. (1999) Food allergy in children. *Pediatric Nursing*, **11**, 328–30.

Gupta. R., Sheikh, A., Strachan, D.P. & Anderson, H.R. (2006) Time trends in allergic disorders in the UK. *Thorax*, doi: 10.1136/thx.2004.038844.

House of Commons Health Committee (2004) *Sixth Report. The Provision of Allergy Services*. London: Stationery Office.

Hourihane, J., Dean, T. & Warner, J. (1996) Peanut allergy in relation to heredity, maternal diet and other atopic diseases: results of a questionnaire survey, skin prick testing and food challenges. *British Medical Journal*, **313**, 518–21.

Nursing & Midwifery Council (2008) *Standards for Medicines Management*. UK: NMC.

Resuscitation Council UK (2008) *Emergency Treatment of Anaphylaxis. Guidelines for Healthcare Providers*. London. www.resus.org.uk

Sampson, H., Metcalfe, D. & Ronald, S. (2003). *Food Allergy: Adverse Reactions to Food and Food Additives*, 3rd edn. Oxford: Blackwell Publishing.

www.allergyinschools.org.uk (accessed August 2010).

www.allergyuk.org/allergy_skintest.aspx (accessed August 2010).

www.medicalconditionsatschool.org.uk (accessed August 2010).

16

Closed Head Injury

Katie Dowdie and Carol McCormick

Scenario

Leah, a ten-year-old girl, who weighs 28 kg lived at home with her parents, Noel and Jane and had a six-year-old brother James.

Leah travelled on the bus each day to school. On a cold frosty November day, Leah as usual caught the bus to school with her brother, James.

Leah chose to sit at the back of the bus beside her school chum.

The school bus continued its journey along the busy road and then prepared to turn right into Leah's school entrance. Due to the frosty conditions the lorry travelling behind the bus braked quickly but unfortunately skidded into the back of the bus. Leah was propelled forward hitting her head of the seat in front and sustained a head injury.

The ambulance was called and Leah was stabilised at the scene.

Leah was then admitted via the accident and emergency department to the paediatric intensive care unit for further management of her closed head injury.

Care Planning in Children and Young People's Nursing, First Edition.
Edited by Doris Corkin, Sonya Clarke, Lorna Liggett.
© 2012 Blackwell Publishing Ltd. Published 2012 by Blackwell Publishing Ltd.

Table 16.1 Mead model.

A Respiratory
B Cardiovascular
C Pain/sedation
D Neurology
E Nutrition/hydration
F Elimination
G (i) Skin/wound care
G (ii) Mobility
G (iii) Hygiene
H (i) Psychological and social/culture
H (ii) Circumstantial

Please see Chapter 1 for further reading.
Adapted from: McClune & Franklin (1987).

Please refer to Table 16.1.

 Questions

1. What is a closed head injury?
2. When using the Mead model, how would the children's nurse safely maintain the airway of a child with a Glasgow Coma Scale (GCS) below 8?
3. Why is pain relief and sedation an important aspect of the care of a child with a closed head injury?
4. (a) Use the Glasgow Coma Scale to assess Leah's neurological status.
   (b) What other observations would you carry out?
5. How would the children's nurse ensure adequate fluid balance?

Answers to questions

Question 1. What is a closed head injury?

A closed head injury (CHI) is defined as non-penetrating injury to the brain and occurs when the head accelerates and then rapidly collides with another object (Steffen-Albert 2010). Trauma causes injury to the brain as a result of a blow to the head, or sudden, violent motion that causes the brain to impact against the skull. No object penetrates through the skull to the brain tissue itself.

Brain injury is classified into phases: primary injury and secondary injury.

The primary injury is the initial brain insult as a result of traumatic impact.

According to Moppett (2007), oedema, capillary leakage and systemic inflammatory response is associated with secondary injury. Furthermore, secondary injury is worsened by hypoxia and hypotension (Pigula *et al.* 1993).

Coup is injury on site of impact and contre-coup is injury on opposite side of impact. This is shown in Figure 16.1.

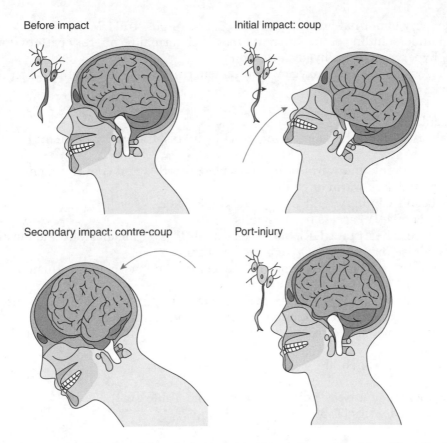

Figure 16.1 Coup and contre-coup injury (collection of L. Henry). Reproduced from Best Practice (http://bestpractice.bmj.com/best-practice/monograph/967/resources/images.html) with kind permission.

Question 2. When using the Mead model, how would the children's nurse safely maintain the airway of a child with a Glasgow Coma Scale below 8?

Respiratory and cardiovascular needs should be looked at (McClune & Franklin1987). Any child presenting with a Glasgow Coma Scale (GCS) <8 is classified as a severe head injury (Moppett 2007; Weinstein 2006). The most important initial interventions are:

- Control of the airway and cervical spine
- Breathing and circulation

Physical needs

Respiratory
Assess: continue to assess Leah's level of consciousness and ability to maintain her: **A**irway, **B**reathing and **C**irculation (ABC).

- Observe her colour – is Leah's skin pink, pale, dusky or cyanosed?
- Check Leah's chest movement – assess rate, depth and rhythm.

- Are there any abnormal breathing sounds, for example stridor?
- Have an understanding of the different types of abnormal respiratory pattern, for example apnoea, hyperventilation/hypoventilation.
- Monitor respiration rate, oxygen requirements, method of administration and pulse oximetry.

Cardiovascular

Assess: this assessment has some overlap with the respiratory assessment:

- Is Leah's skin pink and warm to touch or pale, mottled and cool to touch?
- Are her peripheries warm or cold?
- What is Leah's capillary refill time (normal CRT is 2–3 secs)?
- Has intravenous (IV) access been established?
- Monitor/record heart rate (HR), blood pressure (B/P) (systolic diastolic and mean), respiratory rate, pulse oximetry (SaO_2) and temperature.
- Understand the significance of the HR, BP, central and peripheral perfusion.

It is important to know the cardiovascular stability of the child prior to intubation as the choice of drugs used for induction and intubation can have adverse effects.

These assessments are carried out very quickly and the child is then prepared for intubation and ventilation.

Plan: preparation for child

- Prepare emergency/airway trolley for intubation (Table 16.2).
- Gather required drugs (Table 16.3).

Implement:

- Leah will be admitted to paediatric intensive care Unit (PICU); it is the nurse's responsibility to assist intubation and establishment of central venous access – one nurse to record observations and fluid balance.

Table 16.2 Emergency/airway trolley for intubation.

- Oral and nasal ET tube (required size + a size smaller)
- Introducer and bougie
- Laryngoscope and appropriate blade
- Magill's forceps appropriate size
- Yankauer sucker
- Nasogastric tube and drainage bag
- Elastoplast tape pre-cut
- Dressed applicators
- Friars' Balsam & gallipot
- Sterile lubricating gel and gauze
At the bedside:
- Oxygen and suction supply
- Facemask with bagging set
- Suction catheters
- Equipment to monitor vital signs

Table 16.3 Common drugs used for intubation (see BNFC 2009).

* Thiopentone sodium
Intravenous anaesthetic used for induction of anaesthesia.
Side effects: apnoea, hypotension, arrhythmias, laryngeal spasm. In excessive doses hypothermia and reduction in cerebral function.
* Atracurium
Neuromuscular blocking drug, also known as muscle relaxant.
Side effects – skin flushing, hypotension, tachycardia.
* Suxamethonium
Depolarising neuromuscular blocking drug. Used if fast action and brief duration of action is required.
* Propofol
Intravenous anaesthetic used for induction of anaesthesia.
Side effects: hypotension, tachycardia, less common – thrombosis, pulmonary oedema, hyperkalaemia, cardiac failure.
* Atropine
Antimuscarinic drug used in the treatment of bradycardia.
Side effects: tachycardia, dilatation of the pupils, dry mouth, nausea and vomiting, confusion.
* Adrenaline
Direct acting sympathomimetic agent. Used in CPR, acute anaphylaxis, low cardiac output. Side effects: nausea, vomiting, tachycardia, arrthymias, hypertension, cold peripheries.
* Morphine
Opioid analgesia used to relieve moderate to severe pain.
Side effects: nausea, vomiting, constipation, hypotension, respiratory depression.
* Midazalam
Benzodiazepine used for sedation.
Side effects: gastro-intestinal disturbances, hypotension, heart rate changes, laryngospasm, respiratory depression.
* Sodium chloride 0.9%
Used for drug/line flush.

NB The combination of drugs used will be decided by the anaesthetist, based on the clinical condition of the child.

* Continue to administer 100% oxygen via bag and mask and apply suction when necessary.
* Apply electrocardiograph (ECG) electrodes, B/P cuff and SaO_2 probe to ensure continuous trend of cardiovascular status and oxygenation.
* Pass nasogastric tube (NG), aspirate and attach to drainage bag to prevent aspiration of stomach contents and lung soiling.
* The endotracheal tube (ET) is passed via the nose or orally if basal skull fracture is suspected, and secured firmly with elastoplast.
* Anaesthetist/doctor will auscultate chest for equal air entry and bilateral chest movement.
* Essential to confirm position of tubes (ET & NG) by X-ray.
* Record size and length of ET tube at the lips or nose on observation chart. This is important as it is essential to check regularly for any movement of the position of the ET tube.
* The ET tube is suctioned to assess the type and amount of secretions and a specimen obtained for virology, culture and sensitivity.
* The ventilator is set by the medical staff determined by the arterial blood gas (ABG) result and connected to the ET tube by the intensive care nurse.

Once the airway is established ongoing nursing care involves optimising respiratory function and being aware of potential complications. All ventilator settings are recorded hourly to ensure adequate ventilation and patient safety. Blood gases are checked regularly to ensure ventilation is adequate and ventilator settings changed accordingly. What we should be looking at in the ABG is PaO_2- to ensure oxygen level is adequate to prevent hypoxia. Cerebral hypoxia causes more oedema, leading to raised intracranial pressure (ICP) which further damages brain tissue as described by Williams (2000).

Monitor $PaCO_2$ to prevent hypocapnia /hypercapnia, as this can cause undesirable changes in ICP and cerebral perfusion pressure (CPP).

Leah's airway must be kept patent and she will have suction of her ET tube as indicted by her haemodynamic, respiratory and cerebral stability. Gentle chest physiotherapy can be performed *if* the ICP and CPP are stable. This will prevent stasis of secretions leading to infection, therefore making ventilation more difficult, in turn having an undesirable effect on cerebral perfusion.

Ensure ventilator tubing is positioned to prevent tugging or dragging of the ET tube to prevent displacement or kinking causing loss of or obstruction of the airway. Keep ventilator tubing free from water and ensure water traps are emptied. Once spinal clearance has been documented it will be possible to nurse Leah on alternate sides keeping her head in midline. This also assists in prevention of infection and aids expansion of the lungs. Observation from a cardiovascular perspective will concentrate on HR, BP and SaO_2.

Leah will have continuous monitoring in place with observations recorded hourly. Hypoxia is the most common cause of cardiovascular instability, as mentioned previously. Hypotension is a common complication due to the effects of other treatments such as analgesia, sedation, muscle relaxants and barbiturate therapy. Management is aimed at using correct volume of IV fluids based on BP, central venous pressure (CVP), urine output and fluid balance.

In addition, an inotrope such as dopamine (BNFC 2009) may be required to ensure adequate BP in order to optimise CPP (Table 16.4). Thiopentone lowers metabolism and therefore decreases HR, BP, temperature and may affect pupil reaction. It is important to recognise what may be drug related or a sudden deterioration in Leah's condition. Treatment of head-injured children can be extremely complex; therefore the children's nurse must understand the significance of the observations in order to recognise complications so that changes can be initiated early in management.

Evaluate: use the Mead model of nursing (McClune & Franklin 1987). This framework uses a continuum of care, from being highly dependent moving towards independence.

Question 3. Why is pain relief and sedation an important aspect of care of a child with a closed head injury?

Physical needs

Pain/sedation
In the acute phase of severe head injury, children require sedation and analgesia to prevent unplanned extubation and facilitate ventilation. To ensure invasive lines remain *in situ* and to rest the brain and reduce stimulation, it is important to understand the GCS, as children with low scores can feel pain and become stressed.

Nursing interventions and care are essential for prevention of secondary complications and to promote recovery. However, they can also cause adverse effects, such as raised ICP, reduced CPP, hypoxemia and bradycardia. Therefore it is essential that analgesia and sedation is adequate.

Table 16.4 Drugs which may be used.

- IV fentanyl
Opioid analgesia used to treat moderate to severe pain.
Side effects: abdominal pain, vasodilatation, apnoea, agitation, tremor, laryngospasm.
- Dopamine
Inotropic sympathomimetic. Cardiac stimulant acts on beta receptors in cardiac muscle and increases contractility to increase cardiac output.
Side effects: nausea and vomiting, peripheral vasoconstriction, hypertension, tachycardia.
- IV or oral paracetamol
Non-opioid analgesia used for mild to moderate pain. Also antipyretic properties. Side effects: rare, but rashes thrombocytopenia, leucopenia, neutropenia, hypotension also reported on IV infusion.
Important: liver and renal damage following overdosage.
- Oral or rectal chloral hydrate
Hypnotic, mainly used for sedation.
Side effects: gastric irritation, nausea and vomiting, abdominal distension, headache, dependence.

Please refer to BNFC (2009) regarding drugs above and become aware of possible side effects of each.

Implementation: Leah will be commenced on a morphine intravenous infusion for pain and midazolam infusion for sedation. Atracurium is a neuromuscular blocking agent (NBA), and may be used if Leah has a raised ICP. It is particularly helpful in preventing a cough response to suction, which would further increase ICP. Muscle relaxants do not have sedative or analgesic properties and are not intended to be used without opioids and sedation (Martin *et al.* 1999). Thiopentone is an anaesthetic agent and lowers cerebral metabolism and therefore ICP. This drug causes myocardial depression and vasodilation necessitating inotropic support (BNFC 2009).

Evaluation: how can we assess if Leah is pain free and adequately sedated?

- Look at the HR and BP, is there an increase?
- Is it associated with nursing interventions, or at rest?
- Are there tears and dilatation of the pupils?
- Is there flushing/blotching of the skin? (for example red face)

Evaluation in this group of patients is challenging:

- Is it pain?
- Is it a seizure?

If Leah's analgesia and sedation is adequate you would expect her HR and BP to remain fairly static or show a slight increase in response to interventions but then quickly settle. An unprovoked increase in HR and BP may be associated with seizure activity, usually combined with a drop in SaO$_2$ and increase in pupil size. Muscle relaxants can make assessment difficult. Manifestations of pain may include tearing and pupillary dilation.

Record pain score hourly

There are a variety of pain tools available for use such as FLACC (depending on age of child and dependency level (see Appendix 3 for Chapter 13, RCN Guidelines).

Glasgow coma modified scale

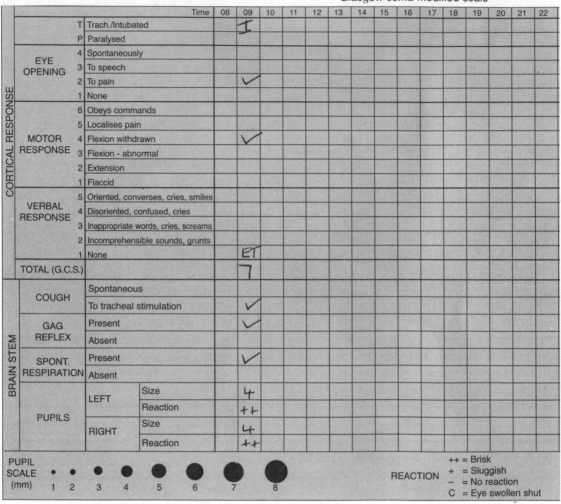

			Time	08	09	10	11	12	13	14	15	16	17	18	19	20	21	22
CORTICAL RESPONSE		T	Trach./Intubated		I													
		P	Paralysed															
	EYE OPENING	4	Spontaneously															
		3	To speech															
		2	To pain		✓													
		1	None															
	MOTOR RESPONSE	6	Obeys commands															
		5	Localises pain															
		4	Flexion withdrawn		✓													
		3	Flexion - abnormal															
		2	Extension															
		1	Flaccid															
	VERBAL RESPONSE	5	Oriented, converses, cries, smiles															
		4	Disoriented, confused, cries															
		3	Inappropriate words, cries, screams															
		2	Incomprehensible sounds, grunts															
		1	None		ET													
	TOTAL (G.C.S.)				7													
BRAIN STEM	COUGH		Spontaneous															
			To tracheal stimulation		✓													
	GAG REFLEX		Present		✓													
			Absent															
	SPONT. RESPIRATION		Present		✓													
			Absent															
	PUPILS	LEFT	Size		4													
			Reaction		++													
		RIGHT	Size		4													
			Reaction		++													

| PUPIL SCALE (mm) | • 1 | • 2 | ● 3 | ● 4 | ● 5 | ● 6 | ● 7 | ● 8 | | REACTION | ++ = Brisk
+ = Sluggish
− = No reaction
C = Eye swollen shut |

Figure 16.2   Royal Belfast Hospital for Sick Children: Paediatric Intensive Care observation sheet.

However, a comprehensive clinical assessment remains the most valuable method of evaluating sedation until the development of a tool is developed in this particular patient population.

Question 4(a). Use the Glasgow Coma Scale (GCS) to assess Leah's neurological status. See Figure 16.2.

Neurology
Assess: according to Williams (2000) the level of consciousness has two parts: arousal and awareness. Leah's GCS will be recorded at least hourly and the assessment is divided into:

1. Cortical response: eye opening, motor response and verbal response.
2. Brain stem: cough, gag reflex and spontaneous breathing.

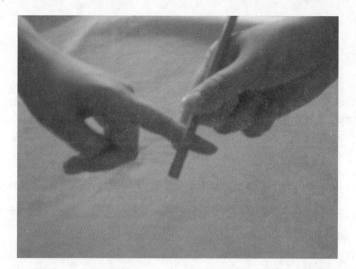

Figure 16.3 Assessing response.

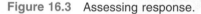

Cortical response

Eye opening (GCS top score is 4)

Check if Leah is able to open her eyes spontaneously (4/4), if not then call out her name, initially softly and then louder (3/4); if there is still no eye opening then apply peripheral painful stimuli by applying pressure with a pen to the lateral outer aspect of the second or third finger (2/4); see Figure 16.3 (Waterhouse 2009).

Gently open Leah's eyes to assess pupil size, reaction and equality. Use a + sign for a reaction or a – sign for no reaction; C is recorded if the eyes are closed due to trauma. Also record if the pupils respond briskly or sluggishly to light, and the size of the pupils (Davies & Hassell 2007). These should be between two and four millimetres in diameter (Williams 2000).

Motor response (GCS top score is 6)

This is to assess the level of consciousness, how deep a coma the patient is in and if simple commands can be obeyed (Waterhouse 2009). Check if Leah obeys simple commands, for example squeezing the nurse's finger (6/6); if she does not respond then central painful stimulus is used to assess the level of consciousness and a response will score 5/6. This can either be by pressing the supraorbital ridge or by using the trapezius squeeze (Waterhouse 2009). The experienced intensive care nurse will be observing Leah for normal or abnormal movements. The lowest score is (1/6) if there is no movement.

Please note: the hand rests on the patient's head and the flat part of the thumb is placed on the supraorbital ridge gradually increasing the pressure for a maximum of 20 seconds. *This is not to be used if there are facial or skull fractures.*

Please note: apply gradual degrees of pressure until the patient attempts to localise pain for a maximum of 20 seconds (not suitable for children under five).

Verbal response (GCS top score is 5)

This provides the children's nurse with information about the patient's speech, ability to understand and functioning areas of the higher, cognitive centres of the brain (Waterhouse 2005).

As Leah is ventilated and sedated she will have an ET tube *in situ*; therefore she can only score (1/5).

Brain stem
Cough
ET suction is an important part of the care in intensive care but this suctioning needs to be kept to a minimal as coughing increases ICP (Tume & Jinks 2008). The nurse can assess the cough reflex during ET suction.

Gag
The gag reflex can be assessed when performing oral suction using a yankauer gently at the back of the throat (Davies & Hassell 2007).

Spontaneous breathing
Breathing indicates that the brain stem is intact. Leah is ventilated, but an experienced intensive care nurse will be able to assess if she has spontaneous breathing.

Question 4(b). What other observations would you carry out?

The following observations are closely monitored to prevent any deterioration in Leah's condition. The heart rate, B/P and respiratory rate are recorded at least hourly. A falling heart rate (bradycardia) and a rising B/P (hypertension) combined with an irregular respiratory rate or apnoea (Cushing's triad) is an indication of a rising ICP. There will also be a decrease in the level of consciousness.

Heart rate range for a 10-year-old
Awake 60–140 (beats/minute) asleep 60–90 (beats /minute)

Systolic blood pressure (mmHg)
Range for a 10-year-old
Normal 90 + 2 × age in years

Lower limit 70 + 2 × age in years

Respiratory rate range for a 10-year-old
Breaths per minute 20–24

As Leah is in intensive care she will have ICP monitoring. Observe closely for any sustained rise in ICP.

Normal range of ICP in a 10-year-old
10–15 mmHg

Cerebral perfusion pressure (CPP)
Cerebral perfusion pressure (CPP) is mean arterial blood pressure (MAP) minus intracranial pressure (ICP). If the ICP is rising the CPP will fall; it is therefore important to maintain a good blood pressure at all times. If the CPP falls the blood supply to the brain is significantly reduced.

An adequate CPP for a 10-year-old is >60 mmHg

The hypothalamus is responsible for controlling body temperature. The importance of recording the body temperature cannot be underestimated; a rise in temperature increases the metabolic rate and therefore increases oxygen consumption. The children's nurse must be able to distinguish between pyrexia caused by infection or caused by a rise in ICP (Suadoni 2009).

Plan: to minimise any further deterioration in the GCS:

- Nurse midline.
- Thirty degree head-up tilt (Feldman *et al.* 1992).
- Ensure good pain relief and sedation
- Maintain $PaCO_2$ at lower end of normal (4.5–5.5 kPa); mild hyperventilation may be required.
- Maintain a blood pressure and a good CPP. To achieve this inotropes may be required, for example dopamine (further reading is required on inotropes – source BNFC 2009).

A neuromuscular blockade, for example vecuronium bromide, may be considered but it does have complications including pneumonia and increasing the stay in intensive care (Tume *et al.* 2008) (further reading required on neuromuscular blockade: source BNFC 2009).

Medical staff will assess fluid requirements and may restrict fluids, but this will depend on blood pressure, perfusion, need for inotropes and if a fluid bolus has been required.

Maintain a normal body temperature. Further brain damage can be associated with hyperthermia (Davies & Hassell 2007).

Consider the use of hyperosmolar therapy if there is a rise in the ICP, for example mannitol (further reading required source: BNFC 2009).

If cervical spine immobilisation is required using a spinal collar, ensure that this is not too tight, obstructing the jugular vein.

If there is a sudden rise in ICP a computed tomography (CT) imaging of the head may be ordered by the neurosurgeons (NICE 2007).

Implicate and evaluate: using the Mead model now ensure all of the above has been effective and then write your evaluation.

Question 5. How would the children's nurse ensure adequate fluid balance?

Nutrition/hydration and elimination
Assess: all children admitted to hospital should have an accurate weight recorded to enable calculation of medications and fluids (NMC 2008). As Leah is critically ill and being admitted to an intensive care unit, it is appropriate to estimate her weight using the following formula.

Child aged 1–10 years
Weight (kg) = (age in years + 4) × 2 (Davies & Hassell 2007)

Ideally, Leah would be nursed on a weighing bed and when she has been stabilised a more accurate weight can be obtained; this would also facilitate a daily weight to be recorded. Maintaining fluid balance is essential to health (Scales & Pilsworth 2008).

Normal fluid requirements for a child weighing 28 kg

Body weight	Fluid requirement per day (ml/kg)
First 10 kg	100 = 1000
Second 10 kg	50 = 500
Subscquent kilograms	20 = 160
Total	1660

Daily fluid requirement will be assessed by the medical staff; however, maintenance fluids will be calculated as per formulae above. Keeping an accurate fluid balance chart is an important part of hydration monitoring. The nurse must take into account all fluid administration when assessing how much fluid is to be administrated on an hourly basis (intravenous fluids, enteral feeds, intravenous drugs). If a fluid bolus has been required this is usually over and above the total 24-hour intake. All fluid administration is regulated by either infusion pumps or drivers and administrated as prescribed. Low intravascular volume is usually indicated by a rising heart rate and falling blood pressure (Cook 2005). In the critically ill it is also assessed by measuring the CVP.

Electrolytes require close monitoring, in particular sodium and potassium. Urea and electrolyte results dictate what type of intravenous fluids are prescribed by the medical staff.

Consider risk management

It is important to avoid hyponatraemia (an electrolyte disturbance) in the acutely ill hospitalised child as this can occur during inappropriate rehydration or with maintenance fluids and may have serious advert effects, such as neurological impairment, and cause death (Jenkins *et al.* 2003). Therefore, it is vital that nursing and medical staff work effectively and efficiently to ensure care planning documentation is consistent, coherent and standardised.

A nasogastric tube will be *in situ*, as enteral feeding is introduced as soon as possible following a traumatic injury, because the body requires an increased amount of calories. Early referral to the dietician is recommended and a high calorie feed commenced; prior to commencing feeds it is necessary to rule out any abdominal injury.

Check regular blood sugars; an insulin intravenous infusion may be required if the blood sugar level is persistently high.

Plan: record the fluid balance chart hourly as accurate intake and output is essential. Calculate the overall balance (intake minus output) at least six hourly. This is to ensure that Leah is neither in a large negative or positive balance. Check regular blood biochemistry (U&E). A urinary catheter will be *in situ*; record output hourly and note how many ml/kg/hour.

Normal urinary output for a 10-year-old: 1 ml/kg/hr

Regular urinalysis should be checked; the specific gravity (SG) will show if a patient's urine is dilute or concentrated (Scales & Pilsworth 2008). Following a head injury there can be a decreased production of the antidiuretic hormone (ADH) resulting in neurogenic diabetes insipidus (Davies & Hassell 2007). Avoid constipation as this can cause a rise in ICP due to straining (Suadoni 2009). A high fibre feed may be required.

Implicate and evaluate: whilst utilising the Mead model ensure all of the above planned care has been effective and then write your evaluation.

References

British National Formulary for Children (2009) *British National Formulary for Children*. London: BNF.

Cook, N.F. (2005) Fundamentals of fluids and hydration in the nursing of the neuroscience patient. *British Journal of Neuroscience Nursing*, **1**(2), 61–6.

Davies, J.H. & Hassell, L.L. (2007) *Children in Intensive Care. A Survival Guide*, 2nd edn. Edinburgh: Churchill Livingstone.

Feldman, Z., Kanter, M. & Robinson, C. (1992) Effects of head elevation on intracranial pressure and cerebral blood flow in head injury patients. *Journal of Neurosurgery*, **76**, 207–211.

Jenkins, J.G., Taylor, B. & McCarthy, M. (2003) Prevention of hyponatraemia in children receiving fluid therapy. *The Ulster Medical Journal*, **72**(2), 69–72. Note: this article incorporates the DHSSPS guidelines.

Martin, L.D., Bratton, S.L. & O'Rourke, P. (1999) Issues and controversies of neuromuscular blocking agents in infants and children. *Critical Care Medicine*, **27**(7), 1358–68.

McClune, B. & Franklin, K. (1987) The Mead model for nursing-adapted from the Roper/Logan/Tierney model for nursing, *Intensive Care Nursing*, **3**(3), 97–105, cited in Viney, C. (1996) *Nursing the Critically Ill*, Edinburgh: Baillière Tindall.

Moppett, I. K. (2007) Trauamatic brain injury: assessment, resuscitation and early management. *British Journal Anaesthesia*, **99**(1), 18–31.

National Institute for Health and Clinical Excellence (2007) *Head Injury: Triage, Assessment, Investigation and Early Management of Head Injury in Infants, Children and Adults*. NICE clinical guideline 56. London: NHS.

Nursing and Midwifery Council (2008) *Standards for Medicines Management*. London: NMC.

Pigula, F.A., Wald, S.L., Shackford, S.R. & Vane, D.W. (1993) The effect of hypotension and hypoxia on children with severe head injuries. *Journal of Pediatric Surgery*, **28**(3), 310–6.

Resuscitation Council (UK) (2007) *Paediatric Immediate Life Support. 2.9*. London: Resuscitation Council (UK).

Scales, K. & Pilsworth, J. (2008) The importance of fluid balance in clinical practise. *Nursing Standard*, **22**(47), 50–57.

Steffen-Albert, K.A. (2010) Management of patients with neurologic trauma, Chapter 63. In: Smeltzer, S.C., Bare, B.G., Hinkle, J.L. & Cheever, K.H. (eds). *Brunner & Suddarth's Textbook of Medical-Surgical Nursing*, 12th edn. Philadelphia: Wolters Kluwer/Lippincott Williams & Wilkins.

Suadoni, M.T. (2009) Raised intracranial pressure: nursing observations and interventions. *Nursing Standard*, **23**(43), 35–40.

Tume, L. & Jinks, A. (2008) Endotracheal suctioning in children with severe traumatic brain injury: a literature review. *Nursing in Critical Care*, **13**(5), 232–40.

Tume, L., Thorburn, K. & Sinha, A. (2008) A review of the intensive care management of severe paediatric traumatic brain injury. *British Journal of Neuroscience Nursing*, **4**(9), 424–31.

Waterhouse, C. (2005) The Glasgow coma scale and other neurological observations. *Nursing Standard*, **19**(33), 56–64.

Weinstein, S. (2006) Controversies in the care of children with acute brain injury. *Curr Neurol Neuroscience Rep*, **6**(2), 127–35.

Williams, A. (2000) Severe head injury in children: a case study. *Emergency Nurse*, **8**(1), 16–19.

www.bestpractice.bmj.com (accessed August 2010).

17

Obesity

Janice Christie

Scenario

Treewood Primary School is located in a deprived inner-city location. Most of the parents with children attending the school have low incomes or are unemployed; many pupils live in single parent households. The surrounding community members often have negative stereotypes of the pupils and the school has a poor local image. Treewood has not performed as well as other local schools in National Curriculum Standardised Tests (SATS) of academic performance.

The school is situated in a large public housing development known as Treeland. There are ten-storey flats and terraced housing in the development. Over the past few years, the area has become increasingly run down, there are many vacant dwellings that have become vandalised. Groups of young people, who have little else to do, break into empty houses or flats to take drugs and alcohol. Many older people, who are fearful of becoming victims of the rising crime rate within the estate, will not leave their homes in the evenings. Parents are reluctant to let their younger children play outside the home due to concerns about harm to their offspring arising from antisocial behaviour. Most people in the estate express hopelessness in their situation; they aim to live for today as they say that they have nothing to aspire to.

Treeland has few local amenities. There is a fast-food outlet that offers mostly fried foods, a small general store that sells staple foods (mostly processed foods) and an off-licence that

Care Planning in Children and Young People's Nursing, First Edition.
Edited by Doris Corkin, Sonya Clarke, Lorna Liggett.
© 2012 Blackwell Publishing Ltd. Published 2012 by Blackwell Publishing Ltd.

sells alcohol. A youth club, for teenagers closed several months ago due to poor attendance and repeated vandalism of the premises. There are several green spaces within Treeland that could be used for play, but these are fouled with dog excrement and broken glass, often children end up playing in the small back gardens of terrace homes or in the corridors of flats. Few people living in Treeland have cars, most are dependent on public transport or private taxi hire for journeys. There is a local bus service that runs every 45 minutes in the evening. The nearest large food store is about a 30-minute walk (ten minutes bus) away and the nearest leisure centre is about a 45-minute walk (or two ten-minute bus journeys).

The local housing authority is aware of problems in the estate and has helped residents form a neighbourhood committee in order to decide how to best tackle locality difficulties. This committee includes local residents as well as professionals (school, police, housing officers, health and social care, etc.) working in the locality. A new headmaster (Mr Jones) was appointed to Treewood school several months ago and he is determined to improve the school's image and increase life chances and academic standards within the school. The teachers in the school are supporting this new school vision.

Jane is a school nurse employed by a primary care trust and attached (provides care) to Treewood primary school. Under the *Healthy Child Programme* (DH 2009), she undertakes measurement of children's height and weight in the reception year (when children are aged 4–5 years) and in year 6 (age 10–11). This assessment has found that 20% and 25% of children in reception year/year 6 (respectively) are obese. Jane knows that many children perform poorly at school; and she has also had to counsel some children who have low self-esteem and who have experienced bullying. The school has a canteen that provides healthy meals, but it is not used by all pupils, some children are given money to buy chips (fried potatoes) from a local fast-food outlet that is near the school. Many children walk to school and have about 30 minutes per week physical education/sporting activity.

Jane has been approached by Jake and his mother. Jake is ten-year-old boy who is obese, and both Jake and his mother are concerned and willing to take action about his recent accelerating weight gain. His two older brothers are both overweight and his mother, who is a single parent, is obese. Jake's mother has a part-time job in a local bakery, starting work at 4 am, and finds she is too tired to cook for her family when she returns home after the end of her shift at 1 pm. All her children have different food preferences and she finds it hard to cater for all their needs, so she buys each a different ready meal. Jake says he never eats fruit or vegetables; his preferred meal is an adult-sized portion of macaroni cheese.

Jake has been showing attention difficulties in school, has poor academic performance and has low self-esteem. His mother has been asking his older brothers to help get him out for school in the morning. As Jake is usually late up out of bed, there usually is no milk for his breakfast cereal and often he leaves home without breakfast. His eldest brother leaves him at school before catching the bus to a local training programme. When he gets to school he finds it difficult to concentrate, especially during morning lessons.

Sometimes Jake's mother has time to make him lunch (usually white bread ham sandwiches, a packet of crisps and a sugary fizzy drink); at other times she gives him money to buy some food at the fast-food shop. She does not want Jake to take free school dinners because of the stigma associated with free meals. Jake lives in a top-floor flat, often the lifts do not work and he uses the stairs to go home. Once at home, there is little to do other than to than to play his video games (his mother worries about the possible negative influence of other friends).

Some helpful additional information

School nurses are responsible for health promotion and health maintenance of school-aged children, both as individual children and as an entire school population; for further information see Christie *et al.* (2009). In this section you will be asked to consider the care for one child and in addition, care for the entire school population of children. The Neuman system model (Neuman & Fawcett 2002) can be used to apply to one person or a group or population of people and therefore, it will be appropriate to devise a one-child and a school care plan using this model.

You may find that your answers (especially for questions 5 and 6) differ from the ones suggested; there are many possible acceptable answers and you should aim to ensure that your response is based on an evidence-based rationale.

 Questions

1. What is obesity and how is it usually defined?
2. What causes obesity?
3. Considering Neuman's system model/grand theory five variables; what are the possible consequences of childhood obesity for pupils that the school nurse, Jane, cares for?
4. This model suggests that the five variables are subject to stressors/pressures. Can you identify for one pupil (Jake) possible stressors and lines of defence or resistance regarding the five variables and their effect on his healthy weight maintenance?
5. Based on the information from questions 2–4, can you develop a healthy weight care plan for Jake?
6. Can you identify the possible stressors and lines of defence or resistance on healthy weight maintenance for the entire Treewood school population? Based on this and the information from questions 2–3, can you develop a healthy weight care plan for the school?

Answers to questions

Question 1. What is obesity and how is it usually defined?

Obesity is a condition that indicates risk to health, associated with excess body fat. It is usually defined according to body mass index (WHO 2000). Body mass index (BMI) is a ratio of a person's weight in kilograms divided by height in metres^2. For adults:

$$\text{BMI} < 20 = \text{underweight}$$

$$20{-}35 = \text{desirable/healthy}$$

$$25{-}30 = \text{overweight}$$

$$>30 = \text{obese}$$

It is currently recommended that BMI is supplemented with waist measurements in adults (NICE 2006) as waist size has closer links to morbidity (disease) and mortality (death) associated with obesity than BMI.

BMI assessment is more complicated to undertake in children as it varies with age and gender. NICE (2006) suggests that young children should be assessed in accordance with standard centile charts that allow comparison of weight for height and that older children are assessed using centile BMI reference charts (see example of boy chart below). Children who are over the 91st centile on these charts are classified as overweight and above the 98th centile as obese. These techniques are useful for assessing individual and population obesity status in the UK. Due to sensitivity about using the term 'obesity', it is recommended that professionals use the term 'overweight' with parents, children and young people (DH 2008).

The International Obesity Task Force (IOTF) (Cole *et al.* 2000), based on information collected from people resident in six different countries, has suggested that BMI of over 25 or 30 (overweight or obese) be used in international epidemiological studies (research comparing rates of obesity in or across populations). Using IOTF criteria, and data from the 2004 Health Survey data in England, it was estimated that 10% of 6–10-year-olds were obese (Butland *et al.* 2007) (Figure 17.1).

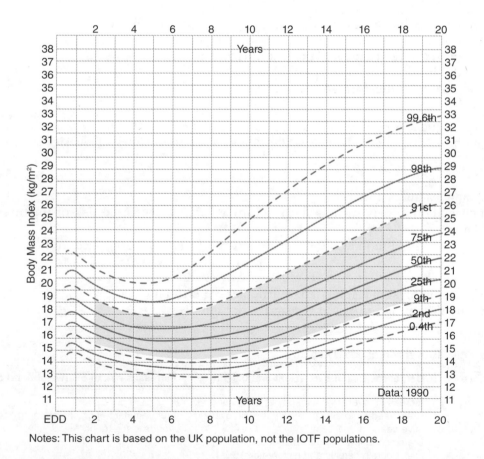

Notes: This chart is based on the UK population, not the IOTF populations.

Figure 17.1   Body mass index chart for boys. © Child Growth Foundation, reproduced with permission, printed charts from www.healthforallchildren.co.uk.

Question 2. What causes obesity?

Obesity arises from an energy imbalance between energy intake (from food and drink) and energy expenditure (internal body processes and physical activity) (RCP *et al.* 2004). Weight gain occurs when energy intake (calories consumed) exceeds total daily energy expenditure for a prolonged period. There are many factors that contribute to this: physiological factors (such as appetite control in the brain), eating habits, activity levels and psychosocial influences (Butland *et al.* 2007). These represent a complex mix of personal, social and environmental factors. Butland *et al.* (2007) suggest that genetics/biology loads the gun of obesity (makes people predisposed to obesity) and the environment factors pull the trigger (brings about the conditions in which obesity happens). Brown *et al.* (2007) summarise the current evidence for prevention of obesity in Table 17.1.

Question 3. Considering Neuman's system model/grand theory five variables; what are the possible consequences of childhood obesity for the pupils that the school nurse, Jane, cares for?

Neuman's system model (Neuman & Fawcett 2002) identifies five client variables:

- Physiological = biochemical, physiological functioning of the body
- Psychological/cognitive = thought processes and emotions
- Socio-cultural = relationships, expectations and activities
- Spiritual = human spirit and spiritual beliefs
- Developmental = lifespan growth

The consequences of obesity (drawn from Swanton & Frost (2007)) will be considered for each of these five client variables. Physiological consequences of obesity in childhood include:

- Sleep apnoea and asthma
- Orthopaedic problems such as flat feet, ankle sprains, increased risk of fractures, knee problems
- Gallstones, NASH (non-alcoholic steatohepatitis) , gastro-oesophageal reflux
- Type 2 diabetes
- Menstrual abnormalities and polycystic ovary syndrome
- Hypertension, dyslipidaemia, left ventricular hypertrophy
- Systemic inflammation/raised C-reactive protein

Table 17.1   Prevention of obesity chart.

Evidence	Decreases risk of overweight and obesity	Increases risk of overweight and obesity
Convincing	Increased (over time) total physical activity	
Probable	Breastfeeding (prevents obesity in child over five years of age)	Frequent, large portions of energy dense foods – sugary drinks
	Diets rich in low energy dense food (wholegrain cereals and dietary fibre)	

Source: Brown *et al.* (2007).

Psychological/cognitive consequences of obesity in childhood include: development of a negative self-image, lowered self-esteem and a higher risk of depression. Socio-cultural consequences of obesity in childhood include: experience of teasing, social exclusion, discrimination and prejudice. Spiritual consequences of obesity in childhood may include: impact on the human spirit in conjunction with psychological or socio-cultural processes resulting in hopelessness. Developmental consequences of obesity in childhood may include a life course impact; obese children are more likely than their non-obese peers to become obese adults. Obese adults are more likely to have morbidity and/or mortality associated with: type 2 diabetes, cardiovascular disease, hypertension, sleep apnoea, cancer, infertility, osteoarthritis, NASH, gallbladder disease, gout, lower back pain, anxiety, depression and stigma.

Question 4. This model suggests that the five variables are subject to stressors/pressures. Can you identify for one pupil (Jake) possible stressors and lines of defence or resistance regarding the 5 variables and their effect on his healthy weight maintenance? It will be useful to review the answer to questions 2 and 3, before completing this question.

Neuman's system model (Neuman & Fawcett 2002) identifies three types of stressors that can act on individual's or groups of individuals' five variables. Stressors can be:

- Intrapersonal: within individuals or population
- Interpersonal: between individuals or populations and groups
- Extrapersonal: these are factors outside the individual or population

Stressors can have actual (overt), potential (covert) or residual effects. The model also identifies that people have lines of defence or resistance that help protect the body from stressors.

Intrapersonal stressors include:

- Biological-genetic and physiological predisposition to weight gain (physiological, potential)
- Erratic eating patterns (no breakfast) (physiological, actual)
- Large/adult food servings (physiological, actual)
- High fat and sugar, low in complex carbohydrate and fruit/vegetables diet (physiological, actual)
- Plays a lot of video games at home (socio-cultural, potential)
- Has low self-esteem (psychological, actual)

Interpersonal stressors include:

- Mother has difficulty finding time to prepare food and needs to cater for Jake's individual food preferences (physiological/psychological, potential)
- Bullying from other children (socio-cultural, residual)
- Jake has little physical activity and plays little with other children when at home (physiological/socio-cultural, potential)
- Other members of family are overweight (influence of family norms, socio-cultural, potential)

Extrapersonal stressors include:

- Limited healthy eating resources outside school (physiological, potential)
- Limited exercise potential outside school (physiological, potential)
- Economic deprivation levels in the surrounding estate (socio-cultural, potential)
- Levels of crime and vandalism in the surrounding estate (socio-cultural, potential)
- Low hope in general community (spiritual, potential)

Jake's lines of defence and resistance are:

- Walking to school and using stairs
- He says he wants to be a healthy weight
- Has some current family support to make change

Question 5. Based on the information from questions 2–4, can you develop a healthy weight care plan for Jake?

Remember to identify the level of nursing intervention (as per Neuman's model) that you will use. Note, we have adapted and modified the Neuman's system model care plan process for the learning aims of this book. A Neuman system model assessment and intervention tool has been developed to help apply the model to the nursing process in practice settings, for more information about this tool please refer to Neuman & Fawcett (2002).

Neuman's system model identifies three levels of nursing interventions:

- Primary prevention occurs before a person or group of people react to a stressor. This can be by strengthening resistance to the stressor and/or by weakening the stressor.
- Secondary prevention occurs when a person or group of people have reacted to a stressor. This can be achieved through strengthening resistance to the stressor and/or removing the stressor.
- Tertiary prevention occurs after a person has had a secondary prevention intervention. It facilitates re-adaptation and prevention of future occurrences.

Jake's care plan

Assessed need	Plan	Type of intervention/ implementation	Evaluation	Rationale
Jake has an imbalanced dietary intake contributing to unhealthy weight	To increase Jake's consumption of healthy foods and drink within a month	Secondary prevention advice to Jake and his mother regarding: Food served on smaller plates to reduce food portions. Regular meals to reduce binge eating. Increase in daily intake of water, also, complex carbohydrates and fruit and vegetables consumption; to decrease sugary drink and fried food/processed intake.	Meet with Jake and his family weekly to discuss Jake's dietary intake and changes made.	Focus on positive eating change rather than negative reduction in foods. Advice to follow NICE (2006) and WHO (2008) guidelines.

Assessed need	Plan	Type of intervention/ implementation	Evaluation	Rationale
Jake has low physical activity, contributing to unhealthy weight	To increase Jake's level of physical activity to 30–60 minutes per day of moderate to vigorous intensity exercise within a month	Secondary prevention: Reduce time playing video games (sedentary behaviour). Encourage walking to school. Family activity at weekends.	Meet with Jake and his family weekly to discuss physical activity undertaken and changes made.	Following NICE (2006) guidelines with eventual aim of achieving WHO (2008) goal of 60 minutes moderate/ vigorous activity per day for school-aged youths.
Jake has low self-esteem and has few friends	To improve self-esteem so that he believes in himself and so that he can achieve a healthy weight within the next six months	Secondary prevention: To repeatedly set realistic, easily achievable, short-term goals. To encourage and praise Jake for achieving goals. Encourage and support Jake in undertaking new activities. Conjointly work on coping strategies for situations and social interaction skills. Referral to school healthy club for peer support.	Meet with Jake weekly and ask about his accomplishments, self-belief and coping. Record monthly BMI readings for next six months.	This follows NICE (2006) guidelines of using psychosocial interventions to help people attain healthy weights.
Jake has previously been bullied and is at continued risk	Within the next three months help Jake to deal with bullying behaviour effectively	Tertiary prevention: Ensure that Jake and his mother are aware of school anti-bully policy procedures and empower and support the family in reporting incidents. Build Jake's self-esteem and teach assertive and communication skills strategies; offering support in line with school policy. Ensure that Jake and his family are aware of additional voluntary support services, such as Childline or ParentLine Plus.	During meetings with Jake and his family during the next three months, enquire about Jake's wellbeing and achievements, as well as relationships with other children.	Applied guidelines of DCSF (2007).

Question 6. Can you identify the possible stressors and lines of defence or resistance on healthy weight maintenance for the entire Treewood school population? Based on this and the information from questions 2–3, can you develop a healthy weight care plan for the school?

Intraschool stressors:

- High levels of obesity (physiological, actual)
- Poor academic achievement, disruptive pupils and bullying (socio-cultural, actual)

- Some pupils with low esteem and attention difficulties (psychological, actual)
- Low use of school canteen (physiological, potential)

Interschool stressors:

- Parents give students money for fatty fast foods (physiological, potential)
- Poor school image by local community (socio-cultural, potential)

Extraschool stressors:

- Limited healthy eating resources outside school (physiological, potential)
- Limited exercise potential outside school (physiological, potential)
- Economic deprivation levels in the surrounding estate (socio-cultural, potential)
- Levels of crime and vandalism in the surrounding estate (socio-cultural, potential)
- Low hope in general community (spiritual, potential)

School lines of defence and resistance:

- Weekly school sport activities
- School involvement with community neighbourhood group
- New headmaster with a vision for school improvement and motivated staff
- Existence of school canteen
- School nurse willing to tackle weight issues in school

School health plan

Assessed need Treewood	Plan	Type of intervention/ implementation	Evaluation	Rationale
School has social, organisational and environmental factors that are contributing to unhealthy food choices by pupils	To help school pupils in making healthy food choices, thereby increasing the intake of fruit and vegetables and increase the amount of high sugar and high fatty foods eaten within the next six months	Primary prevention: Working with headmaster, senior pupils and canteen staff regarding canteen image and marketing healthy foods on the menu. Working with teachers regarding classroom teaching about healthy foods, how to make food choices and how to make basic healthy foods. Working with headmaster, school staff/parent committee and school staff regarding holding family fun events to promote healthy eating and food preparation. Working with Treeland neighbourhood committee to improve local food amenities.	Evaluation of interventions put in place and monitor their effect on reception year and year 6 students by helping students complete a diary of foods eaten during school time and out of school time, in six months time.	Applying principle of multiple interventions aimed at empowering individuals and changing the school and family contexts (Budd and Volpe 2006; NICE 2006; WHO 2008).

Assessed need Treewood	Plan	Type of intervention/ implementation	Evaluation	Rationale
School has social, organisational and environmental factors that are contributing to unhealthy physical activity levels in pupils	To help school pupils to make healthy physical activity and thereby reduce sedentary behaviour and increase activity levels within the next six months	Primary prevention: Working with teachers regarding increasing activity in classrooms, active playground games and additional PE/sports sessions in school week. Working with teachers regarding classroom teaching about healthy activity and increasing physical activity during class. Working with headmaster, school staff/parenting committee and school staff regarding holding family fun events to promote physical activities. Working with Treeland neighbourhood committee to improve local play amenities.	Evaluation of interventions put in place and their effect on reception year and year 6. Monitor school physical activity rates and amount of sedentary behaviour by diary or using accelerometers* (during and outside school hours), in six months time.	Applying principle of multiple interventions aimed at empowering individuals and changing the school and family contexts (Budd and Volpe 2006; NICE 2006; WHO 2008).
Some pupils are overweight or obese	To decrease the percentage of overweight or obese pupils over a school year	Primary prevention dietary and physical activity as above. In addition: Secondary prevention. Healthy club set up after school for children who are overweight, offering professional advice/ support and peer support.	Evaluation of Healthy club outcomes and BMI recording at beginning and end of this school year.	Application of NICE (2006) guidelines.
Some pupils who have been overweight or obese are now healthy weights	To help previously overweight or obese pupils maintain healthier weights over their school career	Tertiary prevention: Ongoing healthy club support for children who have regained normal weight, i.e. offering ongoing professional and peer support.	Evaluation of healthy club outcomes, BMI recording as required during their time at school.	There is a need for ongoing support to ensure long-term programme effects are achieved (Flynn et al. 2002).

*Accelerometers are recording devices that record body movement and distance moved.

Summary

Due to human and economic costs associated with illness, it has been acknowledged that everyone should be encouraged to 'invest' in keeping healthy (Wanless 2004). The Neuman grand theory/model (Neuman &Fawcett 2002) that focuses on 'prevention' ensures that this model is relevant for nurses involved in engaging the public with health matters, and it supports nursing assessment and interventions for both individuals and populations. In addition, the model promotes assessment of psychosocial, physical and developmental needs and this holistic focus means it is useful for nurses caring for younger people and families. Thus, the Neuman model is, potentially, a useful tool for care planning for children's and school nurses, engaged in individual child, young person, family or community focused health promotion.

Activity 17.1

Calculate the BMI for the following children and plot their weights on the BMI chart. To which centiles do these children's BMIs correspond? What action would you take?

Child's name	Gender/age	Weight	Height	BMI	Centile	Action
Ahmed	Boy 6 years	17.5 kg	1 m			
Brendan	Boy 5 years	16 kg	98 cm			
Christopher	Boy 7 years	20.5 kg	110 cm			
Dabir	Boy 8 years	26 kg	1.3 m			
Everton	Boy 9 years	30 kg	1.2 m			

References

Brown, T., Kelly, S. & Summerbell, C.D. (2007) Prevention of obesity: a review of interventions. *Obesity Reviews*, **8**(suppl 1), 127–30.

Budd, G.M. & Volpe, S.L. (2006) School-based prevention: research, challenges, and recommendations. *Journal of School Health*, **76**(10), 485–98.

Butland, B., Jebb, S., Kopelman, P., *et al.* (2007) *Foresight-tackling Obesities: Future Choices*. London: Government Office of Science.

Christie, J., Parkes, J. & Price J. (2009) Public Health Practitioner. In: Hughes, J. & Lyte, G. *Developing Nursing Practice with Children and Young People*. Chichester: J. Wiley and Sons, 87–101.

Cole, T.J., Bellizzi, M.C., Flegal, K.M. & Dietz, W.H. (2000) Establishing a standard definition for child overweight and obesity worldwide: international survey. *British Medical Journal*, **320**, 1240–1246.

Department for Children, Schools and Families (2007) *Safe to Learn Embedding Anti-bullying Work in Schools*. London; Department for Children, Schools and Families.

Department of Health (2008) *Healthy Weight, Healthy Lives Across Government Strategy*. London: DH.

Department of Health (2009) *Healthy Child Programme from 5 to 19 years old*. London: Department of Health and Department for Children, Schools and Families.

Flynn, M.A.T., McNeil, D.A., Maloff, B., *et al.* (2006) Reducing obesity and related chronic disease risk in children and youth: a synthesis of evidence with 'best practice' recommendations. *Obesity Reviews*, **7** (suppl. 1), 7–66.

Neuman, B. & Fawcett, J. (2002) *The Neuman Systems Model*, 4th edn. New Jersey: Prentice Hall.

NICE (2006) *Obesity, Guidance on the Prevention, Identification and Management of Overweight and Obesity in Adults and Children*. NHS: London.

Royal College of Physicians, Royal College of Paediatrics and Child Health, Faculty of Public Health (2004) *Storing up Problems: the Medical Case for a Slimmer Nation*. London: Royal College of Physicians.

Swanton, K. & Frost, M. (2007) *Lightening the Load: Tackling Overweight and Obesity*. London: National Heart Forum.

Wanless, D. (2004) *Securing Good Health for the Whole Population*. Norwich: HM Treasury.

World Health Organisation (2000) *Obesity: Preventing and Managing a Global Epidemic*. Report of a WHO consultation. Technical Report Series 894WHO.

World Health Organisation (2008) *School Policy Framework Implementation of the WHO Global Strategy on Diet, Physical Activity and Health*. Geneva: WHO.

Section 4

Care of Neonates and Children with Respiratory Disorders

18

Neonatal Respiratory Distress Syndrome
Susanne Simmons and Clare Morfoot

Scenario

Arthur is a 27-week gestation preterm infant born by lower segment Caesarean section (LSCS), following maternal pregnancy induced hypertension. His Apgar score (Pinheiro 2009) was 3 at one minute and 7 at five minutes. Following delivery, Arthur was blue, floppy, made weak respiratory effort and had a heart rate less than 100 beats per minute. Arthur was placed in a polythene bag at delivery and a hat was added to prevent heat loss (Resuscitation Council (UK) 2005). Infants less than 30 weeks gestation are at risk of significant heat loss and transepidermal water loss (TEWL). Placing these infants in a polythene bag at delivery, without drying, leaving the head free has been shown to limit/prevent both heat and water loss through the skin. He received five inflation breaths and was electively intubated and received positive pressure ventilation (Fernandez-Alvarez & Bomont 2009). Exogenous surfactant was administered via the endotracheal tube (ETT). Once stabilised, Arthur was transferred to the neonatal unit.

On admission to the unit, Arthur weighed 850 grams and was placed into a closed incubator with 80% humidity. An umbilical arterial catheter (UAC) and umbilical venous catheter (UVC) were sited. A chest X-ray verified the position of the ETT, UAC and UVC and confirmed a diagnosis of respiratory distress syndrome (RDS). Positive pressure ventilation continued and changes to Arthur's ventilator requirements were made in response to improving arterial blood gases. Over the next few days, Arthur's respiratory function improved and he was extubated onto nasal continuous positive airway pressure (nCPAP).

Care Planning in Children and Young People's Nursing, First Edition.
Edited by Doris Corkin, Sonya Clarke, Lorna Liggett.
© 2012 Blackwell Publishing Ltd. Published 2012 by Blackwell Publishing Ltd.

Questions

1. Assessment: how would you assess Arthur's respiratory needs?
2. Planning: what respiratory support will Arthur require?
3. Implementation: what care will Arthur require to optimise his respiratory function?
4. Evaluation: when will Arthur no longer require respiratory support?

This chapter will focus on the respiratory management of a preterm infant with RDS. Although the scenario is based on a premature infant, some of the principles of care outlined in the chapter are also relevant to the term neonate and infant. The neonatal mortality rate has declined significantly since 2000 (CEMACH 2009) with the demand for neonatal care increasing each year (NAO 2007). Approximately one in ten infants born each year will require admission to a neonatal unit, with preterm infants requiring specialist neonatal intensive care.

Answers to questions

Activity of daily living: breathing.

Question 1. Assessment: how would you assess Arthur's respiratory needs?

The lungs *in utero* are filled with foetal lung fluid and the volume of this and amniotic fluid is crucial to normal lung development (Randall 2005). In addition, foetal breathing movements, seen *in utero* from as early as 12 weeks, are also thought to support the development of the diaphragm and chest wall muscles. Lung development is characterised by stages (Moore & Persaud 2008) which overlap and do not occur uniformly within each lung (see Table 18.1). The lungs need to be developed sufficiently to enable the alveoli to be involved in gaseous exchange and this is usually achieved by 32–34 weeks gestation. At 27 weeks gestation, Arthur's lungs will be immature in both structure and the amount of surfactant produced.

Respiratory distress syndrome is a pulmonary disorder caused by a lack of surfactant and is predominantly associated with prematurity. Surfactant is a complex mixture of proteins,

Table 18.1 Overview of the stages of lung development.

Pseudoglandular stage (6–16 weeks)	The trachea, bronchi and bronchioles are formed. Connective tissue, muscle and blood vessels start to develop.
Canalicular stage (16–6 weeks)	The bronchioles continue to branch and the vascular network develops alongside the airways. Type 2 cells begin to secrete small amounts of surfactant. The cells lining the alveolar are cuboidal, epithelial cells and are thick.
Terminal saccular stage (26 weeks to birth)	The alveoli develop and multiply. The alveolar epithelial lining thins (squamous epithelium) which allows closer contact with the capillaries. There is a surge of surfactant produced at 32–34 weeks gestation.
Alveolar stage (32 weeks to childhood)	This stage continues after birth and into childhood. The alveoli develop further and mature. There are approximately 50 million alveoli present in the full-term infant and this reaches adult values of 300 million during childhood.

lipids and phospholipids and spreads across the liquid lined surface of the alveoli (Randall 2005). It reduces surface tension and prevents the collapse (atelectasis) of the alveoli on expiration, therefore maintaining a positive pressure in the airways (functional residual capacity). The liquid lined surface of the alveoli facilitates normal gaseous exchange.

It is known that during a normal vaginal delivery the release of adrenaline promotes the switch of lung cells from producing foetal lung fluid to absorbing it. In addition, the pressure applied to the infant's ribcage during the delivery 'squeezes' the lung fluid out through the mouth and nose. As the infant takes its first breath a high intrathoracic pressure is generated which pushes the lung fluid into the pulmonary vascular and lymphatic system (Moore & Persaud 2008). As Arthur was delivered by an emergency LSCS, this process did not occur. Antenatal corticosteroids, given in time to have an effect, cross the placenta and appear to accelerate lung development (Sweet *et al.* 2007). However, Arthur's mum did not receive antenatal steroids prior to delivery. Arthur is therefore challenged at delivery in terms of his respiratory function.

Respiratory assessment of Arthur: airway and breathing

Airway
Neonates are predominantly nose breathers for the first few months of life. Arthur's airways are extremely narrow and his large tongue in relation to his small jaw can allow the tongue to fall back and obstruct his upper airway. In addition, the gag reflex is underdeveloped and the large occiput of the neonate's head can push the chin downwards onto the chest when lying supine and cause airway obstruction. Due to surfactant deficiency his alveoli are collapsed (atelectasis) and a chest X-ray (Figure 18.1) reveals the lung fields have a 'ground glass appearance', with air bronchograms (the air-filled left and right main bronchi stand out black against the collapsed 'white' lung fields).

Breathing
A normal respiratory rate for the neonate is below 60 breaths per minute. Without respiratory support, Arthur will demonstrate signs of respiratory distress due to surfactant deficiency. These signs include nasal flaring, subcostal (underneath ribcage) recession, intercostal (in-between ribs) recession, sternal recession, tracheal tug and an expiratory grunt. Grunting occurs when an infant breathes out against a partially closed glottis in order to prevent alveoli collapse and preserve lung volume. Due to his compliant ribcage and small airways, Arthur also uses accessory abdominal muscles to ensure effective air entry. Therefore, a diaphragmatic breathing pattern is observed.Atelectasis results in ineffective gaseous exchange which means that Arthur would be hypoxic and hypercarbic (high carbon dioxide). Oxygen saturation monitoring and blood gas analysis is important in assessing respiratory function and metabolic parameters (Lynch 2009). Arthur's initial arterial blood gas on admission revealed a respiratory acidosis: pH 7.19, $PaCO_2$ 8.9, PaO_2 6.0, base excess –2, standard bicarbonate 20.

Question 2. Planning: what respiratory support will Arthur require?

In RDS the lack of surfactant causes the alveoli to collapse and high ventilator pressures are then needed to ensure the alveoli can participate in adequate gaseous exchange. These high pressures cause inflammatory changes and protein to leak onto the alveolar surface and form hyaline membranes. In uncomplicated RDS, surfactant production increases from approximately 36–48 hours and the infant's respiratory function then improves (Jollye &

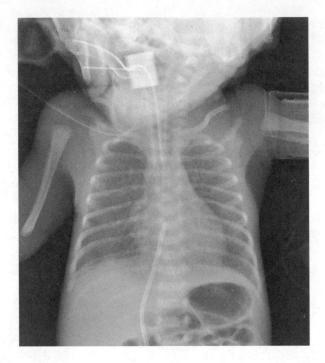

Figure 18.1   Chest X-ray.

Summers 2010). The plan of care for Arthur is therefore to provide respiratory support until this occurs.

The primary cause of Arthur's respiratory distress is due to surfactant deficiency. Administration of exogenous surfactant has improved the outcome for neonates with RDS. Currently, animal-based surfactants such as porcine derived Curosurf® are the treatment of choice as they reduce surface tension more effectively (McDonald & Ainsworth 2004). In preterm infants, particularly below 30 weeks gestation, it would seem that improved outcomes are achieved if surfactant is given prophylactically rather than as a rescue treatment (Stevens *et al.* 2007). Prophylactic surfactant administration with early extubation onto nCPAP can be used to manage RDS in very preterm infants. However, nCPAP at delivery has also been shown to be an effective alternative to intubation and ventilation in treating preterm infants if the infant demonstrates good respiratory effort (Morley *et al.* 2008).

Currently, exogenous surfactant is administered via an ETT, necessitating the infant undergoing the invasive procedure of intubation (BNFC 2010). Arthur received surfactant at delivery in the labour ward. This was undertaken by an experienced practitioner skilled in neonatal resuscitation who was able to verify the correct position of the ETT without a chest X-ray. Following this initial dose of surfactant, Arthur required a further dose at 12 hours of age as he was still requiring ventilatory support and oxygen.

The aim of ventilatory support is to maintain the pressures at which oxygen and carbon dioxide are dissolved in arterial blood within safe limits (Figure 18.2). This support should reduce the work of breathing for the infant and minimise the risk of lung injury. Advances in respiratory technology have resulted in the development of newer methods of mechanical ventilation (Gupta & Sinha 2007). Modern neonatal ventilators have the facility to synchronise the ventilator breath with the respiratory pattern of the infant. Therefore, the infant does not receive a ventilator breath when they are breathing out.

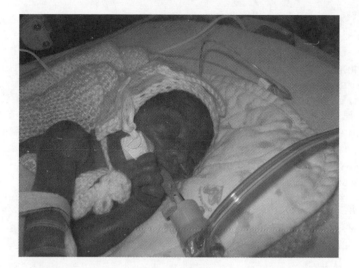

Figure 18.2   Ventilated neonate.

Mechanical ventilation can cause lung injury and contributes to the development of chronic lung disease (CLD) (oxygen requirement at 36 weeks). The plan of care is therefore to provide respiratory support until Arthur's lungs recover and to reduce the risk of CLD. Minimal ventilation is used to promote satisfactory lung inflations for gaseous exchange to occur, as high positive pressures are known to cause 'barotrauma' and high volumes of gas may cause 'volutrauma'. The amount of oxygen administered is carefully controlled as oxygen toxicity can cause lung damage. In infants less than 32 weeks' gestation, constant shifts in oxygenation are thought to be a contributing factor in the pathogenesis of retinopathy of prematurity (ROP) (Coe 2007).

Ventilator requirements will be dependent on arterial or capillary blood gases. Blood gases may need to be taken frequently in the first 24–48 hours and this can contribute to iatrogenic blood loss, necessitating a replacement blood transfusion (Bell 2008). As mechanical ventilation is known to cause lung injury the aim is to extubate Arthur as soon as possible onto nCPAP. This reduces the work of breathing for the infant and is a non-invasive method of respiratory support. The continuous pressure splints the infant's upper airway, reducing obstruction and apnoea, and providing a positive end expiratory pressure (PEEP) which promotes recruitment of alveoli and may also promote chest wall stability (Davis *et al.* 2009).

There are a number of ways of delivering CPAP, but normally it is given via bi-nasal prongs. In bubble CPAP the CPAP pressure is generated by placing the distal limb of the CPAP circuit under a known depth of water, for example $6\,cmH_2O$ (Glynn 2004). In variable flow CPAP there is an integrated nasal interface and pressure generator; the pressure is generated by the increased resistance as the gas leaves the nasal device and enters the infant's nasopharynx (Davis *et al.* 2009).

Question 3. Implementation: what care will Arthur require to optimise his respiratory function?

Airway

It is important to ensure that Arthur has a patent and secure airway. There are a number of ways of securing the ETT, all with the aim of reducing the risk of accidental extubation.

Whilst ventilated, the ETT provides an artificial airway, but its presence can cause problems. The size of the ETT should be big enough to allow effective amounts of gas to enter the lung but not so big that it causes pressure damage to the delicate epithelial lining of the pharynx, larynx and trachea. A small tube will create resistance to the flow of gas and increase the amount of gas leak around the ETT, therefore compromising effective ventilation. The presence of the ETT reduces the normal mucocillary action within the respiratory tract.

Warming and humidifying ventilator gases are vital in loosening secretions and reducing the risk of drying and damage to the mucosa. Secretions will need to be suctioned to maintain an open airway. Suction should only be given if needed and not as a routine procedure and avoided if possible for at least 12 hours following administration of surfactant. Ideally it should be performed by two people and Arthur will need support throughout (see Chapter 12). The type and amount of secretions obtained should be documented. The patency of the ETT can be assessed by observing Arthur's chest for equal movement on both sides, listening in to breath sounds with a stethoscope and ensuring that his oxygen saturations are within normal limits.

Once Arthur no longer requires ventilation, the ETT can be removed. Again, this procedure requires two people, one to carry out the procedure and one to support Arthur (see Chapter 12). The ETT may be suctioned prior to removal and any care that Arthur requires may be carried out beforehand. This means that once Arthur has been extubated he can be left to settle after the procedure. The nasogastric tube should be aspirated and resuscitation equipment readily available. The CPAP device should be ready by the cotside so that Arthur can be placed onto nCPAP just before the ETT is removed, thereby minimising alveolar collapse. The tip of the ETT should be sent to the microbiology laboratory for microscopy, culture and sensitivity (M, C and S).

The size of the nasal prongs and hat required by Arthur are measured using the manufacturer's template and adhering to the manufacturer's and local unit guidelines. It is important to ensure that the bi-nasal prongs fit comfortably in the nares without causing pressure, as erosion of the nasal septum has been documented and is attributed to poor fixation. Observation of the nose is essential and is carried out when care is given. If redness is present the use of a CPAP mask or appropriate hydrocolloid dressing may be indicated.

Ensuring patency of the airway is important. As CPAP may contribute to increased amounts of oral and nasal secretions, assessment of the need for nasal suctioning should be carried out regularly. Gentle suctioning of mouth and then the nares should be given. Loss of CPAP pressure may occur if the neonate's mouth is open. Use of a CPAP dummy (with parental consent) or a chin strap may help minimise this loss of pressure.

Breathing

Arthur's temperature, pulse, respirations, blood pressure and oxygen saturations will be continuously monitored and recorded every hour. At the beginning of each shift the monitor alarm parameters will be set so that if there is an increase or a decrease in Arthur's vital signs the monitor will alarm. The position of the oxygen saturation probe is changed at least every four hours (or more often if instructed by the manufacturer) and documented to reduce the risk of thermal injury and tissue damage (MHRA 2001).

Arthur's respiratory function will be assessed by observing his respiratory pattern, auscultation of the chest and blood gas analysis. Improvements in blood gases mean that Arthur's respiratory function is improving and therefore the ventilation he is receiving can be reduced. The amount of oxygen administered to Arthur will depend on his oxygen saturations and can be increased or decreased according to his needs. In order to promote comfort and synchrony with the ventilation he is receiving, Arthur is given a continuous infusion of morphine (BNFC 2010) whilst ventilated (Bellù *et al.* 2008). He also receives non-pharmacological pain relief throughout his stay on the neonatal unit (see Chapter 12).

The ribcage in the neonate is mostly cartilage rather than bone and so is very compliant. The ribs are horizontal rather than downward sloping and therefore the rigid 'bucket handle' action provided by the ribcage in the child and adult is missing (Randall 2005). It is known that the prone position can reduce the work of breathing for neonates and improve respiratory function. This effect is thought to be due to the mattress creating stability for the compliant ribcage. Arthur is nursed prone and his parents are assured that this position is safe in the acute phase of his illness, as he is being continuously monitored. However, once monitoring is no longer needed, Arthur will be nursed supine (DH 2009).

When extubated onto nCPAP the gastric tube can be left on free drainage and aspirated to reduce the gastric distension caused by air entering the stomach from CPAP. The neonate's abdominal muscles are immature and therefore the neonatal abdomen distends easily. Abdominal distension can cause respiratory compromise and assessment of the abdomen should be undertaken to ensure that it is soft, bowel sounds are present and stools are being passed.

Apnoea of prematurity is common in neonates of less than 32 weeks' gestation. It can be obstructive, central or mixed. It is demonstrated by frequent apnoeas and bradycardias, which may be reversed by gentle stimulation or, if life threatening, may require resuscitative measures, such as lung inflations. Caffeine is administered once daily either orally or intravenously as this medicine stimulates the respiratory centre of the brain (BNFC 2010). As Arthur's respiratory centre is immature, caffeine is prescribed to promote his respiratory drive. He is given a loading dose of caffeine and then receives a daily dose. Apnoeas and bradycardias can also be an indication of a blocked ETT, sepsis or gastro-oesophageal reflux.

Question 4. Evaluation: when will Arthur no longer require respiratory support?

Once Arthur has been stable on nCPAP with good blood gases then the decision may be made to gradually wean him off nCPAP. This can be achieved by taking Arthur off nCPAP for short periods of time or weaning pressures. During this time Arthur will be observed for signs of respiratory distress. High flow nasal cannula oxygen may also be used to support weaning (Armfield & West 2009).

It is likely that Arthur will remain on the neonatal unit until close to his expected date of delivery, i.e. 13 weeks. Indications for discharge will depend on local unit guidelines. Discharge planning should commence on admission and Arthur's parents should be encouraged to participate in his care as soon as possible and throughout his stay on the unit (POPPY 2009). As a premature infant, Arthur is at increased risk of sudden infant death syndrome (SIDS) and therefore his parents will be taught infant cardiopulmonary resuscitation (CPR) prior to discharge (Parsons & MacKinnon 2009). Long-term studies of children born very prematurely suggest that prematurity can have wide-ranging physical and cognitive effects (EPICURE/EPICURE 2). Therefore, Arthur will be followed up closely over his first two years of life and may require frequent readmissions to the children's ward with continuing respiratory needs.

References

Armfield, M. & West, G. (2009) Use of Vapotherm for respiratory support with neonates. *Paediatric Nursing*, **21**(1), 27–30.

Bell, E.F. (2008) When to transfuse preterm babies. *Archives of Disease in Childhood Fetal and Neonatal Edition*, **93**, F469–F473.

Bellù, R., de Waal, K.A. & Zanini, R. (2008) Opioids for neonates receiving mechanical ventilation. *Cochrane Database of Systematic Reviews* Issue 1.

BNFC (2010) *British National Formulary for Children.* London: BMJ Group.

Coe, K. (2007) Nursing update on retinopathy of prematurity. *Journal of Obstetric, Gynecologic and Neonatal Nursing (JOGNN)*, **36**(3), 288–92.

Confidential Enquiry into Maternal and Child Health (CEMACH) (2009) *Perinatal Mortality 2007.* London: CEMACH.

Davis, P., Morley, C. & Owen, L. (2009) Non-invasive respiratory support of preterm neonates with respiratory distress: continuous positive airway pressure and nasal intermittent positive pressure ventilation. *Seminars in Fetal and Neonatal Medicine*, **14**, 14–20.

Department of Health (2009) *Reduce the Risk of Cot Death.* London: DH.

EPICURE/EPICURE 2 Population based studies of survival and later health status in extremely premature infants. www.epicure.ac.uk/ (accessed 30 June 2010).

Fernandez-Alvarez, J.R. & Bomont, R.K. (2009) Algorithm for the management of preterm infants less than 35 weeks gestation at birth. *Infant*, **5**(4), 112–14.

Glynn, G. (2004) A low technology type of device for nasal CPAP: Bubble CPAP. *Journal of Neonatal Nursing*, **10**(4), 108–110.

Gupta, S. & Sinha, S.K. (2007) Newer modalities of mechanical ventilation in the extremely premature infant. *Paediatrics and Child Health*, **17**(2), 37–42.

Jollye, S. & Summers, D. (2010) *Management of respiratory disorders.* In: Boxwell, G. (ed.), 2nd edn. *Neonatal Intensive Care Nursing.* London: Routledge.

Lynch, F. (2009) Arterial blood gas analysis: implications for nursing. *Paediatric Nursing*, **21**(1), 41–44.

McDonald, C. & Ainsworth, S. (2004) An update on the use of surfactant in neonates. *Current Paediatrics*, **14**, 284–9.

Medicines and Health Products Regulatory Agency (MHRA) (2001) *Tissue Necrosis Caused by Pulse Oximeter Probes.* SN 2001 (08). London: MHRA.

Moore, K.L. & Persaud, T.V.N. (2008) *The Developing Human: Clinically Oriented Embryology*, 8th edn. Pennsylvaia: Elsevier Science.

Morley, C., Davis, P., Doyle, L., Brion, L., Hadcoet, J. & Carlin, J. (2008) Nasal CPAP or intubation at birth for very preterm infants. *New England Journal of Medicine*, **358**, 700–8.

National Audit Office (2007) *Caring for Vulnerable Babies: the Reorganisation of Neonatal Services in England.* London: HMSO.

Parsons, S. & MacKinnon, R.J. (2009) Teaching parents infant resuscitation. *Infant*, **5**(3), 77–80.

Pinheiro, J.M.B. (2009) The Apgar cycle: a new view of a familiar scoring system. *Archives of Disease in Childhood Fetal and Neonatal Edition*, **94**, F70–F72.

POPPY (Parents of Premature Babies Project) (2009) *Family-centred Care in Neonatal Units.* London: National Childbirth Trust.

Randall, D. (2005) Development of the respiratory system and respiration. In: Chamley Chamley, C., Carson, P. & Randall D. (eds) *Developmental Anatomy and Physiology of Children.* UK: Elsevier Churchill Livingstone.

Resuscitation Council (UK) (2005) *Newborn Life Support.* London: Resuscitation Council (UK).

Stevens, T., Blennow, E., Myers, E. & Soll, R. (2007) Early surfactant administration with brief ventilation vs. selective surfactant and continued mechanical ventilation for preterm infants with or at risk for respiratory distress syndrome. *Cochrane Database of Systematic Reviews* 2007 Issue 4.

Sweet, D., Bevilacqua, G., & Carnielli, V., *et al.* (2007) European consensus guidelines on the management of neonatal respiratory distress syndrome. *Journal of Perinatal Medicine*, **35**(3), 175–86.

19

Cystic Fibrosis

Hazel Mills and Mary MacFarlane

Scenario

James is an eight-year-old boy with cystic fibrosis (CF) admitted to hospital for intravenous antibiotics. He is an only child and lives at home with his parents Patrick and Sarah. James was diagnosed with CF at six weeks of age, by neonatal screening. He was admitted to hospital at that time for five days to initiate treatment and teach his parents the management of CF.

Cystic fibrosis is an inherited, multi-system disorder affecting infants, children and adults as a result of a defect in the cystic fibrosis transmembrane conductance regulator (CFTR) gene (Rosenstein & Cutting 1998). It results in dysfunction of the exocrine glands affecting particularly the respiratory tract, digestive tract, pancreas and sweat glands (CFF 2006).

The hallmark of cystic fibrosis is excessive mucus production, chronic respiratory infection, leading to airway inflammation and progressive lung disease, which is regarded as having the greatest role in morbidity (Chmiel *et al.* 2002). Other manifestations include pancreatic insufficiency, leading to fat malabsorption, failure to gain weight and poor absorption of fat soluble vitamins, high levels of electrolytes in sweat and later complications of biliary cirrhosis and diabetes (De Boeck *et al.* 2006).

The clinical presentation may vary between individuals (Rosenstein & Cutting 1998). Cystic fibrosis can present early, with meconium ileus on the first day of life, or later in life with infertility in otherwise healthy males. The most common presentation of CF is with malabsorption, failure to thrive and chronic cough. The lower airways of patients with CF are typically infected with, initially, *Staphylococcus aureus*, later with *Haemophilus influenzae* and ultimately with *Pseudomonas aeruginosa* (PA) (Khan *et al.* 1995).

Care Planning in Children and Young People's Nursing, First Edition.
Edited by Doris Corkin, Sonya Clarke, Lorna Liggett.
© 2012 Blackwell Publishing Ltd. Published 2012 by Blackwell Publishing Ltd.

Pseudomonas has been cultured from cough swabs since James was three years old. Initially this was successfully treated with a three-month course of oral ciprofloxacin and nebulised colistin. When James was four years old PA grew again and this time the eradication therapy failed to clear the pseudomonas, resulting in regular admissions for intravenous antibiotics. James is reviewed 2–3 monthly at OPC where, if required, admissions or a change of treatment is arranged. Intravenous antibiotics are usually required when James' cough and sputum production increases, appetite and energy levels decrease and there is a decline in lung functions.

Peripheral venous access eventually became difficult so James had a TIVAD (totally implantable venous access device) inserted when he was five years old. James finds accessing of the TIVAD frightening and uncomfortable despite much reassurance. Admissions are generally for 10 to14 days during which time James is confined to his room.

 Questions

1. How is CF diagnosed?
2. Discuss the medication prescribed to James, the newly diagnosed baby with CF.
3. What is a totally implantable venous access device (TIVAD)?
4. How would the children's nurse plan care to reduce James' anxiety during the accessing of the TIVAD?
5. Discuss how the children's nurse would devise a care plan to meet James' needs in relation to respiratory function.
6. What is the role of the community CF nurse specialist?

Answers to questions

Question 1. How is CF diagnosed?

Based on the presence of clinical features CF is confirmed by several different investigations. CF can present from birth through to adulthood and severity can vary from mild to severe. In the CF population 10–15% of babies will present with meconium ileus within 24–48 hours (failure to pass first stool). This may result in abdominal distension and vomiting. These babies should then be transferred to the regional infant surgical unit, for further treatment and investigations. Initially rectal gastrograffin may be tried under radiological conditions. Gastrograffin draws fluid into the bowel and helps to expel faecal matter. If unsuccessful a surgical laparotomy will be required to relieve the obstruction. Bloods should be sent for genetic mutation analysis for CF.

What is immune reactive trypsin (IRT)?

Trypsinogen is a naturally occurring substance produced in the pancreas. In CF babies the mucus they produce can prevent the trypsinogen from leaving the pancreas and reaching the small bowel. This then allows the trypsinogen level to build up in the blood.

When is the IRT test carried out?

A sample of blood is collected from the heel of a baby aged 5–8 days. This blood is placed on a special card which when dry is sent to biochemistry laboratory for analysis.

In August 2009, a national screening programme was rolled out across the UK. Prior to this Northern Ireland had screened all babies born for CF on the routine heel prick test from 1983. The following route for screening is now been carried out:

1. Normal in full (IRT) → CF not suspected
2. Raised IRT → genetic analysis→no mutation → repeat IRT → normal limits → CF not suspected
3. Raised IRT → genetic analysis → two mutations identified → CF suspected → sweat test → confirmed diagnosis
4. Raised IRT → genetic analysis → one mutation identified → repeat IRT → raised IRT→ sweat test → confirmcd diagnosis or carrier for CF gene
(Northern Ireland Bloodspot Screening Programme DHSSPSNI 2009)

Question 2. Discuss the medication prescribed to James, the newly diagnosed baby with CF.

1. From time of diagnosis all patients will be commenced on an anti-staphylococcus prophylactic antibiotic, usually flucloxacillin. This will help to reduce staphylococcal infection and subsequent inflammation during the time of lung development when the lung is most vulnerable (BNFC 2010–2011).
2. Multivitamins are administered on a daily basis: vitamin E and multivitamins containing A+D. The rationale for giving these specific preparations is the malabsorption due to the pancreatic insufficiency in the CF person. Dosage varies according to age and plasma levels. Plasma levels should be checked annually as most children with CF have problems with malabsorption. To ensure these children reach optimum vitamin levels to promote health and wellbeing all children are prescribed fat soluble vitamins on a daily basis. Therefore levels are checked to ensure an adequate dose is being prescribed and administered.
3. Pancreatic enzyme supplements are required by approximately 90% of the CF population. This is due to an inadequacy of their own pancreatic secretions. Pancreatic enzyme replacement should be started as soon as pancreatic insufficiency is established. Dosage should be adjusted according to weight gain, number and consistency of bowel movements. Enzyme replacement capsules, for example Creon 10,000, are administered immediately prior to all feeds (BNFC 2010–2011). They are opened and the small microspheres are placed on a spoon and delivered to the baby.

Question 3. What is a totally implantable venous access device (TIVAD)?

Totally implantable venous access devices were developed to overcome the problems associated with repeated venous access in patients needing long-term intravenous therapy. The implantable port requires surgical placement under general anaesthetic. It is placed completely under the skin, usually the chest or arm, and consists of two components (Figures 19.1 and 19.2):

1. A portal chamber made of titanium and a silicone septum (injection area).
2. A radio-opaque silicone catheter which is introduced into the cephalic, jugular or subclavian veins.

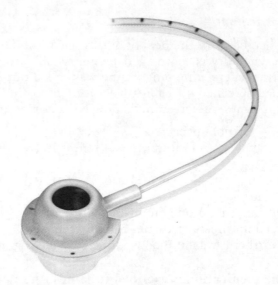

Figure 19.1   A totally implantable venous access device. Image provided by Vygon (UK) Ltd and used with kind permission.

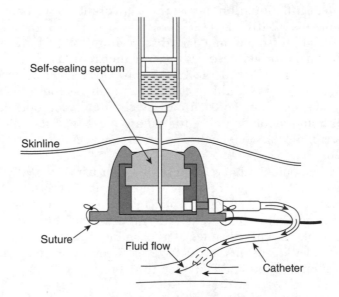

Figure 19.2   Diagram showing a needle inserted through the skin and silicone septum into the portal chamber. Image provided by Vygon (UK) Ltd and used with kind permission.

Medication is given into the TIVAD by inserting a non-coring needle through the skin into the portal chamber and injecting or infusing the drugs, which will travel along the catheter into the veins (Vygon 2009). A sterile, transparent, semi-permeable adhesive dressing is used to secure the needle in place. The intravenous system must be flushed and a heparin lock established following each usage and at least every four weeks between uses (Weblock 2009).

Table 19.1 Advantages and disadvantages of TIVAD devices.

Advantages of TIVAD device	Disadvantages of TIVAD device
Fully implantable	Need to use special needle
Reduced risk of infection compared to a central line	Device is expensive
Less interference with everyday activities – child is able to bath/shower/swim	Surgery required for insertion
Low maintenance – requires infrequent flushing	Two people required for flushing
Less risk of displacement compared to a central line if not treated promptly	Infections can be life threatening
Can be cosmetically placed	Other possible complications – access difficulties, blockage, leakage or difficulty with removal of catheter, if required

For further reading, seek local regional or trust guidelines: *Care of the Child with a Totally Implantable Venous Access Device and Procedure for Flushing a Port-a-cath.* See Table 19.1.

Question 4. How would the children's nurse plan care to reduce James' anxiety during the accessing of the TIVAD?

Problem: communication (Roper *et al.* 2000).
   James is anxious about having his TIVAD accessed.
   Goal: to minimise James' anxiety.

Nursing action

- Assess level of anxiety.
- Plan strategies to help reduce anxiety. A procedure preparation programme which involves the use of strategies such as role play, distraction and reassurance may be effective (Jelbert *et al.* 2005)
- James should be settled into a child and family friendly environment, be made comfortable with his surroundings and introduced to his named nurse on admission.
- A family-centred approach should be adopted to include the family's participation in aspects of care.
- If possible, give James a choice of where the procedure is carried out, for example treatment room or own side ward.
- Ensure James is in a comfortable position on examination couch/bed.
- Consider James' privacy needs during the procedure.
- Facilitate questions James or his parents may have regarding the procedure.
- Following discussion with the play therapist regarding information already communicated to James and his parents the children's nurse should give a brief explanation of the procedure including:
  — The use of local anaesthetic cream, for example Emla™, Ametop™
  — Cleansing of the injection site with antiseptic solution as this is an aseptic procedure
  — The port will be held in place whilst the needle is inserted
  — A slight pricking sensation may be felt as the needle passes through the skin

— Saline and heparin flushes will be administered through the TIVAD
— The needle will be taped in place with a suitable dressing material
- If possible allow James to decide when he is ready for the procedure to begin.
- Reassure James during the procedure.
- Keep James and his parents informed of what is happening during the insertion of the TIVAD needle.
- At the end praise and reward James for completing the procedure.

Evaluation: document all care, recording the strategies which were most useful at reducing anxiety.

Question 5. Discuss how the children's nurse would devise a care plan to meet James' needs in relation to respiratory function.

Problem: breathing (Roper *et al.* 2000).
  James has been admitted for treatment of a chest infection.
  Goals:

1. To relieve symptoms of respiratory distress
2. To safely administer medication to treat Infection

Nursing action

1. Record vital signs – temperature, pulse, respiratory rate and oxygen saturations.
2. Report any deviation from within normal limits to doctor or nurse in charge.
3. Observe rate, rhythm and depth of breathing.
4. Observe for coughing and note colour and consistency of sputum.
5. Ensure James has sputum cartons to allow expectoration of sputum.
6. Nurse sitting upright beside suction and oxygen.
7. Inform physiotherapists of admission to initiate chest physiotherapy and carry out lung function tests.
8. Encourage oral fluids to maintain hydration and help reduce viscosity of sputum.
9. Administer medication as prescribed; observe for effects and side effects.

Evaluation: record and report to James and his parents, in suitable terms, changes in:

- Vital signs
- Cough and mucus production
- Energy levels
- Appetite and weight

Problem: maintaining a safe environment (Roper *et al.* 2000).
  James has a TIVAD *in situ*.
  Goal: to ensure safe administration of intravenous antibiotics and patency of line.

Nursing action

1. Access the device using aseptic technique.
2. Two registered nurses to check each antibiotic, name, dose, route of administration.

3. Check patient details on drug Kardex® and patient armband – name, date of birth and hospital number.
4. Inform James of administration and alleviate any anxieties.
5. Administer antibiotics using the protocol for TIVADS.
6. Observe site for redness, swelling, and pain – stop administration if James experiences any problems and report immediately to doctor or nurse in charge.
7. Record administration of medication.
8. Observe for any side effects and report immediately to doctor or nurse in charge and take appropriate action.
10. Nurse beside working oxygen and suction in case of emergency.

Evaluation:

• Record and report changes in respiratory function.
• Observe port site for redness and swelling when needle removed at end of IV course.

Question 6. What is the role of the community CF nurse specialist?

In Northern Ireland, all children with CF attend the Regional Paediatric Centre in Belfast. Between the regular check-up visits or hospital stays the community CF nurse visits the home to provide assessment of health, advice and support to both children and their parents. Treatments can also be initiated at home, which reduces hospital attendance. Home visits can allow parents, who are often anxious, to ask appropriate questions that they may feel unable to do in a hospital environment. At time of diagnosis the CF nurse links closely to the child's other health providers, for example GP and health visitor, educating them on the individual treatment and management of the CF child. The community CF nurse will liaise with schools at time of starting, transferring or at other times when issues may arise, to ensure the child with CF is given every aid as required with their education. Indeed throughout the child's years until they transfer to the adult services the CF nurse is there to provide all possible assistance that these families and children may need. The community CF nurse is fortunate to be part a dedicated team of professionals who look after these children and can contact colleagues for advice when required.

References

BNFC (2010–2011) *British National Formulary for Children*. London: BMJ Group.
Chmiel, J.F., Berger, M. & Konstan, M.W. (2002) The role of inflammation in the pathophysiology of CF lung disease. *Clin Rev Allergy Immunol*, **23**, 5–27.
Cystic Fibrosis Foundation (2006) *Cystic Fibrosis Foundation Patient Registry, 2006*. Annual data report. Bethesda, MD: Cystic Fibrosis Foundation.
De Boeck, K., Wilschanski, M., Castellani, C., *et al.* (2006) Cystic fibrosis: terminology and diagnostic algorithms. *Thorax*, **61**, 627–35.
Jelbert, R., Caddy, G., Mortimer, J. & Frampton, I. (2005) Procedure preparation works! An open trial of twenty-four children with needle phobia or anticipatory anxiety. *The Journal of the National Association of Hospital Play Staff*, **36**, 14–18.
Khan, T.Z., Wagener, J.S., Bost, T., Martinez, J., Accuroso, F.J., & Riches, D.W. (1995) Early pulmonary inflammation in infants with cystic fibrosis. *Am Journal Respiratory Critical Care Med*, **151**, 1075–82.

The Department of Health, Social Services and Public Safety Northern Ireland (DHSSPSNI) (2009) *Northern Ireland Bloodspot Screening Programme, MCADD and Revised CF Screening Implementation, April 2009*. Northern Ireland: DHSSPSNI.

Roper, N., Logan, W.W. & Tierney, A.J. (2000) *The Roper-Logan Tierney Model of Nursing: Based on Activities of Living*. http://books.google.co.uk/books?id=RJ211KAZQQ4C. Edinburgh: Elsevier Health Sciences.

Rosentein, B.J. & Cutting, G.R. (1998) The diagnosis of cystic fibrosis: a consensus statement. *Journal Pediatr*, **132**, 589–95.

Vygon (2009) *Patient Information for Sitimplant Implantable Port System*. Vygon (UK) Limited, Bridge Road, Cirencester, Gloucestershire, UK.

Weblock, K. (2009) *The Use of Totally Implantable Access Devices in Cystic Fibrosis*. www.cftrust.org.uk/aboutcf/publications/factsheets/ports.

20

Asthma

Barbara Maxwell

Scenario

George is a five-year-old boy (weighing 19 kg), who lives at home with his eight-year-old sister and both parents (smokers). George's sister, Daisy, suffers from eczema and was diagnosed three years ago with exercise-induced asthma and often self-administers a dry powder bronchodilator prior to playing hockey.

George's previous history included bronchiolitis when he was a five months old, when he required hospital admission. Since then George has been susceptible to intermittent 'wheezy' episodes. His mum administers a bronchodilator metered dose inhaler (MDI) to George as and when required. To date he has never needed inhalers at school. However, over the past two years George has generally needed his bronchodilators more frequently during the summer months.

Today, as part of his summer school trip, George went to visit a local farm where he and his friends met and stroked farmyard animals. When George's mum picked him up from school at 3 pm he was slightly breathless, complaining about tightness in his chest and unable to tell his mum about his school trip. George's mum brought him to be assessed by his GP.

On oscultation the GP observed George to have an inspiratory wheeze accompanied by marked respiratory effort. He prescribed ten puffs of a bronchodilator (100 mcg per dose) via a yellow aerochamber. George's symptoms did not improve so he was referred to his local children's hospital.

In A&E, the triage nurse noted George to have an audible wheeze, nasal flaring and that he was unable to complete sentences. His respiratory rate was 56, heart rate 128 and oxygen saturations 88% in room air.

Care Planning in Children and Young People's Nursing, First Edition.
Edited by Doris Corkin, Sonya Clarke, Lorna Liggett.
© 2012 Blackwell Publishing Ltd. Published 2012 by Blackwell Publishing Ltd.

Activity 20.1

Please read the British Thoracic Guidelines (2005) in relation to asthma management.

Questions

1. What is asthma?
2. Discuss the importance of monitoring vital signs.
3. What are the risk and trigger factors of asthma?
4. Explain the importance of asthma medication and education.
5. Plan George's discharge from hospital.

Answers to questions

Question 1. What is asthma?

Asthma is a common and chronic inflammatory disorder of the airways and it can affect both adults and children of all ages (Price *et al.* 2004).

During an exacerbation of asthma, bronchoconstriction causes obstruction in the airways and therefore limits airflow. The obstruction in the airway is partially or completely reversible and this occurs either spontaneously or due to therapeutic interventions. The smooth muscle goes into spasm; there is also increased mucus secretion and cellular infiltration of the airway walls mainly by eosinophils, which leads to epithelial damage (Scullion 2005).

The tightness George felt in his chest was as a direct result of his airways narrowing and spasm of the smooth muscle, probably as a result of the exposure to the farmyard animals.

Activity 20.2

Blow out a candle until you have expelled all the air in your lungs. Inhale approximately 50% of air back into your lungs. Fully exhale again and once more inhale 50% of what you've just exhaled back into your lungs. If you keep repeating this task for a few minutes, the sensation you feel should be one of a 'tight' chest.

Reflect upon the scenario: apply Roper *et al.* (1996) model of care.
Activity of living: breathing.

In A&E the doctor prescribed ten puffs (100 mcg/puff) of salbutamol. Terbutaline is also a commonly used bronchodilator. An MDI device was chosen to administer the drug via a yellow aerochamber. It was administered by a member of the nursing team in accordance with Nursing and Midwifery Council guidelines (NMC 2008). Doses prescribed were based on the British Guidelines on the Management of Asthma (2008/2011) (see Appendix 6).

George's condition did not improve and he was beginning to feel agitated and frightened because of his breathing difficulties. He was reassured by the doctors and nurses. After 15 minutes he was reassessed by the medical team. The same prescribed dose of bronchodilator was administered again on two further occasions, unfortunately with no obvious improvement. George was also commenced on an oral steroid (prednisolone 30 mg). It was decided at this point that he needed to be admitted to the paediatric medical ward.

✎ Activity 20.3

Write a care plan based on the Roper *et al.* (1996) model in relation to breathing, then compare with Appendix 7.

Question 2. Discuss the importance of monitoring vital signs.

Activity of living: maintaining a safe environment.

On admission to the acute medical ward, George was tachypnoeic (respiratory rate: 52) and tachycardic (heart rate: 128). George was using his accessory muscles. Use of accessory muscles is indicated by nasal flaring, sternal recession and over-inflation of the chest wall. These symptoms are due to the respiratory system having to compensate for the narrowing of the airways.

George was pale, his oxygen saturations (SaO_2) were 88% in room air. Normal oxygen saturations are usually >95%, a reading of <93% will require oxygen (O_2) therapy.

Oxygen passes through the alveolar capillary interface of the lungs into the circulation during respiration and is then transported to the tissues of the red blood cells attached to haemoglobin (Hb). Each molecule of Hb can potentially carry four O_2 molecules, which form oxyhaemaglobin. In conditions where the level of O_2 in the tissues is low, oxyhaemaglobin breaks down and releases O_2 to the tissues (Boooker 2008).

SaO_2 is the percentage of Hb absorbed with the O_2 and measured in the arterial blood. SpO_2, meanwhile, is the process used for measuring pulse oximetry. Pulse oximetry, when performed correctly, is accurate to within plus or minus 3% of SpO_2 at higher ranges, but reflects SaO_2 less accurately when SpO_2 falls below 80% (Jubran 1999).

As part of good practice, paediatric nurses must assess the child holistically and not just rely on monitors, for example observing vital signs, monitoring patient's use of accessory muscles, shortness of breath and skin colour. Signs of pallor or cyanosis as well as low SpO_2 are all indicators that O_2 therapy may have to be prescribed and administered. In George's case two litres O_2 therapy was commenced via nasal specs, resulting in his SpO_2 rising from 88% to 95%.

When attaching the saturation probe to an infant's/child's thumb or toe, the light sensor needs to be attached directly opposite the probe to give a true reading (Booker 2008). It is also worth noting that nail varnish can interfere with SpO_2 readings and therefore needs to be removed where applicable (Booker 2007a).

A quick and easy way to assist in the diagnosis of asthma is to measure peak expiratory flow (PEF). This is a simple, cheap test which measures lung function. It is measured in litres/minute and occurs early in a forced expiration to within the first tenth of a second (Booker 2007b). Booker (2007b) also states that calculation of a patient's percentage of reference value for PEF is the formula:

$$\frac{\text{PEF recording}}{\text{patient's best recording}} \times 100$$

If the patient feels well enough to perform PEF he/she should stand, take in a deep breath and expel all the air from their lungs in one simple puff. This exercise should be repeated on three occasions and the best of the three readings taken into consideration. Peak expiratory flow is generally used in the over five years age bracket; however, George found the exercise too difficult pre- and post-administration of bronchodilators so it was not recorded after two attempts. If it had been successful a change of around 15–20% pre- and post-bronchodilator administration is indicative of asthma (Scullion 2005).

Spirometry testing in children >5 years assesses airway obstruction. It is rarely useful during exacerbations of asthma, except where air leaks are suspected. However, it is useful when a diagnosis other than asthma is suspected (Townshend *et al.* 2007a).

Question 3. What are the risk and trigger factors of asthma?

It is important for medical and nursing staff to take a detailed history of symptoms during any consultation in a hospital ward/outpatients or a GP surgery.

In George's case he had a higher probability of developing asthma compared to his peers. Family history included George's sister, Daisy, who was known to suffer from asthma and eczema. Both parents were smokers and Daisy had had a previous history of bronchiolitis.

A risk factor increases the probability of a person developing asthma, whereas a trigger factor may be the instigating factor during an exacerbation of asthma.

Risks: family history of atopy/allergy, gender (more common in males than females), passive smoking, certain foods and recurrent chest infections.

Triggers: viruses, house dust mites, cat allergens, pollens, exercise, emotions (e.g. stress), drugs (e.g. NSAIDs) and cold air (Scullion 2005).

Both of George's parents were smokers. Smoking during pregnancy increases the child's risk of respiratory conditions by 35%. Also, children whose parents smoke face a 50% increased risk of developing asthma (Asthma UK 2005).

George's sister Daisy also had a history of eczema. Atopic conditions such as eczema and rhinitis increase the probability of asthma (British Guideline on Management of Asthma 2008/2011).

Daisy's asthmatic symptoms became worse when playing outdoor sports. In George's case his symptoms became worse once he was exposed to farmyard animals. Skin prick testing could confirm George's allergens. If positive, George would then avoid known trigger factors.

One reason why atopic asthma patients wheeze with viruses is due to the fact that they are born with smaller airway dimensions than those who do not wheeze (Townshend *et al.* 2007b).

Question 4. Explain the importance of asthma medication and education.

George's symptoms improved with the assistance of various medications:

1. Bronchodilators: open up the airways
2. Steroids (inhaled and oral): reduce airway inflammation
3. Montelukast: leukotriene receptor antagonist

George's respiratory symptoms initially did not improve with the aid of an MDI via spacer device. He was prescribed and administered bronchodilators via a nebuliser device which was attached to the O$_2$ mains by his bedside. Nebulisers are instruments designed to atomise liquid drugs into fine mists for inhalation into the lungs (Booker 2007a). Booker (2007a) also states that nebulisers require a driving gas flow rate of 6–8 litres. Nebulisation of normal volume of drug (2–4 ml) should be complete in about ten minutes. Realistically it may be necessary to reduce the time to around five minutes when administering nebulisers to infants. Toddlers often find the mist from nebulisers quite scary and generally do not like to be held for long periods.

The mist of the drug can only be delivered to the lungs once the patient has inhaled. Therefore the nebulised drug is wasted during exhalation (Booker 2007a). Since so much of the drug is wasted it is important to keep the nebuliser mask sealed to the child's face and not wafting from a short distance from the face to ensure that maximum dose is administered.

Nebulised salbutamol 2.5 mg was prescribed half-hourly for one hour. Initially no improvement was noted so ipratropium bromide 0.25 mg (a B2 agonist) was added in. As George's symptoms improved, the frequency of nebuliser therapy was increased from one to four hourly. His mum noticed that George's hands had started to shake.

Side effects of bronchodilators include fine tremor of the hands, tachycardia and hypocalcaemia (BNFC 2010–2011). Around 12% of the nebulised drug which leaves the chamber enters the lungs, but the majority of the drug stays in the apparatus (Rees 2005).

Once George's symptoms improved and vital signs settled to within normal limits, i.e. heart rate 98, respiratory rate 28 and SpO$_2$ 95% in room air he was changed to an MDI via a yellow spacer device. Aerochambers generally fit all forms of MDIs. They are available in three different sizes:

• Brown: has mask attached, suitable for children <1 year.
• Yellow: has mask attached, suitable for children aged 1–6 years.
• Blue: has mouthpiece attached, suitable for children and adults who can control breathing.

Activity 20.4

Describe how you would demonstrate to a child the most effective way to administer inhalers. See photos of children using an MDI with aerochambers (Figures 20.1 and 20.2).

When an MDI is used correctly, approximately 10% of the drug reaches the airways below the larynx. The rest of the drug is deposited no further than the oropharynx and is ultimately swallowed (Rees 2005). When using a spacer, tidal breathing (normal breathing rate) is equally as effective as deep breaths. Please note: if MDI or dry-powdered devices are prescribed then the patient will be required to take a sharp intake of inspiration. If used with a spacer device, MDIs are easier and more effective to use. All children aged less than five years should use an MDI with a spacer (Newell & Hume 2006).

George's nurse taught him and his parents the correct way to administer his MDI via his yellow spacer and correct breathing technique. When administering each dose the MDI

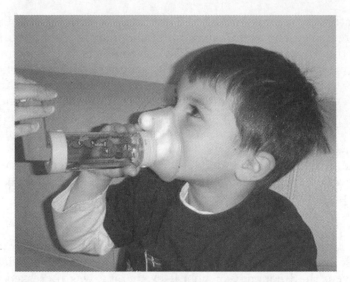

Figure 20.1   Child using an aerochamber with mask.

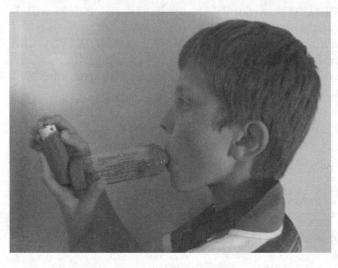

Figure 20.2   Medication via aerochamber.

should be shaken, attached to the aerochamber and the mask fitted properly to George's face.

George was encouraged to breathe normally and his mum advised to count to ten in between each dose. If further doses are required, the MDI should be removed from the aerochamber and shaken in between each use. George's mum was also taught to rinse out the aerochamber once weekly in warm soapy water and to leave it to air dry. Aerochambers should be replaced every 6–12 months (Rees 2005).

Older patients have the option of using a MDIs or dry powdered inhalers such as turbohalers and accuhalers. The dry powder inhalers may make patients cough. Patients who are prescribed inhaled steroids should be encouraged to rinse their mouths after each use to prevent the common side effect candidiasis (BNF 2010–2011).

George's doctor prescribed a bronchodilator for QID (four times daily) use for four days post-discharge and then to be administered on a PRN basis only. He was also to complete a three-day course in total of oral steroids (1–2 mg/kg).

Question 5. Plan George's discharge from hospital.

Activity of living: communication (Casey 1988; Roper *et al.* 1996).

According to the BTS/SIGN guidelines (2005) all people with asthma should have access to primary care which is delivered by doctors with appropriate training in asthma management (Scullion 2005).

People with asthma need the NHS to provide two main approaches of care:

1. *'Proactive'*, i.e. routine appointments with doctors and nurses for reviews, repeat prescriptions and personal written asthma plans.
2. *'Reactive'*, i.e. emergency care in hospital or with a doctor to regain control of worsening symptoms (Asthma UK 2004).

Planning the discharge for any child from a paediatric ward should begin from admission. The BTS guidelines (2005) recommend that all patients with asthma should have a written, individualised asthma management plan (Townsend *et al.* 2007b).

Appendix 8 shows an example of written asthma guidelines used at a regional children's hospital. The details include name of patient, GP, hospital consultant, as well as emergency contact telephone numbers in the event of an asthma attack. Each treatment card should include clear concise information and advice in regards to treatment and include a list of possible trigger factors, early/late signs and symptoms of asthma, as well as personalised treatment plans. The plans should include prescribed medication on a day-to-day basis as well as increased dosages required during an exacerbation of asthma. Parents and children should be aware that 'blue' inhalers are relievers (bronchodilators) and 'brown' inhalers are preventers (steroids which aim to prevent exacerbations of asthma). Please refer to the BNFC (2010–2011) to increase knowledge of short and long-acting inhaled bronchodilators and inhaled steroids.

Austin *et al.* (2005) has stated that children with asthma miss more days off school than their peers. Since George was only five years old, he still enjoyed school especially his school trips and was not keen to miss playing with his friends.

As part of discharge planning, the multidisciplinary team need to educate children as well as parents. Health professionals often talk to the carers instead of children, which can make children feel intimidated. Parents tend to see their role as carer and advocator (Iley 2007). Children need to take a certain amount of responsibility for their condition so that they recognise the warning signs because their parents will not always be with them. Parents also need to inform other people, for example teachers, grandparents or friends about medication and action required during asthma attacks. Educating the family unit will benefit the whole family (Casey 1988). Children with asthma frequently tend to have a nocturnal cough. A child's cough can be distressing and also have a significant impact on their sleep, school performance and play (Shields *et al.* 2008). Therefore effective therapeutic treatments will contribute to the whole family having undisturbed sleep.

While in the hospital ward, George and his mum were advised to avoid trigger factors such as farmyard animals. George was to be referred back to the hospital for skin prick testing to confirm potential allergens (Whaley & Wong 1999). George's mum and dad were also advised to stop smoking. Many parents are under the illusion that if they smoke 'out the back' they are not exposing their children to nicotine; this is not the case as cigarette smoke lingers on clothing for many hours.

George was discharged from hospital and was to be reviewed by his GP within two weeks. At each further consultation, whether at a GP centre or asthma clinic, each asthmatic patient should have their inhaler technique reviewed to ensure the maintenance of good inhaler technique (BTS & SIGN 2005). By acting as conscientious and dedicated health professionals and through ongoing education and support during each consultation with child and parent, asthmatic children should lead a relatively normal lifestyle.

References

Asthma UK (2004) *Where Do We Stand, Asthma in the UK Today.* 1–15. London: Asthma UK.

Asthma UK (2005) *A Moving Picture, Asthma in Northern Ireland Today.* 1–11. Belfast: Asthma UK.

Austin, J.B., Selvaraj, S., Godden, D. & Russell, G. (2005) Deprivation, smoking and quality of life in asthma. *Archives of Disease in Childhood*, **90**(3), 253–7.

BNF for Children (2010–2011) *BNF for Children.* London: BMJ Publishing group.

Bowlby, J. (1953) *Child Care and the Growth of Love.* Harmondsworth: Penguin.

Booker, R. (2007a) Correct use of nebulisers. *Nursing Standard*, **22**(8), 39–41.

Booker, R. (2007b) Peak expiratory flow measurement. *Nursing Standard*, **21**(39), 42–3.

Booker, R. (2008) Pulse oximetry. *Nursing Standard*, **22**(30), 39–41.

British Guideline on the Management of Asthma (2008, revised 2011) *Thorax*, **63**, supplement iv, iv1–iv121.

British Thoracic Society and Scottish Intercollegiate Guidelines Network (2005) *British Guideline on the Management of Asthma: a National Clinical Guideline.* London: BTS.

Casey, A. (1988) A partnership with child and family. *Senior Nurse*, **8**(4), 8–9.

Iley, K. (2007) The impact of asthma on children's lives: a social perspective. *Primary Health Care*, **17**(8), 25–9.

Jubran, A. (1999) Pulse oximetry. *Critical Care*, **3**(2), 11–17.

Newell, K. & Hume, S. (2006) Choosing the right inhaler for patients with asthma. *Nursing Standard*, **21**(5), 46–8.

Nursing and Midwifery Council (2008) *The Code – Standards of Conduct, Performance and Ethics for Nurses and Midwives.* London: NMC.

Price, D., Foster, J., Scullion, J. & Freeman, D. (2004) *Asthma and COPD.* London: Churchill Livingstone.

Rees, J. (2005) ABC of asthma, methods of delivering drugs. *British Medical Journal*, **331**, 504–6.

Roper, N., Logan, W. & Tierney, A. (1996) *The Elements of Nursing*, 4th edn. Edinburgh: Churchill Livingstone.

Scullion, J. (2005) A proactive approach to asthma. *Nursing Standard*, **20**(9), 57–65.

Shields, M.D., Bush, A., Everard, M.L., McKenzie, S., Primhak, R. and on behalf of the British Thoracic Society Cough Guideline Group (2008) Recommendations for the assessment and management of cough in children. *Thorax*, **63**, 1–15.

Townshend, J., Hails, S. & McKean, M. (2007a) Management of asthma in children. *British Medical Journal*, **335**, 253–7.

Townshend, J., Hails, S. & McKean, M. (2007b) Diagnosis of asthma in children. *British Medical Journal*, **335**, 198–202.

Whaley, L.F. & Wong, D.L. (1999) *Nursing Care of Infants and Children*, 6th edn. St Louis: Mosby.

Section 5

Care of Infants and Young Persons with Cardiac Conditions

21

Cardiac Catheterisation
Pauline Carson

Scenario

David is 13 years old and has a history of pulmonary valve stenosis and asthma. When he was three years old David underwent a balloon pulmonary valvuloplasty to relieve the stenosis, and has had routine yearly cardiac follow up since then. During his last clinic visit some restenosis of his pulmonary valve was identified and it was decided that a second balloon pulmonary valvuloplasty was required to relieve the stenosis and he has now been admitted for cardiac catheterisation and a balloon pulmonary valvuloplasty. David's asthma was diagnosed when he was six, it is well controlled with inhalers and he has not required hospitalisation since his initial diagnosis. He administers his own inhalers but often has to be reminded to do so by his parents.

David is in his second year at senior school, where he has lots of friends who he enjoys spending time with. He enjoys playing football and cricket, swimming and playing on his Xbox with friends and is a sociable and active teenager. Apart from becoming wheezy when he plays football neither of his conditions has restricted his education or his involvement in sports. On admission to the ward David is very quiet, his parents answer most of the questions and also tell you that David has recently started to argue with them all the time. On talking to David afterwards he tells you that his parents think he should not play football and they do not allow him to stay over with friends or go on overnight trips with school because of his heart and asthma problems and that's what causes the arguments. He says his older brothers tend to protect him although he does not want to be different from his friends and wants to do all the things they do. David also says he is worried about being in hospital and having an 'operation' as he does not remember the first one and he is also concerned that his friends will not be allowed in to visit.

Care Planning in Children and Young People's Nursing, First Edition.
Edited by Doris Corkin, Sonya Clarke, Lorna Liggett.
© 2012 Blackwell Publishing Ltd. Published 2012 by Blackwell Publishing Ltd.

> **Questions**
>
> 1. What is congenital heart disease and how are defects classified?
> 2. What is pulmonary stenosis and how is it treated?
> 3. What is a cardiac catheterisation?
> 4. What is transitional care?
> 5. Using the nursing process and Orem's self-care model, how would the nurse assess and plan care to alleviate David's anxiety?
> 6. David has reached an age where he now needs not only to begin taking control of his medical conditions, but also to start the transition process which will lead to transfer to the adult service in a few years' time. Using Orem's model and the nursing process, how can David and his parents be supported in this?

Answers to questions

Question 1. What is congenital heart disease and how are defects classified?

Congenital heart disease is an overall term used to describe congenital heart defects. It affects approximately 5–8 children per 1000 live births, the severity of which depends on the complexity of the defect, some children are born with multiple and or very complex defects (Hockenberry & Wilson 2007).

Defects have previously been thought of in terms of simple or complex; cyanotic or acyanotic. However, a more useful classification system now used is based on the blood flow and divides the above into:

- Obstructive defects
- Increased pulmonary blood flow or left to right shunts (acyanotic)
- Decreased pulmonary blood flow or right to left shunts (cyanotic)
- Complex mixed blood flow defects

Question 2. What is pulmonary stenosis and how is it treated?

Pulmonary stenosis is one of the most common obstructive defects, where there is narrowing or stenosis above (supravalvular), below (subvalvular) or at the site of the pulmonary valve itself (valvular). The degree of stenosis can vary from mild to severe, with treatment either non-surgical or balloon valvuloplasty, or surgical, such as pulmonary valvotomy, depending on the severity and degree of stenosis present (Jones *et al.* 2009). In the scenario above David is scheduled to have a balloon valvuloplasty in the catheter laboratory.

Question 3. What is cardiac catheterisation?

Cardiac catheterisation is an invasive procedure used for therapeutic interventions, electrophysiological evaluation and treatment and diagnostic purposes. However, as echocardiography and other non-invasive diagnostic imaging methods advance the latter is decreasing, although it is still a necessary procedure if pressure measurement is required (Dhillon *et al.* 2009). Procedures performed during interventional catheterisation include creation and device closure of atrial and septal defects, device closure of ventricular septal defects, coil occlusion of a patent ductus arteriosus and balloon valvuloplasty for pulmonary and aortic valvular stenosis. The procedure itself is carried out in the cardiac catheterisation laboratory and in children and young people usually under general anaesthetic; therefore they will not be allowed to eat or drink prior to the procedure.

During the procedure a radio-opaque catheter is inserted through a peripheral blood vessel, usually a femoral vessel, allowing pressures in the heart chambers to be recorded, angiography contrast material to be delivered and defects to be corrected using occlusive devices and balloons. After the procedure the catheter is removed and pressure is applied to the site. Close observation is required for 24 hours for any side effects or adverse reaction to the contrast medium or for complications such as bleeding, haematoma, arrhythmias, thrombosis, cardiovascular accident, perforation, cardiac tamponade, and/or cardiac arrest.

Activity 21.1

Review the pathophysiology and related care for other cardiac defects in:
Hockenberry, M.J. & Wilson, D. (2007) *Wong's Nursing Care of Infants and Children*, 8th edn. St Louis: Mosby.
Cook, K. & Langton, H. (2009) *Cardio-thoracic Care for Children and Young People*. Chichester: Wiley-Blackwell.

Question 4. What is transitional care?

Transition is described as 'a young-person-centred, multidimensional, multidisciplinary, holistic active process that attends to the medical, psychosocial and educational/vocational needs of adolescents as they move from child to adult-centred services' (McDonagh 2007, p161). The need for planned and effective transition from children's to adult services for young people with chronic illnesses and/or disabilities is well documented (DfCSF 2006; 2008). Child and adult healthcare services are very different; therefore it is important that young people and their families are adequately prepared for this beforehand. Evidence suggests, however, that the transfer to adult services for many young people is often not a positive event (Shaw *et al.* 2004; While *et al.* 2004). There are several factors that are key to the effectiveness of a young person's transition to adult services: namely starting early; consulting with the young person and their family; communication and collaboration between child and adult services and last, the timing of the transfer to the adult service itself (Sloper *et al.* 2011).

Question 5. Using the nursing process and Orem's self-care model, how would the nurse assess and plan care to alleviate David's anxiety?

Assessment

Box 21.1 Assessing and planning care			
	Normal self-care/ dependent care ability	**Current self-care**	**Self-care deficit**
Universal self-care requisite			
Maintenance of a balance between solitude and social interaction. Promotion of normalcy.	David has lots of friends. He plays football and cricket, swims and enjoys playing on his Xbox by himself and with his friends. Usually very happy and doesn't worry about anything. David's parents do not allow him to stay over with friends or go on overnight trips with school and restrict the amount of time they allow him to play football.	In hospital and away from his social network of friends. Very quiet, anxious and apprehensive about procedure. David is in the early phase of adolescent development, peer group connections are becoming very important to him and he will not want to be seen to be different.	Feelings of isolation in an unfamiliar environment and unable to maintain normal contact with his friends and peer group. Lacks knowledge about procedure and is very anxious and apprehensive about undergoing cardiac catheterisation and having a general anaesthetic. David feels that he is different from his friends and is beginning to resent his parents for restricting the activities he can do with his friends.
Developmental self care requisite			
	Parents have been responsible for meeting all of David's needs, including his healthcare needs, since his birth.	David has now entered adolescence and will be starting to move towards achieving independence from his parents.	David's knowledge and understanding of his asthma and pulmonary stenosis needs to be developed. Parental input into meeting David's healthcare needs will begin to decrease as he gains independence.

Planning

Maintenance of a balance between solitude and social interaction.

Problem: David is feeling isolated in an unfamiliar environment and is unable to maintain normal contact with his friends and peer group.

Goal/aim: David will become familiar with the ward environment and also be able to maintain contact with his friends and peer group. Nursing Interventions will include:

- Allocate David a bed space with other adolescents, preferably in a designated adolescent bay if available.
- Familiarise David with the ward environment and ensure he knows where the bathroom facilities and kitchen facilities are; where he can use his mobile phone and where the adolescent activity/games room is, if available.
- Introduce David to the ward/hospital youth worker if one is available.
- Inform David and his parents of the visiting times and reassure him that his friends are able to come and visit him while he is in hospital.
- Make David aware that there are PlayStations, Xboxes and DVD players available for him to use and that he can bring in his own games and DVDs for them.

Nursing action: educative/supportive (Orem 1995; Pearson *et al.* 2005).

Promotion of normalcy

Problem: David lacks knowledge about procedure and is therefore very anxious and apprehensive about undergoing cardiac catheterisation and having a general anaesthetic.

Goal/aim: David will know and understand what the procedure entails will feel less anxious about it.

Nursing interventions:

- Encourage David to express his concerns and take time to listen to what he has to say.
- Explain the cardiac catheterisation procedure to David in terms he will understand.
- Provide literature and use online resources aimed at adolescents which explain cardiac catheterisation.
- Arrange a preliminary visit to the cardiac catheterisation laboratory.
- Arrange for David to meet with the adolescent cardiac liaison nurse.
- Reassure David that the medical and nursing staff will explain any procedures to him before they carry them out and that it is all right for him to ask questions if he is unsure about what they are going to do.
- Explain the pre-operative procedure and ensure David understands what it entails.
- Explain the postoperative procedure, i.e. the observations that will be carried out and the length of time he will have to remain in bed and ensure he understands why this is necessary.
- Reassure David that his parents can accompany him to the catheterisation laboratory, stay with him until he goes to sleep and be with him when he wakes up.

Nursing action: educative/supportive (Orem 1995; Pearson *et al.* 2005).

Problem: David feels that he is different from his friends and is beginning to resent his parents for restricting the activities he does with his friends.

Goal/aim: David will equate himself with his peers and will not feel he is different to them just because he has asthma and pulmonary stenosis.

Nursing interventions:

- Talk to David's parents to establish what their understanding is with regard to asthma and pulmonary stenosis and the activities David can participate in.
- Explain to David's parents that while it is normal for them to want to protect David with regard to his asthma and pulmonary stenosis he is at an age and stage of development where it is important for him to be able to spend time with his friends.
- Encourage David and his parents to identify activities that he and his friends can do together which his parents will be less apprehensive about him doing.
- Arrange for David and his parents to meet with the cardiac liaison nurse and asthma specialist nurse to discuss how best to manage David's activities when he goes home so that he does not feel he is any different to his friends.
- Provide David's parents with information on parent support groups.
- Provide David with information about the adolescent support group within the GUCH (grown up congenital heart) support group and adolescent asthma support groups and asthma camp.

Nursing action: educative/supportive (Orem 1995; Pearson *et al.* 2005).

Question 6. David has reached an age where he now needs not only to begin taking control of his medical conditions, but also to start the transition process which will lead to transfer to the adult service in a few years' time. Using Orem's model and the nursing process, how can David and his parents be supported in this?

Developmental self-care requisite

Problem: David needs to become more independent in managing his asthma and pulmonary stenosis but his knowledge and understanding of both is very limited.

Goal/aim: David will become more independent in meeting his own healthcare needs as he begins the process of transition which will eventually lead to the transfer over to adult services when he is older.

Nursing interventions:

- Explain to David and his parents what the term transition means and what it will involve for both David and his parents.
- Allow both David and his parents the opportunity to ask questions and express any fear, anxiety or apprehensiveness they may have regarding this process, i.e. why it starts at such an early age.
- Arrange for David and his parents to meet with the transition nurse to begin to plan David's transition.

Nursing action: educative/supportive.

Activity 21.2

Access and read the following documents.

What key principles of transition can you identify?

Department for Children Schools and Family (2008)*Transition Moving on Well*. London: Department of Health.
Royal College of Nursing (2004) *Adolescent Transition Care*. London: RCN.
Royal College of Nursing (2008) *Adolescence: Boundaries and Connections an RCN Guide for Working with Young People*. London: RCN.
McDonagh, J. (2007) Transitions for young people with complex health needs. In: Coleman J., Hendry, L.B. and Kloep, M. (eds). *Adolescence and Health*. Chichester: John Wiley and Sons Ltd.

References

Cook, K. & Langton, H. (2009) *Cardio-thoracic Care for Children and Young People*. Chichester: Wiley-Blackwell.
Department for Children Schools and Family (DfCSF) (2006) *Transition: Getting it Right for Young People*. London: Department of Health.
Department for Children Schools and Family (DfCSF) (2008) *Transition Moving on Well*. London: Department of Health.
Dhillon, R., Sharland, G., Robinson, AM. , Clay, C. & Bearne, C. (2009) Presentation and diagnosis. In: Cook, K. & Langton, H. (eds). *Cardio-thoracic Care for Children and Young People*. Chichester: Wiley-Blackwell.
Hockenberry, M.J. & Wilson, D. (2007) *Wong's Nursing Care of Infants and Children*, 8th edn. St Louis: Mosby.
Jones, T., Cook, K., Dhillon, R., *et al.* (2009) Treatment options/management. In: Cook, K. & Langton, H. (eds). *Cardio-thoracic Care for Children and Young People*. Chichester: Wiley-Blackwell.
McDonagh, J. (2007) Transitions for young people with complex health needs. In: Coleman J., Hendry, L.B. & Kloep, M. (eds). *Adolescence and Health*. Chichester: John Wiley and Sons Ltd.
Orem, D.E. (1995) *Nursing: Concepts of Practice*, 5th edn. St Louis: Mosby.
Pearson, A., Vaughan, B. & FitzGerald, M. (2005) *Nursing Models for Practice*, 3rd edn. Edinburgh: Elsevier.
Royal College of Nursing (2004) *Adolescent Transition Care*. London: RCN.
Royal College of Nursing (2008) *Adolescence: Boundaries and Connections: an RCN Guide for Working with Young People*. London: RCN.
Shaw, K.L., Southwood, T.R. & McDonagh, J.E. (2004) Users' perspectives of transitional care for adolescents with juvenile idiopathic arthritis. *Rheumatology*, **43**, 770–78.
Sloper, P., Beecham, J., Clarke, S.,Franklin, A., Moran, N. & Cusworth, L. (2011) Transition to adult services for disabled young people and those with complex health needs. Research Works, 2011–02, Social Policy Reasearch Unit, University of York, York.
While, A., Forbes, A., Ullman, R., Lewis, S., Mathes, L. & Griffiths, P. (2004) Good practices that address continuity during transition from child to adult care: synthesis of the evidence. *Child: Care, Health and Development*, **30**(5), 439–52.

22

Infant with Cardiac Failure
Anne Finnegan

Scenario

Dora (seven months old) is being admitted to the ward via the walk-in centre accompanied by her parents, Jane and Paul. Her older sister, Lily, is at nursery school. The referral letter gives a provisional diagnosis of congestive cardiac failure, stating that Dora's respirations are 45 per minute, apex 184 beats per minute, temperature 37.4°C and oxygen saturations 92%.

Dora's parents took her to the walk-in centre because she has been restless and irritable during the night. They were unable to see the GP today but have been consulting the doctor frequently about their worries over Dora's faltering growth. Her birth weight was 3.2 kg and she is now 4.5 kg. Mum, Jane, stopped breastfeeding when Dora was 12 weeks, worried that she had insufficient milk. Dora now has formula feeds, can take 45 minutes to finish a bottle, sometimes falling asleep during the feed and has started a weaning diet four weeks ago, which she has twice a day.

Dora is a restless sleeper, waking frequently, often seems distressed and does not settle when offered a night feed. She was a full-term baby delivered vaginally and did not require admission to special baby care. On admission Dora is awake but lethargic and looks pale. She has good head control, but cannot sit unaided. Movement in all four limbs is noted but they are mottled and cool to touch. Eye contact is present and Dora turns to locate the source of any sound. She smiled when offered a toy, grasped it with both hands, moving it from one hand to another.

Jane works as a hotel manager so she is worried about missing work whilst Dora is in hospital. Dad, Paul, is a transport manager at a local firm. Dora's grandmother provides childcare. Dora is being admitted for further investigation of congestive cardiac failure (CCF).

Care Planning in Children and Young People's Nursing, First Edition.
Edited by Doris Corkin, Sonya Clarke, Lorna Liggett.
© 2012 Blackwell Publishing Ltd. Published 2012 by Blackwell Publishing Ltd.

Questions

1. Using Roper, Logan and Tierney's model of nursing (Holland *et al.* 2008):
   (a) Review the scenario and highlight any information which is relevant to Dora's holistic assessment.
   (b) Note the additional assessment information needed about Dora to ensure safe and effective nursing care during her first 24 hours in hospital. Think about observation, interviewing and measurement during this process and how a genogram might contribute to the assessment.
2. Cardiac failure is a symptom and always has an underlying cause. List some possible causes of Dora's cardiac failure.
3. Some children with CCF are cyanosed. Explain why cyanosis occurs in heart disease.
4. Write a holistic care plan for Dora's first 24 hours in hospital, giving a rationale for the prescribed nursing actions.
5. Explain the immediate investigations that Dora may need to establish the possible cause of her cardiac failure.

Dora's initial assessment should provide sufficient information to highlight her immediate problems, establish a plan of care and commence treatment. It is a challenging activity because Dora lacks the verbal skills to guide the nurse, and her physical immaturity may mean that rapid and serious deterioration is possible. Her parents may be distressed, anxious and unable to answer some initial enquiries.

A calm and sympathetic environment will benefit Dora, with an initial visual assessment providing further useful information about Dora's physical condition, level of consciousness and behaviour. It should be performed prior to physical contact and the use of medical devices, because the use of equipment may upset Dora, causing her to cry and changing baseline measurements.

A systematic approach should help to prevent omissions from the assessment.

Answers to questions

Question 1. Using Roper, Logan and Tierney's model of nursing (Holland *et al.* 2008):

(a) Review the scenario and highlight any information which is relevant to Dora's holistic assessment.

Breathing

At the walk-in centre, Dora's respiratory and apex rates exceeded the normal range for her age group (Miall *et al.* 2007, p12–13), whilst her oxygen saturation rate is below the usual rate of 95–98% (Sims 1996). These rates need to be re-assessed to provide baseline measurements and should be performed whilst Dora is relaxed and calm.

A visual assessment of Dora's respiratory effort should be made, checking for signs of distress, such as head bobbing, nasal flaring, sternal or intercostal recession. Although, not typical in babies with cardiac failure, these signs would indicate that she has some acidosis with low cardiac output or high blood flow through the lungs (Duderstadt 2006). Whilst observing the chest area, it might be possible to see Dora's apical pulse because she is thin, but any other visible pulsations and/or diffuse heaves and thrills should be noted. These signs can be evident in CCF, with a visible heave indicating right ventricular enlargement (Engel 2002).

Observe Dora for evidence of central cyanosis on the conjunctiva, lips, mucous membranes and tongue; if it is evident are there signs of accompanying polycythaemia and/or finger clubbing? Polycythaemia indicates prolonged tissue hypoxia and can be present in cyanotic heart disease, indicating an increase in circulating red blood cells (Wong 1999, p1605). It is characterised by a deep reddish-purple colouring over the cheeks, and signs of jaundice, including yellowing of the skin, eyes and mucous membranes. Chronic hypoxia even if it is mild would also explain any clubbing of the nail beds provided it had been present for six months or more (Lehrer 2003, p43). Whilst looking at Dora's nails check for any splinter haemorrhages because these fine vertical dark red lines can be a sign of bacterial endocarditis (Rushforth 2009).

At the same time, listen for signs of wheeze and coughing which might indicate lung oedema. Does the cough sound dry and hacking or is it causing copious secretions? Remember, secretions may not be obvious because a child of Dora's age is likely to swallow them. Grunting or gasping respirations should be reported immediately because they denote severe distress (Bethel 2008).

Whilst Dora is calm count her respirations, which are likely to be high because tachypnoea is a common feature of CCF. Then measure her apex rate, listening for a full minute to ensure an adequate length of time for irregularities of rhythm to be evident (Wong 1997 in Trigg & Mohammed 2006, p88). The apex beat should be located at the fourth intercostal space to the left of the mid-clavicular line in a child of Dora's age, with a lower more lateral position indicating heart enlargement (Engel 2002, p26). Tachycardia is always present when a child has CCF. However, it will still be necessary to take a peripheral pulse to ensure consistency with the apex rate and to provide additional information about the volume, rhythm and character.

Rushforth (2009, p45) states that volume can be classified as:

- Absent pulse – where no impulse can be palpated.
- Weak or thready pulse – where it is hard to feel a pulse and light finger pressure eliminates the impulse.
- Normal pulse – the pulse is easy to feel but needs strong finger pressure to eliminate the impulse.
- Bounding pulse – easy to feel but difficult to eliminate with finger pressure.

A weak and thready pulse may indicate that compensatory mechanisms within Dora's heart and circulatory system are weakening and her condition is deteriorating (Lehrer 2003).

Capillary refill should be assessed and would normally be within two seconds; however, a slower capillary refill would not be unusual where poor cardiac perfusion is present (Mackway-Jones 1997). The forehead or sternum should be used as Dora's limbs are cool to the touch, affecting the result.

Mackway-Jones (1997) would define Dora's oxygen saturations as low, so re-check them. Some congenital heart lesions can cause differential oxygen saturation levels in the upper and lower limbs, so take measurements in both the upper and lower body (Duderstadt 2006).

Measurement of blood pressure may provide additional information and if attempted should be taken electronically (Cook & Montgomery 2006 in Trigg & Mohammed 2006, p89). However, changes to blood pressure are a late indicator of problems in young children. It is likely that Dora will move around during this procedure, affecting the result and limiting the value of any reading.

Temperature control

Dora's temperature of 37.4°C is within the normal range for her age group but she may feel clammy and sweaty. This happens as a result of sympathetic nervous system stimulation as the heart tries to compensate for falling cardiac output (Hockenberry & Wilson 2007, p1447) and additionally may have caused Dora to have cradle cap.

Lack of pyrexia indicates that Dora does not have an active infection, but ask her parents about recent contacts with anyone who has had an infectious illness because her problems could be the result of recent, acquired infection.

Sleep

Dora wakes during the night and is difficult to settle, indicating that orthopnoea/dyspnoea maybe a problem, whilst falling asleep during feeds indicates fatigue, poor exercise tolerance and might be contributing to her poor weight gain.

Dora's sleep pattern may have affected her parents' ability to get enough sleep, impacting upon their ability to recognise Dora's needs and respond appropriately.

Nutrition

Dora's history indicates she is being offered an appropriate amount of formula feed for weight (Figari & Fearon 2006 in Trigg & Mohammed 2006, p166) and commenced a weaning diet as recommended by the Department of Health (DH 2004 (online)). However, Dora's weight has decreased by a centile since birth and is now below the 15th centile (WHO Child Growth Standards 2006 (online)), indicating that she is failing to thrive (Maill *et al*. 2007, p13). Unfortunately, the true extent of poor weight gain may not be evident due to presence of generalised oedema, caused by water and sodium retention, a common feature of CCF. Also, acute fluid retention may cause ascites, which could make Dora seem pot-bellied (Hockenberry & Wilson 2007).

Dyspnoea and tachypnoea may have contributed to Dora's poor growth because these symptoms make sucking difficult, as well as increasing Dora's metabolic rate and calorie requirements (Moules & Ramsay 2008).

The swallowing of mucus may mean that Dora is prone to vomiting, further affecting weight gain, so ask her parents if, when and how much vomiting occurs.

Enquire about Dora's normal feeding pattern, the amount of formula offered and the foodstuffs offered as weaning diet. Her parents may want to continue to give her feeds, so discuss their preferences.

Finally, Dora should be weighed again to establish a baseline measurement, allowing clinicians to monitor the effects of prescribed therapy and feeding regimes.

Mobility

Dora might be expected to be sitting unaided by this age and her inability to do so may stem from the effects of illness. Children with cardiac failure often exhibit delays in gross motor skills because they lack energy to practice them and for physical activity (Hockenberry & Wilson 2007). However, her ability to transfer a toy from one hand to another would indicate that fine motor skills are developmentally appropriate (Cook & Montgomery 2006 in Trigg & Mohammed 2006, p84).

Dora's limbs may look mottled and seem cool to touch due to stimulation of the sympathetic nervous system and the release of catecholamines (Hockenberry & Wilson 2007).

Safety

At seven months, Dora has low levels of immunoglobulins, making her vulnerable to opportunistic infection (Neill & Knowles 2004), so ask if Dora has had any infections. In particular, the presence of mucus in the lungs would provide an ideal environment for respiratory infection, further compromising her respiratory effort. However, vulnerability to some infections would be minimised by immunisation and a full history of vaccinations should be recorded.

Ask her parents about known allergies, but remember Dora will still be meeting new substances. Her reaction to them cannot be predicted. Find out if Dora has been given any medications, either prescribed, over the counter or herbal.

Dora should be weighed to allow for the accurate calculation of prescribed medications and feeds, and to facilitate the monitoring of the effectiveness of any prescribed diuretic therapy.

Communication

Dora lacks the ability to verbalise her needs but her behaviour indicates that she is conscious of the visual and auditory information around her. She is old enough to feel and express a range of emotions, including distress, pleasure, sadness, disgust and anger (Slater & Lewis 2007, pp220–25) and to have a sense of object permanence. Dora may feel frightened by strangers and experience distress if separated from her parents (Birch 1997, pp68, 28 and 19; Rana & Upton 2009, p170). She may well have been examined and treated by clinicians before, and remember upsetting events such as injections (Levy 1960). Consequently, Dora's facial expressions and crying patterns should be observed for signs of anxiety or increasing distress. At the same time, observing Dora's facial features will highlight any dysmorphic features. Children with a range of syndromes are more likely to have cardiac problems (Greydanus *et al.* 2008).

Dora's communication skills should include turn taking in 'conversation' and the ability to babble to attract and maintain the attention of others, but any sounds may seem hoarse due to the pressure of secretions on the largyngeal nerve (Hockenberry & Wilson 2007).

Elimination

Ask about the number of wet and dirty nappies Dora normally has each day and find out if there have been any recent changes to frequency, consistency or smell of urine or faeces. It is probably advisable to test Dora's urine to exclude infection and this can be done using a urine collection pad. Whilst inserting the pad take the opportunity to check the napkin area for signs of irritation or nappy rash.

Cleansing and dressing

Ask the parents about bath times, and clothing preferences. Dora's parents may want to meet her hygiene needs, so note their choices.

The generalised oedema which is often present in CCF increases the likelihood of skin breakdown so observe Dora's skin, particularly the pressure points for evidence of redness or breaks, noting at the same time any rashes or bruising (Hockenberry & Wilson 2007).

Playing

Discuss Dora's play preferences and abilities. Dora may have favourite toys and her parents could be encouraged to bring them to the hospital, providing an essential link with home, and aiding normality. Discuss some quiet play activities with the parents to help minimise regression whilst Dora is in hospital (Weaver & Groves 2010 cited in Glasper *et al.* 2010, p73) and decrease Dora's oxygen requirements related to vigorous activity.

Sexuality

Dora is too young to understand the biological differences between females and males but her parents may have definite ideas about gender differences, so establish if Dora's parents have any specific preferences related to clothing and toys.

Death and dying

Dora will lack any concept of death but her parents may have fears about the possibility of Dora dying, because many people associate heart problems with early death. Conversely, Jane and Paul may not have considered this possibility, so limit discussion to any current fears or anxieties. Further discussion can be initiated by clinicians when more concrete information about the cause of Dora's problems is known.

Question 1. Using Roper, Logan and Tierney's model of nursing (Holland *et al.* 2008):

(b) Note the additional assessment information needed about Dora to ensure safe and effective nursing care during her first 24 hours in hospital. Think about observation, interviewing and measurement during this process and how a genogram might contribute to the assessment.

A detailed family history might provide further relevant information about Dora's likely diagnosis. The completion of a genogram facilitates discussion of such issues (Whyte 1997) and provides information about miscarriages, genetic illnesses, or sudden infant or adult deaths which might have been caused by heart problems (Duderstadt 2006). Parents who have had a congenital heart malformation themselves or who already have had an affected child are at increased risk of having a child with cardiac problems (Attard-Montalto & Saha 2006).

Table 22.1 Causes of congestive cardiac failure.

Common congenital heart malformations*	Acquired heart problems	Decreased efficiency/ contractibility of the heart muscle	Increased cardiac demands
Acyanotic			
Patent ductus arteriosus	Infective endocarditis	Low levels of	Severe anaemia
Atrial septal defect	Myocarditis	potassium, calcium,	Hyperthyroidism
Ventricular septal defect	Rheumatic fever	magnesium or	Sepsis
Coarctation of the aorta	Kawasaki disease/syndrome	glucose	
Aortic stenosis	Bacterial endocarditis	Acidaemia	
Pulmonary stenosis	Henoch-Schönlein purpura	Cardiomyopathy	
Cyanotic			
Tetralogy of Fallot			
Tricuspid atresia			
Transposition of the great arteries			

*Pang & Newson (2005).

Question 2. Cardiac failure is a symptom and always has an underlying cause. List some possible causes of Dora's cardiac failure.

Congestive cardiac failure occurs when the heart is unable to pump sufficient blood around the body to meet its metabolic demands for nutrients, the transport of blood gases and electrolytes (Hockenberry & Wilson 2007). There is always an underlying cause (see Table 22.1). The most common cause of CCF in the child is a congenital heart malformation. Something happens during foetal life to disrupt the normal development of the heart structures and/or the vessels leading to or from the heart. This might be a missing heart valve or chamber, a hole between two chambers, or a narrowing in a valve, artery or vein. Such problems can occur singly or in combination. Pang & Newson (2005) state that there are more than one hundred different cardiac malformations but a small number of defects cause the majority of cases.

Acquired heart problems develop after birth as a result of autoimmune disorders, infection, environmental or familial factors. They can happen at any age but are rare during infancy (Greydanus *et al.* 2008).

Occasionally, a child can develop CCF which is unrelated to the functioning of the heart. A condition develops which increases the demands on the heart, which it cannot meet or something happens which prevents the myocardium contracting efficiently (Attard-Montalto & Saha 2006).

Question 3. Some children with CCF are cyanosed. Explain why cyanosis occurs in heart disease.

Cyanosis is a bluish discolouration which can affect the limbs and mouth of any child. It is unusual but usually benign (Greydanus *et al.* 2008). More worrying is central cyanosis where the mucous membranes are affected because this sign is often an indicator of cardiopulmonary disease.

Central cyanosis can be caused by the presence of deoxygenated blood in the arterial circulation in excess of 5 g per dl (Pang & Newson 2005). This blood enters the arterial system from the right side of the heart without going to the lungs to collect oxygen, due to a malformation or abnormal opening in the heart or its surrounding vessels, for example where the child has one ventricle instead of two.

Question 4. Write a holistic care plan for Dora's first 24 hours in hospital, giving a rationale for the prescribed nursing action (see Chapter 10).

See Box 22.1.

This care plan is based on Dora's history given at the beginning of the chapter highlighting those activities of daily living which differ from normal and can be supported in the acute setting. The nursing actions described are often required by children with cardiac failure, and will often form the basis of any initial care plan. However, children in cardiac failure will require further supportive therapy depending on the additional assessment information collected, the cause of the cardiac failure, the medical plan of care and the wider needs of the family.

Box 22.1   Care plan

Problem	Goal	Nursing action
Breathing		
Dora is breathless with tachycardia, possible dyspnoea and orthopnea.	To ensure a respiratory rate between 30–40 breaths per minute (Miall *et al*. 2007, p12). To ensure a resting apex/pulse rate of 110 and 160 (Miall *et al*. 2007, p13).	Ensure Dora is nursed in a sitting position using a baby chair when awake (45 degrees). Tilt cot when Dora is sleeping (45 degrees). Monitor and record apex and respiratory rate every four hours using auscultation/ manual palpation techniques. Use continuous bedside monitoring for oxygen saturations and ECG trace. Observe and report any undue pallor or cyanosis. Administer humidified oxygen if prescribed. Consult the physiotherapy team and perform chest physiotherapy and suction prior to feeds if required.

Rationale

Dyspnoea/orthopnoea is relieved by placing the child in the sitting position, which lowers the pressure of the abdominal contents on the diaphragm and decreases venous return to the heart by allowing blood to pool in the lower limbs (Hockenberry & Wilson 2007). Dora will feel more comfortable and should be able to sleep with greater ease.

The apex/pulse and respiratory rate should be measured for a full minute, noting any abnormalities. Gormley-Fleming (2010 cited in Glasper *et al*. 2010, p116) suggests that the

continued

Box 22.1 *(Continued)*

apical route gives the most accurate measurement for the child under two years of age because of their rapid heart rate and difficulties associated with manual palpation techniques. However, manual palpation of the pulse should not be omitted because it enables assessment of volume, rhythm and character (Duderstadt 2006). The brachial pulse is likely to be easily accessible and palpable.

A low oxygen saturation level is not usual in children with heart conditions, and Dora might normally function with a lower rate than normal but it is important to establish her 'norm', so that any change or deterioration is recognised at an early stage (Giles 2006 cited in Trigg & Mohammed 2006, p259).

Children with cardiac conditions can require oxygen therapy to reduce heart and respiratory rates and decrease the work of breathing (Glasper *et al.* 2010), but oxygen administration is regarded as a therapy and should always be prescribed on the child's medicine chart by a doctor (British National Formulary 2010–2011). Humidification will prevent drying of the upper respiratory tract.

Chest physiotherapy and suction is needed when children cannot clear chest secretions on their own, or when the work of breathing is increased with a high respiratory rate and effort, or when oxygen saturation rates decrease (Dixon 2006 cited in Trigg & Mohammed 2006, p386). These problems will in turn increase the effort involved in feeding.

Temperature control

Dora's temperature regulation is physiologically immature.	Dora's body temperature remains 36–37.5°C. Dora is free of the signs of fever or hypothermia.	Monitor temperature four hourly using the tympanic or axillary route and report any pyrexia. Investigate and treat pyrexia. Wrap warmly if cold.

Rationale
Pyrexia and low body temperature both increase the consumption of oxygen (Hockenberry & Wilson, 2007, p1453; Moules & Ramsay, 2008, p566).

Safety

Dora is at risk of hospital acquired infection. Dora maybe commenced on medication to improve cardiac function.	Dora will remain free of infection throughout her stay in hospital. To administer medication as prescribed. Monitor and report any side effects of prescribed medications.	Nurse in single cubicle with the door closed. Explain and demonstrate infection control measures to parents, including hand washing technique, appropriate disposal of nappies, towels and bedding. Ensure nameband *in situ* and checked prior to all administration episodes. Calculate, check doses and record administration according to local policy. Ensure no known allergy to administered substances. Note and report any possible side effects.

Box 22.1   (*Continued*)

Rationale

Nursing Dora in a cubicle should decrease the number of people in her immediate environment who are symptomless carriers or have contaminated hands or clothing and therefore reduces her exposure to air-borne infection (Dougherty & Lister 2008). The use of infection control measures reduces the risks of transmission via hands and clothing.

Dora could be prescribed a range of medications to improve the function of her heart and/or reduce the fluid retention associated with cardiac failure and checking procedures should diminish the chance of inaccurate calculation or administration whilst ensuring that the requirements of the Nursing and Midwifery Council are met (NMC 2010).

Communication

Dora is pre-verbal and cannot make her needs known.

Dora's parents may be anxious about her hospital admission.

Dora's mother worried about missing work time.

Dora will not be distressed by separation and stranger anxiety.

Dora will maintain developmental milestones during admission.

Explain all procedures and interventions to parents, negotiating their role. Encourage parents to hold and speak to Dora during nursing/medical interventions.

Replicate home routines where possible.

Allocate nursing staff consistently and minimise number of practitioners working with her.

Provide toys and play materials as discussed with parents.

Explain parental residence and visiting policy to parents.

Negotiate the parent's role in Dora's daily living activities.

Negotiate parent's level of participation in nursing interventions.

Establish which friends and family might visit Dora and whether they will be providing any daily care activities when parents cannot be present.

Rationale

The presence and support of parents and family members should be soothing for Dora, preventing separation anxiety. Her parents will be able to provide informed consent for any further investigations or treatments.

Negotiation related to visiting and care activities will help parents to prioritise activities and balance other commitments such as Lily's care and their employment.

continued

Box 22.1 (*Continued*)

Nutrition

| Dora is having difficulty feeding with poor weight gain. | Dora will gain weight. | Offer feeds three hourly for a maximum of 30 minutes. Introduce top-up NG feeds if Dora remains unable to finish feeds. Consult dietician about feeding supplements and calorie dense weaning foods. Weigh daily at same time on same scale. Complete a daily fluid balance chart. |

Rationale

Dora may find frequent, smaller feeds easier to finish which will facilitate weight gain. However, frequency of feeding should not be less than three hourly to allow sufficient rest and sleep (Hockenberry & Wilson 2007). However, if feeds remain incomplete, NG feeding will increase the calorie intake associated with milk feeds.

A daily weight will provide information about the success of the feeding regime. The fluid balance chart will highlight any fluid retention. Combined scrutiny of this information will assist the medical practitioner's decisions about ongoing treatment.

Sleep

| Dora's sleep is disturbed. Parental tiredness | Dora will sleep soundly overnight and have a short nap(s) during the day. | Cluster daily activities and nursing care to ensure rest periods of 2–3 hours and an unbroken sleep pattern. Involve family members in comforting activities to try to minimise crying. Negotiate regular breaks with parents. Encourage adoption of routines which facilitate sleep. |

Rationale

Dora may be less tired and more able to feed if given frequent rest periods. Preventing episodes of crying will decrease the work of respiration and use of calories.

Encouraging the parents to take adequate breaks should help them maintain their physical fitness and ability to recognise Dora's needs.

Cleansing and dressing

| Dora is at risk of skin breakdown due to possible oedema and sweating. | Dora's skin will remain intact throughout her hospital admission. | Daily bath. Change nappies prior to all feeds. Inspect pressure points for redness and abrasions during hygiene procedures and following daily weight. Change Dora's position following feeds. |

Rationale

Cleansing skin and changing Dora's position will diminish the chances of pressure sores caused by tissue compression or friction on any particular area of the body (Willock 2010 cited in Glasper *et al.* 2010, p325).

Question 5. Explain the immediate investigations that Dora may need to establish the possible cause of her cardiac failure.

Initially Dora will be assessed by the medical staff who will take a detailed history about Jane's pregnancy and Dora's birth. The history will include information about the mother's health because there are strong links between long-term health conditions in the mother and heart disease in babies. Mothers who suffer from lupus or diabetes mellitus (Greydanus *et al.* 2008) or are taking prescribed medications including lithium, thalidomide or phenytoin are more likely to have affected infants (Lehrer 2003). Jane will be asked if she had infections during pregnancy, particularly rubella, or if she has used recreational drugs, including alcohol (Pang & Newson, 2005).

The doctor will listen to Dora's heart and lung fields. Ascultation will provide information about the presence and timing of any heart murmurs, any fluid in the lungs or associated chest infection (Duderstadt 2006).

The chest X-ray will provide information about the size and shape of the heart, demonstrating any enlargement and any congenital problem which has changed the silhouette (Lehrer 2003).

An ECG will provide a permanent record of the electrical activity of the heart, showing its wave pattern on graph paper. This permanent record highlights any enlargement, conduction problems, damage to the myocardium/pericardium, and electrolyte imbalances. These problems alter the normal PQRST complex in a predictable ways (Dougherty & Lister 2008).

Echocardiography will provide visual information about the structure of the heart and surrounding vessels. It will highlight areas of stenosis in vessels or valves, and abnormal openings. Where an abnormality exists, it is possible to see the effect of the problem on the flow of blood (Miall *et al.* 2007).

Blood tests will include haematocrit, haemoglobin and red cell count, giving further information related to oxygenation (Lehrer 2003). Sodium, potassium and calcium levels may be assessed.

Follow-up action plan

Dora's case history has given an introduction to the problems of an infant with cardiac failure but the practitioner will need to broaden their knowledge. Further study is recommended related to:

1. The anatomy and physiology of the normal heart.
2. Signs and symptoms associated with the disorders listed in Table 22.1.
3. The pathophysiology of congestive cardiac failure in all age groups.
4. Medications which are used to support children with cardiac problems, including cardiac glycosides, angiotensin-converting inhibitors and diuretics.

References

Attard-Montalto, S. & Saha, V. (2006) *Paediatrics: a Core Text with Self Assessment*. Edinburgh: Churchill Livingstone.

Bethel, J. (2008) *Paediatric Minor Emergencies*, 1st edn. Cumbria: M. & K. Publishing.

Birch, A. (1997) *Developmental Psychology from Infancy to Adulthood. Introductory Psychology Series*, 2nd edn. London: Macmillan.

British National Formulary (2010–2011) *British National Formulary.* London: BMJ Publishing Group Ltd and RPS Publishing.

Cook, K. & Montgomery, H. (2006) *Assessment,* Chapter 3. In: Trigg, E. & Mohammed, T.A. (eds). *Practices in Children's Nursing. Guidelines for Hospital and Community,* 2nd edn. Edinburgh: Churchill Livingstone, Elsevier.

Department of Health (2004) *Birth to Five: Your Complete Guide to Parenthood and the First Five Years of Your Child's Life.* www.dh.gov.uk

Dixon, M. (2006) Suctioning, Chapter 31. In: Trigg, E. & Mohammed, T.A. (eds). *Practices in Children's Nursing. Guidelines for Hospital and Community,* 2nd edn. Edinburgh: Churchill Livingstone, Elsevier.

Dougherty, L. & Lister, S. (2008) *The Royal Marsden Hospital Manual of Clinical Nursing Procedures,* 7th edn. Oxford: John Wiley & Sons.

Duderstadt, K.G. (2006) *Pediatric Physical Examination. An Illustrated Handbook.* St Louis: Mosby.

Engel, J. (2002) *Mosby's Pediatric Assessment,* 4th edn. St Louis: Mosby.

Figari, T. & Fearon, J. (2006) Feeding, Chapter 10. In: Trigg, E. & Mohammed, T.A. (eds). *Practices in Children's Nursing. Guidelines for Hospital and Community,* 2nd edn. Edinburgh: Churchill Livingstone, Elsevier.

Giles, R. (2006) Oxygen therapy, Chapter 7. In: Trigg, E. & Mohammed, T.A. (eds). *Practices in Children's Nursing. Guidelines for Hospital and Community,* 2nd edn. Edinburgh: Churchill Livingstone, Elsevier.

Glasper, A. Aylott, M. & Battrick, C. (2010) *Developing Practical Skills for Nursing Children and Young People.* London: Hodder Arnold.

Gormley-Fleming, E. (2010) Assessment and vital signs: a comprehensive review, Chapter 9. In: Glasper, A., Aylott, M. & Battrick, C. (eds). *Developing Practical Skills for Nursing Children and Young People.* London: Hodder Arnold.

Greydanus, D.E., Feinberg, A.N., Patel, D.R. & Homnick, D.N. (2008) *The Pediatric Diagnostic Examination.* McGraw Hill Medical: New York.

Hockenberry, M.J. & Wilson, D. (2007) *Wong's Nursing Care of Infants and Children,* 8th edn. St Louis: Mosby Elsevier.

Holland, K., Jenkins, J., Solomon, J. & Whittam, S. (2008) *Applying the Roper, Logan & Tierney Model in Practice.* 2nd edn. Edinburgh: Churchill Livingstone.

Lehrer, S. (2003) *Understanding Paediatric Heart Sounds,* 2nd edn. Philadelphia: Saunders.

Levy, D.M. (1960) The infant's earliest memory of inoculation. *Journal of Genetic Psychology,* **96**(3), 46–50.

Mackway-Jones, K. (1997) *Emergency Triage: Manchester Triage Group.* Plymouth: BMJ Publishing Group.

Miall, L. Rudolf, M. & Levene, M. (2007) *Paediatrics at a Glance,* 2nd edn. London: Blackwell Publishing.

Moules, T. & Ramsay, J. (2008) *The Textbook of Children's and Young People's Nursing,* 2nd edn. Oxford: Blackwell Publishing.

Neill, S. & Knowles, H. (2004. *The Biology of Child Health. A Reader in Development and Assessment.* New York: Palgrave Macmillan.

Nursing and Midwifery Council (2010) *Standards for Medicine Management.* www.nmc.uk.org

Pang, D. & Newson, T. (2005) *Paediatrics. Crash Course,* 2nd edn. Edinburgh: Mosby.

Rana, D. & Upton, D. (2009) *Psychology for Nurses.* Harlow: Pearson Education.

Rushforth, H. (2009) *Assessment Made Incredibly Easy,* 1st edn. London: Lippincott, Williams & Wilkins and Walter Kluwer Health.

Sims, J. (1996) Making sent of pulse oximetry and oxygen dissociation cure. *Nursing Times,* **92**(1), 34–5.

Slater, A. & Lewis, M. (2007) *Introduction to Infant Development,* 2nd edn. Oxford: Oxford University Press.

Trigg, E. & Mohammed, T.A. (2006) *Practices in Children's Nursing. Guidelines for Hospital and Community,* 2nd edn. Edinburgh: Churchill Livingstone, Elsevier.

Weaver, K. & Groves, J. (2010) Play provision for children, Chapter 7. In: Glasper, A. Aylott, M. & Battrick, C. (eds). *Developing Practical Skills for Nursing Children and Young People*. London: Hodder Arnold.

Whyte, D. (ed.) (1997) *Explorations in Family Nursing*. London and New York: Routledge.

Willock, J. (2010) Skin health care, Chapter 19b. In: Glasper, A., Aylott, M. & Battrick, C. (eds). *Developing Practical Skills for Nursing Children and Young People*. London: Hodder Arnold.

Wong, D. (1999) *Whaley & Wong's Nursing Care of Infants and Children*, 6th edn. St Louis: Mosby.

World Health Organisation (2006) *Child Growth Standards*. www,who.int.en/

Section 6

Care Planning – Surgical Procedures

23

Tonsillectomy

Kathryn O'Hara and Doris Corkin

Scenario

Mark weighs 40 kg, is eleven years of age and is in the concrete-operational stage of development (Bee & Boyd 2007). He is an only child and lives with his mum, Anna, and dad, Patrick. Mark has no known health problems, apart from mild asthma which is well controlled using Seretide® 50 mcg two puffs twice daily and Ventolin 100 mcg two puffs as required. He is allergic to ibuprofen which exacerbates his asthma. Other than that, Mark has no known allergies. He has never been in hospital and has never had a general anaesthetic.

For the past two years Mark has suffered from recurrent tonsillitis, requiring antibiotic treatment at least five or six times a year. As a result Mark has missed long periods off school and this is affecting his overall academic performance. His GP referred him for an ENT consultation. At this consultation the specialist advised that Mark have his tonsils removed. The surgeon explained to Mark and his parents what the surgical procedure would entail and possible complications. Mark's mum signed his consent form and Mark's name was placed on the waiting list for a tonsillectomy.

This surgical procedure requires a short admission to hospital and a general anaesthetic. It can be very painful postoperatively and is occasionally complicated by bleeding.

Mark and his parents were invited to attend the pre-admission clinic, one week before his hospitalisation. At this clinic both parents and child are prepared for what is to happen both pre-operatively and postoperatively and they are given the time to ask questions. Furthermore, it also gives them the opportunity to meet both the nurses and doctors who will be involved in their care. However, Mark's mum is very anxious about the surgery.

Care Planning in Children and Young People's Nursing, First Edition.
Edited by Doris Corkin, Sonya Clarke, Lorna Liggett.
© 2012 Blackwell Publishing Ltd. Published 2012 by Blackwell Publishing Ltd.

Activity 23.1

Please refer to British National Formulary for Children (BNFC 2010–2011).

1. As ibuprofen is a non-steroidal anti inflammatory drug should Mark be prescribed this medication?
2. Using appropriate formula, what should the prescribed dose of paracetamol be for Mark, who weighs 40 kg? (see care planning in Chapter 27, for example of formula).
3. What should the prescribed dose of codeine be for Mark?

Questions

1. What is a tonsillectomy?
2. Having reflected upon the nursing process and models of care, how would the children's nurse prepare this young boy, Mark, and his family pre-operatively?
3. Describe the nursing care of Mark on his return to the ward during the immediate postoperative period (first 24 hours).
4. What discharge advice will be given to Mark and his parents?
   Mark has been readmitted to ward with history of secondary postoperative bleeding. Blood results (Hb <7 g/dl; GAIN, 2009) and history from his mum indicate a significant blood loss.
5. Discuss the nursing care of Mark when receiving a blood transfusion.

Answers to questions

Question 1. What is a tonsillectomy?

Tonsils are oval shaped masses of lymphatic tissue located on either side of the back of the throat. Their function is to prevent the entry of bacteria and viruses into the body via the nose and throat, thus protecting the gastrointestinal system from infection (McConochie 2001).

A tonsillectomy is a surgical procedure carried out to remove the tonsils. Some of the indications for this can be: following recurrent throat infections, suspected malignancy, sleep apnoea, or peritonsillar abscess.

Each year in the UK thousands of children under fifteen years of age have their tonsils removed.

Question 2. Having reflected upon the nursing process and models of care how would you the children's nurse prepare this young boy Mark and his family pre–operatively?

Assess/plan/pre-operative implementation and evaluation.

Models of care (Casey 1995; Roper *et al*. 1996).

- On arrival at the ward Mark and his family are taken to his bed. He is shown were to put his belongings and how to activate his television. Mark is introduced to his 'named nurse'.
- A family-centred approach (Casey 1995) is adopted and Mark and his family are encouraged to participate in his care. They are shown around the ward, toilets, parent's facilities, theatres and where the recovery ward is located.
- All available biographical details are confirmed with Mark's parents and when correct his patient identification armband is applied.
- Mark has baseline observations taken: temperature, pulse, respirations (TPR), oxygen saturation levels and blood pressure (BP). These are recorded as per ward pre-operative checklist.
- Mark's weight of 40 kg and height are recorded on his anaesthetic chart and medicine chart.
- A full medical history is taken and Mark's allergy to ibuprofen is highlighted on his medicine chart and anaesthetic chart. The nurse will establish if he has any current throat infections or head colds. If he does the anaesthetist must be informed and Mark's surgery would possibly be cancelled due to the higher risk of postoperative infection and bleeding.
- A family medical history is taken to establish any problems with general anaesthetic or bleeding.
- Mark and his family are introduced to the multidisciplinary team, consultant anaesthetist, consultant surgeon, ward doctor, nurses and play therapist.
- Check that the consent form has been signed and dated by one of Mark's parents and they are fully aware what they have consented to.
- Check pre-operative fasting times are adhered to: normally two hours for clear fluids and six hours for solids (RCN 2005), but as per anaesthetist's instructions.
- Apply anaesthetic cream to venous site as prescribed by doctor.
- Give full, clear explanation to parent and Mark regarding what will happen in anaesthetic room. If it is hospital policy, a parent and 'named nurse' should be able to accompany the child until they are asleep.
- Pre-operative checklist: confirm Mark's details are correct against his armband and both medical and nursing notes. Weight, baseline observations, allergies, any loose teeth (crowns or braces) should be noted. Confirm signed consent form, and pre-medication administered if ordered by anaesthetist. Also check fasting times were adhered to and offer parents the opportunity to accompany Mark to theatre.
- Prepare Mark's bed space for his return. Ensure working oxygen and suction in case of emergency. Have pulse oximetry monitor ready and nursing care documentation. Also a box of disposable tissues and emesis bowl should Mark feel sick.

Question 3. Describe the nursing care of Mark in relation to the immediate postoperative period (first 24 hours), having returned to the ward.

Assess and plan postoperative intervention.

Activity of living: maintaining a safe environment (Roper et al. 1996).

- Family-centred care approach (Casey 1995), if hospital policy, parents will be brought into recovery to be with Mark as he is waking. Mark and his parents will be involved in all aspects of his care. They will accompany him back to his bed space on the ward.

Implement post-operative intervention.

- If Mark is still asleep, attach him to monitor, explaining its purpose to his parents.
- Read medical and nursing notes and adhere to anaesthetist and surgeon's instructions.
- Document in nursing care plan medications and analgesia's Mark has received in theatre and recovery.
- Monitor and record Mark's TPR, oxygen saturations and BP on return to ward, according to hospital policy and as often as patient's condition dictates. Observations should be monitored at least half hourly for the first four hours.
- Mark should be observed for any bleeding from his mouth or nose; findings should be reported to the surgeon immediately. Blood loss can sometimes be difficult to measure as the tonsil bed can ooze slowly over a long period of time and may be swallowed.
- Mark should also be observed for excessive swallowing and or pallor, as children will often swallow blood postoperatively.
- Tell parent/Mark about the operation and provide reassurance.
- Hospital policy must be adhered to regarding care of intravenous (IV) cannula.
- If vomiting occurs, monitor and record amount, content and frequency, observing for any sign of fresh bleeding. Administer anti-emetic as prescribed and monitor and record effect/side effects.
- Any fresh blood in vomit must be reported immediately to surgeon in case Mark needs to return to theatre.
- Administer analgesia as prescribed and monitor and record effect/side effects.
- When fully conscious and there are no obvious signs of bleeding Mark can be given sips of water to drink initially. If tolerated then progress to free fluids and a light diet.
- It is important that Mark should drink and eat a normal diet postoperatively when considered appropriate. This aids healing by keeping the throat clean and moist.
- It is also important that Mark be given analgesia at least half an hour before meal times. If his throat is sore he will be reluctant to eat or drink, and there is then a greater risk of infection and postoperative bleeding.
- Ensure Mark's IV cannula is removed prior to discharge.

Question 4. What discharge advice will be given to Mark and his family?

Activity of living: communication (Roper *et al.* 1996).

Discharge advice

- Mark and his family will be advised of the importance of taking regular analgesia as prescribed. Try to take pain relief about half an hour before meals. The throat tends to be sorest first thing in the morning and at fifth day postoperatively.
- It is very important that Mark eats and drinks when he goes home so that he is well hydrated. This helps keep his throat moist and clean and aids healing.
- Some earache is normal; however, if pain is excessive see GP.
- At any sign of bleeding/haemorrhage either from the nose or throat Mark needs to be seen by an ENT doctor immediately. Parents are advised to contact the ward immediately, so that the doctor can be made aware of their impending arrival at A&E department.
- Mark is advised to stay off school for two weeks and stay indoors for the first two to three days, avoiding smoky atmospheres.
- Parents are given the ward contact number and told to phone at any time if they require advice.

There are two types of haemorrhage that may occur following a tonsillectomy:

* Intermediary
* Secondary

Intermediary haemorrhage occurs within the first 24 hours of surgery as a result of BP stabilisation (Chambers 1999). Secondary haemorrhage usually occurs within the first week or two after surgery and is associated with sloughing of the eschar (dead tissue) on the tonsil bed and/or an infection in the tonsillar fossae (Coleman 1992).

Question 5. Discuss the nursing care of Mark when receiving a blood transfusion.

Activity of living: communication/maintaining a safe environment (Roper *at al.* 1996).

Activity 23.2

Access and review the following resources:

Royal College of Nursing (2006) *Right Blood, Right Patient, Right Time: RCN Guidance for Improving Transfusion Practice.* London: RCN.
Serious Hazards of Transfusion (SHOT 2009) http://www.shotuk.org
Thompson, C.L., Edwards, C. & Stout, L. (2008) Blood transfusions 2: signs and symptoms of acute reactions. *Nursing Times*, **14**(3), 28–9.
Montgomery, H. & Kumar, J. (2008) Safe administration of blood and blood products, Chapter 25. In: Kelsey, J. & McEwing, G. (eds). *Clinical Skills in Child Health Practice.* Edinburgh: Churchill Livingstone, Elsevier.
http://www.learnbloodtransfusion.org.uk/ e-learning for safe, effective and appropriate transfusion practice.

Please note: it is very important that nurses adhere to hospital policy when administering blood to patients.

* Mark and his family should be fully informed by the doctor of his need for a blood transfusion, the likely duration of it and consent must be obtained and recorded in his medical records.
* Mark's pre-infusion observations should be taken and recorded: T, P, R and BP.
* Ensure that Mark is wearing an identification armband, stating his name, date of birth and hospital number.
* Blood must be prescribed by a doctor on the blood prescription sheet. This sheet must also have Mark's name, date of birth and hospital number on it. The doctor must prescribe the blood product, infusion rate, start and finish times and it must be transfused within four hours.
* Two registered nurses must check that Mark's details, blood group, expiry date and laboratory number do correspond with his prescription sheet, blood bag and blood component form.

- Ensure two nurses bring all this documentation to Mark's bedside and then ask him to clarify his name and date of birth. This will be double checked by asking the child's parents the same details.
- Again, two nurses check Mark's name, date of birth and hospital number against his wristband.
- Only when all checks are correct is blood administered.
- Sodium chloride 0.9% is first flushed through the blood infusion set, before connecting blood transfusion.
- Mark and his parents are asked to inform the nurse should he experience any of the following symptoms:
  — Sweating
  — Mottled appearance
  — Dizziness
  — Rash
  — Flushed appearance
  — Pyrexia
  — Tachycardia
  — Nausea

  Mark will be closely observed for any of these signs of an adverse reaction and will not be left unattended for the first 15 minutes of the blood transfusion or as policy dictates.
- Mark will also be observed for any major adverse reactions:
  — Rigors
  — Breathlessness/wheeze
  — Chest pain
  — Back or loin pain
  — Loss of consciousness
  — Collapse
- Should Mark experience any of these symptoms the blood transfusion should be stopped immediately and medical assistance called.
- Marks observations T, P, R and BP should be taken after the first 15 minutes of the blood transfusion commencing and again at the end of the transfusion or more frequently should his condition require.
- His infusion site should be checked at least hourly for any redness, swelling, tenderness or leakage.
- When the blood transfusion is completed the children's nurse should ensure Mark's nursing notes are accurately recorded.

Activity 23.3

Answer these questions about blood transfusion.

1. When should a blood infusion be started following removal from refrigerator?
   (a) 15 minutes
   (b) 20 minutes
   (c) 25 minutes
   (d) 30 minutes

2. Which of the following do BCSHguidelines.com/ (2009) recommend that the blood unit should be checked with:
   (a) Doctor prescription
   (b) Compatibility report
   (c) Patient ID
   (d) All of the above
3. Prior to administering blood, the giving set should be primed with:
   (a) 0.5% dextrose
   (b) 0.9% glucose
   (c) 0.5% sterile water
   (d) 0.9% sodium chloride
4. Current guidelines recommend that for every blood component transfused the following vital signs should be recorded *before* the start of each transfusion:
   (a) Temperature, pulse and respiration
   (b) Temperature and pulse
   (c) Temperature, pulse, respiration and blood pressure
   (d) Temperature, respiration and blood pressure
5. Adverse reactions usually occur within
   (a) First five minutes
   (b) First 15–20 minutes
   (c) First 60 minutes
   (d) After transfusion complete
6. In prolonged transfusion of consecutive units the giving sets must be changed:
   (a) After 2–6 hours
   (b) After 8–12 hours
   (c) After 12–16 hours
   (d) No need to change giving set
7. A blood transfusion should be completed within
   (a) 4 hours
   (b) 3 hours
   (c) 5 hours
   (d) 8 hours
8. On completion of transfusion each/all packs must be kept at ward level for
   (a) 12 hours
   (b) 24 hours
   (c) 48 hours
   (d) 72 hours

References

Bee, H. & Boyd, D. (2007) *The Developing Child*, 11th edn. London: Pearson.

British Committee for Standards in Haematology (BCSH) (2009) *The Administration of Blood Components*. www.bschguidelines.com/

British National Formulary for Children (BNFC) (2010–2011) *British National Formulary for Children*. British Medical Journal. London: PS Publishing.

Casey, A. (1995) Partnership nursing: influences on involvement of informal carers. *Journal of Advanced Nursing*, **22**, 1058–62.

Chambers, N. (1999) Wound Management. In: Hogston, R. & Simpson, P. (eds). *Foundations of Nursing Practice*. pp240–66. Basingstoke: Macmillan.

Coleman, B. (1992) *Diseases of the Nose, Throat and Ear and Head and Neck*, 14th edn. London: Churchill Livingstone.

Guidelines & Audit Implementation Network (GAIN, 2009) *Better Use of Blood in Northern Ireland: Guidelines for Blood Transfusion Practice*. Belfast, DHSSPS. (GAIN, formerly known as CREST) www.gain-ni.org.

McConochie, J (2001) Pathophysiology of tonsils, post-tonsillectomy bleed, treatment and nursing care. In: Sadik, R. & Campbell, G. (eds). *Client Profiles in Nursing: Child Health*. London: Greenwich Medical.

Montgomery, H. & Kumar, J. (2008) Safe administration of blood and blood products. Chapter 25. In: Kelsey, J. & McEwing, G. (eds). *Clinical Skills in Child Health Practice. Edinburgh*: Churchill Livingstone, Elsevier.

Roper, N., Logan, W. & Tierney, A.J. (1996) *The Elements of Nursing*, 4th edn. Edinburgh: Churchill Livingstone.

Royal College of Nursing (2005) *Perioperative Fasting in Adults and Children: an RCN Guideline for the Multidisciplinary Team*. London: RCN.

Royal College of Nursing (2006) *Right Blood, Right Patient, Right Time: RCN Guidance for Improving Transfusion Practice*. London: RCN.

Serious Hazards of Transfusion (SHOT 2009) www.shotuk.org

Thompson, C.L., Edwards, C. & Stout, L. (2008) Blood transfusions 2: signs and symptoms of acute reactions. *Nursing Times*, **14**(3), 28–9.

www.learnbloodtransfusion.org.uk/ e-learning for safe, effective and appropriate transfusion practice.

Answers to activities

Answers to activity 23.1

1. Ibuprofen should not be prescribed as the patient is allergic to it.
2. Paracetamol 15–20 mg/kg 4–6 hourly per day. No more than four doses in 24 hours. Mark could be prescribed 800 mg per dose.
3. Codeine is prescribed 0.5–1 mg/kg 4–6 hourly. Mark could be prescribed 20 mg per dose.

Answers to activity 23.3

1. (d) 30 minutes.
2. (d) All of the above.
3. (d) 0.9% sodium chloride.
4. (c) Temperature, pulse, respiration and blood pressure.
5. (b) First 15–20 minutes.
6. (b) After 8–12 hours.
7. (a) Four hours.
8. (c) 48 hours.

24

Appendicectomy

Lorna Liggett

Scenario

Catarina, a seven-year-old girl, is admitted to the children's surgical ward with a history of vomiting and abdominal pain for the past six hours. Following a nursing assessment and medical examination Catarina is prepared for theatre to have an appendicectomy preformed.

Catarina and her parents have recently come to the UK from Portugal. Catarina's father works in a local factory which involves 12-hour shifts and her mother works part time as a waitress in a local restaurant. Both can speak relatively good English and do not need an interpreter for everyday situations. Catarina attends the local primary school and is progressing well for her age.

The operation notes indicate that the appendix was slightly inflamed and therefore removed. The wound was sutured with six dissolvable sutures and a simple dressing was applied. Pain relief was given in theatre. After a short period in the recovery ward, Catarina was transferred to the ward where her mother was waiting for her.

Two aspects of care postoperatively will be addressed; these are wound care and communication.

The proposed scenario incorporates two nursing models for planning care, i.e. Roper *et al.* (2000) and Casey (1988). The author recommends the student to undertake additional reading.

Care Planning in Children and Young People's Nursing, First Edition.
Edited by Doris Corkin, Sonya Clarke, Lorna Liggett.
© 2012 Blackwell Publishing Ltd. Published 2012 by Blackwell Publishing Ltd.

> ## Questions
>
> 1. Explain the pathophysiology of appendicitis.
> 2. What are the stages of wound healing and types of dressings?
> 3. How does the children's nurse plan the care for Catarina in relation to personal cleansing and dressing?
> 4. Discuss how the children's nurse would utilise a family-centred approach to Catarina and her mother to explain the postoperative care in relation to wound care.

Answers to questions

Question 1. Explain the pathophysiology of appendicitis.

In acute appendicitis there is a compromised blood supply due to obstruction of the lumen, whereby it becomes very vulnerable to invasion by bacteria normally found in the gut.

Obstruction of the appendix lumen can be caused by hard impacted faeces, enlarged lymph nodes, worms, a tumour, or indeed a foreign object, which brings about a raised intra-luminal pressure that causes the wall of the appendix to become distended. Normal mucus secretions causes further build up of intra-luminal pressures and distension, which in turn cause compression and ischaemia of the mucosal walls.

Because there is a reduced blood supply to the wall of the appendix there will be little or no nutrition and oxygen to the appendix. It also means a reduced supply of white blood cells and other natural fighters of infection found in the blood being made available to the appendix. At this point the appendix will become necrosed and perforation of the appendix may occur. Pus formation, which is a combination of dead white cells, bacteria and dead tissue, occurs when nearby white blood cells are recruited to fight the bacterial invasion. The contents of the appendix are then released into the abdominal cavity causing peritonitis (Axton & Fugate 2003).

These events occur quite rapidly, possibly within one to three days, so this is why delay can be fatal.

Pain in appendicitis is caused initially by the distension of the wall of the appendix, and later when the grossly inflamed appendix rubs on the overlying inner wall of the abdomen and then with the spillage of the content of the appendix into the general abdominal cavity (peritonitis). The pain is usually noted in the right lower quandrant of the abdomen with associated abdominal tenderness, guarding and vomiting.

Fever is brought about by the release of toxic materials following the necrosis of the wall of the appendix, and later by pus formation.

Question 2. What are the stages of wound healing and types of dressings?

Revise the stages of wound healing:

- Inflammatory stage
- Destructive stage
- Proliferative stage
- Maturation stage

Table 24.1 Types of wound dressings.

Types of dressing	Examples	Use
Simple dressing	Mepore	Used for straightforward surgical wound, clean wounds. Skin-friendly, water-based, solvent-free adhesive for gentle and secure fixation. Soft, elastic non-woven for better patient comfort. Viral and bacterial proof backing film for protection of the wound from outer contamination.
Adhesive film dressing	Opsite Tegaderm	This is a transparent, vapour permeable dressing which acts as a barrier to bacteria and water. Transparent allowing wound checks. Suitable for shallow wound with low exudates.
Medicated and non-medicated dressings	Inadine Jelonet	These are normally soft-weave cotton dressings with soft paraffin, antibiotics or antiseptics and used for infected wounds or burns/scalds.
Hydrogels	Aquafoam	Composed mainly of water in a complex network or fibres that keep the polymer gel intact. Water is released to keep the wound moist .This provides a moist environment and is used in dry necrotic, granulating wounds. A secondary dressing is necessary.
Foam dressings	Flexipore Trufoam Lyofoam Mepilex	Designed to absorb large amounts of exudates. Maintain a moist wound environment but are not as useful as alginates or hydrocolloids for debridement.
Hydrocolloids	Tegasorb Hydrocol	Available in many forms (adhesive or non-adhesive pad, paste, powder), but most commonly as self-adhesive pads. Provides a moist environment for wounds which are necrotic, infected or granulating. Alginates or enzymatic (elase) removal of slough.

From Hess (2007).

For further reading please see Cardwell (2009), Chapter 32.

When undertaking wound care it is important to consider wound assessment, cleansing solutions and type of dressing (see Table 24.1). Following an assessment of the wound, health professionals should consult with the multidisciplinary team and as to which approach would be the most appropriate.

Assessing the postoperative wound

When a child returns from theatre with a wound the nurse must make an initial assessment of the wound and check if there is a dressing or drain in place. The children's nurse should always read the operation notes to ascertain how the procedure went and any special instructions to be followed.

- Appearance: if a wound dressing is in place it is important not to disturb this, other than to inspect the wound dressing for signs of intermediary bleeding. If no dressing is in place the nurse must continue with assessment of the wound.
- Size: the children's nurse must note the size of the wound and location of any dehiscence.
- Drainage: the children's nurse must observe location of wound, colour, exudate and odour.

- Exudate: fluid arising from the wound due to increased permeability of the capillaries; this will influence dressing type.
- Odour: an offensive odour is a sign of infection that needs to be assessed to identify an appropriate wound dressing.
- Inflammation: the children's nurse must observe for swelling and redness, though some slight swelling is normal in early stages of wound healing.
- Infection: needs to be addressed as it can affect the wound healing. Swabs should be taken for microbiology to assess what is causing the infection.
- Pain: expect a child to complain of pain around the area for several days. It is important to use an appropriate pain scale to assess pain intensity (Hockenberry & Wilson 2009).
- Drains/tubes: if any, what type, amount and colour of drainage.

Wound cleansing solutions

Children's nurses must be aware of the advantages and disadvantages of the different solutions available. Sodium chloride 0.9% is currently recommended as the solution of choice for wound cleansing (Cunliffe & Fawcett 2002). The advantages are that it is non-toxic to human tissues and does not give rise to sensitivity reactions. Also, it is non-expensive and as an isotonic solution it minimises the risk of cell damage. There is no documentation of disadvantages in the literature.

Activity 24.1

Name three other cleansing solutions you have seen being used for wound cleansing and ascertain the advantages and disadvantages of these.
   Refer to Chapter 4 in Bastin & Newton (2007).

Care planning for child following an appendicectomy: in-depth focus

Question 3. How does the children's nurse plan the care for Catarina in relation to personal cleansing and dressing?

Activity of daily living: personal cleansing and dressing.
Potential problem: Catarina's wound is at risk of becoming infected (NICE 2008).
Goal: to promote wound healing and prevent infection.
Nursing intervention:

- Explain to Catarina and her mother that the wound will be cleansed and redressed, to ensure they understand the intervention.
- Ensure strategies, such as pain assessment tools and distraction therapy, are in place to minimise wound pain before commencing, to ensure successful outcomes (Independent Advisory Group 2004).
- Educate Catarina and her mother regarding the importance of not removing the dressing until wound has healed.

- Discuss the process of wound cleansing with Catarina and her mother.
- Prepare child, equipment, environment and self to undertake aseptic technique.
- Carry out aseptic technique using non-touch technique (Glasper *et al.* 2010).
- Report and record on completion in order to promote continuity of care and collaboration between all professionals.
- Ensure Catarina is comfortable at all times.
- Encourage Catarina to ask questions and respond to these in an age appropriate manner.
- Educate Catarina and her mother when it is appropriate to shower or have a bath.

Evaluation: the purpose of this stage of the nursing process is to evaluate the progress towards the set goal in the care plan. If progress is not being made or is slow then the nurse must report and document this. Then the care plan may require to be modified accordingly. If goals have been achieved then the care can stop. Any new problems which arise can be identified at any stage and measurable goals must be negotiated and agreed with Catarina and her family.

All documentation must be available to members of the multidisciplinary team to perform the agreed care and update if necessary. Examples of questions the nurse could ask herself:

- Is the wound healing?
- What is the status of the wound?
- What are the priorities for caring for Catarina?
- Is her condition stable?
- What are her clinical observations?
- Is she progressing, i.e. drinking, mobile, relatively pain free?
- When will she be discharged, who will be at home with her?

The collection of data to determine the extent to which the set goals are achieved is crucial to the evaluation.

Question 4. Discuss how the children's nurse would utilise a family-centred approach to Catarina and her mother to explain the postoperative care in relation to wound care.

Activity 24.2

Review the key components of family-centred care.
  (See Chapter 1)
  Peate & Whiting (2006) Chapter 3
  Moules & Ramsey (2008) p280

Good communication is essential when working with children, young people and their families since it assists in building up trust and encourages them to feel comfortable in seeking advice. Children, young people and their families have the right to be fully informed and involved in all decisions about their treatment and plan of care (Wales *et al.* 2008). The nurse must always communicate with children and young people in an age appropriate manner and appreciate personal circumstances and the needs of the person. In order to build a good rapport the nurse must show respect, understanding and be honest throughout as this will have a positive impact on their lives (DfCSF 2010).

In 2009 the Nursing Midwifery Council (NMC) undertook a review of pre-registration nursing education (RPNE) which focused on the future and how nursing programmes across the UK would need to look in order to enable nurses to meet the needs of patients safely and effectively. Under the domain of communication and interpersonal skills the field standard of competence statement for children's nursing states: 'children's nurses must also take account of individual differences, including the child's, young person's developmental stage, their ability to understand, their culture, any learning or communication difficulties and their health status. They must communicate effectively with parents and carers' (nmc. uk.org). This statement clearly indicates the importance of communication when working with children and their families and identifies the need for development through training, education and experience in order to communicate effectively.

✎ Activity 24.3

Reflect upon your practice using the Gibbs (1988) reflective cycle as seen below in Figure 24.1.

   Consider a recent experience in caring for a young person whilst in practice.
   Explore your communication with the young person.

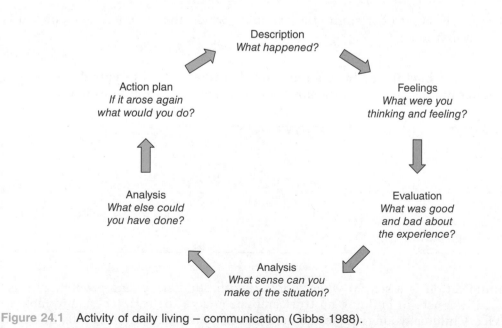

Figure 24.1   Activity of daily living – communication (Gibbs 1988).

Activity of daily living: communication (Gibbs 1988).

Potential problem: Catarina and her mother may not fully understand the information given to them and the medical terminology used. This could lead to misinterpretation and advice and guidance not being followed through.

Goal: to ensure Catarina and her mother fully understand the information given to them.

Nursing intervention: the children's nurse must:

- Take account of the Catarina's cognitive ability (Boyd & Bee 2010).
- Use a family-centred approach throughout to promote collaboration and partnership (Casey 1988).
- Sit down with Catarina and her mother and speak slowly to ensure understanding.
- Appreciate the mother's ability to understand and contact a translator if necessary so that the information is accurate.
- Determine Catarina and her parents' level of understanding regarding the surgery and subsequent care.
- Give time for them to ask questions, listen to them and respond appropriately to ensure no misinterpretation.
- Reassess their understanding on a regular basis.
- Share all information with parent and child regarding progress, to promote understanding.
- Recognise the family's strengths and methods of coping.
- Encourage and facilitate parent-to-child support.
- Provide information leaflets to reinforce verbal information.
- Incorporate the developmental needs of Catarina to promote her independence.
- Provide play/distraction therapies.

Evaluation: this is an important aspect of nursing care which can be productive, satisfying and rewarding. Evaluation of the care plan provides a tool to reflect on current practices, identify ways to improve care and services to patients and also builds a solid foundation for continuous quality improvement initiative. Evaluation helps the nurse to learn how to meet the child and family's needs more efficiently and to follow progress over time. It also helps to identify things which are going well and provides positive feedback to the child and family.

The nurse should select each point from the plan of care and report and record outcome/progress.

- The children's nurse should explain the operation to Catarina's mother when Catarina returns to the ward.
- When Catarina awakes from the anaesthetic the nurse should explain that she has returned to the ward and her mother is there.
- Ensure Catarina is comfortable and relatively free from pain.
- The nurse will seek consent from Catarina to look at the wound site.
- The nurse should take time to explain the ongoing care of Catarina to her mother: when she can have oral fluids, if she can sit up in bed or walk to the toilet and how long she may be in hospital for.
- Negotiate with Catarina's mother what aspects of care she wishes to be involved in.
- When Catarina is fully awake, relatively pain free and clinical observation all within normal limits the nurse should reassess her progress and report and record.

- Arrange for a play therapist to visit Catarina.
- Select appropriate leaflets for both to read.

References

Axton, S. & Fugate, T. (2003) *Paediatric Nursing Care Plans for the Hospitalised Child*, 3rd edn. Upper Saddle River, NJ: Pearson, Prentice Hall.

Bastin, J. & Newton, H. (2007) Wound care, Chapter 4. In: Chambers, M. & Jones, S. (eds). *Surgical Nursing of Children*. Edinburgh: Butterworth Heinemann.

Boyd, D, & Bee, H. (2010) Chapter 14. *The Growing Child*. London: Allyn and Bacon, Pearson.

Cardwell, P. (2009) Chapter 32. In: Glasper, A. McEwing, G. & Richardson, J. (eds). *Foundation Skills for Caring*. UK: Palgrave Macmillan.

Casey, A. (1988) The development and use of the partnership model of nursing care. In: Glasper, E. A, & Tucker, A. (eds) (1993). *Advances in Child Health Nursing*. London: Scutari Press. pp 183–93.

Cunliffe, P.J. & Fawcett, I. (2002) Wound cleansing: the evidence for the techniques and solutions used. *Professional Nurse*, **18**(2), 95–9.

Department for Children, Schools and Families (2010) *Effective Communication with Children, Young People and Families. Every Child Matters*. London: DfCSF. www.dcsf.gov.uk/everychildmatters/strategy/deliveringservices/commoncoreofskills

Gibbs, G. (1988) *Learning by Doing: a Guide to Teaching and Learning Methods*. Oxford: Further Education Unit, Oxford Brookes University.

Glasper, A, Aylott, M, & Battrick, C. (2010) *Developing Practical Skills for Nursing Children and Young People*. London: Hodder Arnold.

Hess, C.T. (2007) *Clinical Guide to Wound Care*, 6th edn. Philadelphia: Lippincott. Williams and Wilkins.

Hockenberry, M.J. & Wilson, D. (2009) *Wong's Essentials of Paediatric Nursing*. St Louis: Mosby.

Independent Advisory Group (2004) *Best Practice Statement Minimising Trauma and Pain in Wound Management*. Wounds-UK and Moinlycke Health Care.

Moules T. & Ramsey, J. (2008) *The Textbook of Children's and Young People's Nursing*, 2nd edn. Oxford: Blackwell Publishing.

National Institute for Health and Clinical Excellence (2008) *Surgical Site Infection: Prevention and Treatment of Surgical Site Infection*. London: NICE.

Peate, I. & Whiting, L. (2006) *Caring for Children and Families*. Chichester: Wiley.

Roper, N., Logan, W.W. & Tierney, A.J. (2000) *The Roper-Logan-Tierney Model of Nursing: Based on the Activities of living*. Edinburgh: Elsevier Health Sciences.

Wales, S. Crisp, J. Moran, P. Perrin, M. Scott, E. (2008) Assessing communication between health professional, children and families. *Journal of Children's and Young Peoples Nursing*, **2**(2), 77–83.

www.nmc.uk.org (accessed 2 August 2010).

Section 7

Care of Infants and Young Persons with Orthopaedic Conditions

25

Ilizarov Frame

Sonya Clarke

Scenario

Patrick is 14 years old and lives in a two-storey town house with his parents and five-year-old sister Annie. As an active seven-year-old Patrick regularly cycled in the local park. However, as he attempted to cross the busy road that leads to the park a car collided with him due to poor visibility. Patrick was taken to A&E, where his condition was stabilised and a diagnosis of a growth plate arrest injury confirmed, he was then transferred to the children's ward. Post-discharge Patrick's condition continued to be monitored long term under the care of an orthopaedic consultant. But over time the road traffic accident (RTA) resulted in a 6 cm leg length discrepancy (LLD), where one leg became shorter than the other due to the growth plate arrest.

A child with LLD walks on the toes of the short leg, with the heel never touching the ground, whereas the adult walks with a heel toe gait on short side and vaults over the long leg. The result is excessive up and down motion of the pelvis and trunk. Long-term effects include scoliosis, hip adduction and flexion or recurvatum on the long side and equinus deformity on the short side. Patrick was subsequently monitored regarding his LLD.

Patrick now wears a 'shoe raise' which he hates as it makes him appear 'different', even though it equalises his leg length and aids mobility. During a consultation with his orthopaedic surgeon it was agreed for Patrick to be admitted to hospital for elective surgery which involves application of an Ilizarov frame to his right tibia (see Figure 25.1) in order to correct the 6 cm leg length discrepancy. Limb lengthening will be achieved via osteogenesis distraction with the frame in situ for approximately six months (see Table 25.1 for principles of limb lengthening). Successful limb equalisation would mean Patrick would be able to wear normal shoes and trainers like his peers following removal of the frame.

Care Planning in Children and Young People's Nursing, First Edition.
Edited by Doris Corkin, Sonya Clarke, Lorna Liggett.
© 2012 Blackwell Publishing Ltd. Published 2012 by Blackwell Publishing Ltd.

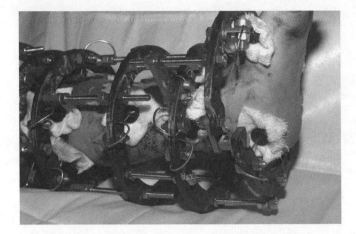

Figure 25.1 Ilizarov frame (from Clarke and Richardson (2008), reproduced with permission. Copyright Elsevier).

Table 25.1 Principles of limb lengthening.

A three-phase process – delay, distract and consoldiate
Minimal disturbance of the bone

- Delay before distraction: this allows osteogenesis formation to begin
- Rate of distraction: 1 mm a day
- The duration of the consolidation phase depends on the amount of bone to be lengthened 6 cm = 6 months' consolidation

 Questions

1. What is an Ilizarov frame/Ilizarov technique?
2. Reflecting upon the nursing process and a model of care how would the children's nurse prepare this young person and his family for application of an Ilizarov frame?
3. Discuss the nursing care of Patrick in relation to the immediate postoperative period (first 24 hours), having returned to the ward.
4. In an attempt to prevent pin site infection Patrick will be taught pin site management. Discuss the methods currently used within the UK.
5. How would the children's nurse prepare Patrick and his family for discharge, following application of an Ilizarov frame?

The proposed answer plans offer 'lists of potential responses' with limited rationale. It is therefore recommended for the individual student/healthcare professional to explore the issues through further reading.

Answers to questions

Question 1. What is an Ilizarov frame/Ilizarov technique?

Ilizarov frame/fixation is used for fracture fixation and stabilisation, limb reconstruction, deformity correction and limb lengthening, using wires instead of pins and a circular frame instead of bars (Santy *et al.* 2009).

Ilizarov technique: a bone-fixation technique using an external fixator for lengthening limbs, correcting pseudarthroses and other deformities, and assisting the healing of otherwise hopeless traumatic or pathological fractures and infections, such as chronic osteomyelitis. The method was devised by the Russian orthopaedic surgeon Gavriil Abramovich Ilizarov (1921–1992) (http://128.240.24.212/cgi-bin/omd?Ilizarov+technique).

Question 2. Reflecting upon the nursing process and a model of care how would the children's nurse prepare this young person and his family for application of an Ilizarov frame?

Activity of living: maintaining a safe environment.

Assess: determine the child's and parents' level of knowledge in relation to all aspects of hospitalisation care.

Plan: the children's nurse must ensure Patrick and his parents are given appropriate preoperative preparation at ward level, which will involve physical and psychological care, the induction of a general anaesthetic (GA), pain management, the actual surgical procedure and what to expect post-surgery regarding application of the Ilizarov frame (as shown in Table 25.2). All planned care should adopt an appropriate model of nursing, for example Casey (1988; 1995) and Roper *et al.* (2005). Although Roper *et al.* (2005) address 12 activities of daily living (refer to Chapter 1) this chapter will only address the problems in pre- and postoperative care in relation to maintaining a safe environment.

Implement/preoperative interventions:

- Patrick should be settled into his bed space, be comfortable with the ward surroundings and introduced to his nominated 'named nurse'.
- A family-centred care approach should be adopted to include the family during all aspects of care, in addition to open visiting, tea-making and overnight facilities for a parent if required.
- Explain what an Ilizarov frame is, show pictures, models and if possible introduce Patrick and parents to another child with a frame *in situ*.

Table 25.2 Phases of treatment.

- Pre-operative
- Latency period: initial postoperative period
- Distraction (approx 1/3 of time in frame)
  Starts about 5–7 days postoperatively
  1 mm day divided into four increments or 0.25 cm every six hours
- Consolidation (approx 2/3 of time in frame)
- Removal of frame (6–12 months approx)
- Rehabilitation

- Facilitate Patrick and his parents to raise any concerns they have regarding application of the frame, complications and the effects of altered body image for a 14-year-old boy.
- Complete and record base line observations – temperature, pulse, respirations (TPR) and blood pressure (BP).
- Complete ward urinalysis, if nothing abnormal detected (NAD) record and proceed, otherwise report and send mid-stream specimen of urine (MSSU) to laboratory for organism and sensitivity (O&S).
- Record weight and height accurately.
- Apply patient identification armband(s).
- Complete baseline venapuncture (may be undertaken by nurse or doctor) and send to laboratory as ordered by anaesthetist, full blood picture (FBP) and urea and electrolytes (U&E), plus 'group and hold' (blood for transfusion usually not ordered as operation carried out using tourniquet with minimal blood loss).
- Teach an appropriate pain assessment tool, 0–10 would be appropriate for a 14-year-old boy, where 0 is 'no pain' and 10 is the 'most imaginable pain' (Clarke 2003a).
- Discuss potential pain management options:
    — Patient controlled analgesia (PCA)
    — Continuous epidural infusion (Clarke 2003b; Wheetman 2006)
    — Intravenous paracetamol (Clarke & Richardson 2007) and step-down medication
- Record full medical history, known allergies, establish if smoker/non-smoker, any family problems with a GA, etc.
- Facilitate informed consent (medical responsibility) through verbal, written and visual display of an Ilizarov frame.
- Multidisciplinary approach and introduction to team: anaesthetist, consultant, named nurse, physiotherapist, occupational therapist (OT), and specialist Ilizarov nurse.
- Information on maintaining an Ilizarov frame, i.e. pin site care.
- Risk assessment using a dedicated tool, for example Waterlow (1998) score, and placed on appropriate pressure relieving device (bed and mattress).
- Plan discharge date.
- Pre-operative fasting times as per anaesthetist's instructions (normally two hours for fluids and six hours for solids), patient shower, clean bed, gown *in situ* and premedication administration if prescribed.
- Check out system; confirm patient details are correct, weight, allergies noted, notes, blood results and X-rays available, confirm signed consent form, and pre-medication administered if ordered. Also record if fasting times adhered to and offer parents to escort Patrick to theatre.
- Prepare Patrick's bed space to ensure a safe environment following his return from surgery – collect appropriate documentation, check oxygen and suction equipment is working, and gather any necessary monitoring or infusion devices.

Evaluate all nursing interventions and document.

Question 3. Discuss the nursing care of Patrick in relation to the immediate postoperative period (first 24 hours), having returned to the ward.

Activity of living: maintaining a safe environment.
  Assess and plan postoperative interventions:

- Family-centred care approach, involve the parents when collecting Patrick from recovery and return Patrick to his prepared bed space. Patrick and parents to be involved in all aspects of care.

Implement postoperative interventions:

- Attach Patrick to appropriate monitoring and infusion equipment as per hospital policy.
- Read medical and nursing notes, adhering to anaesthetist and surgeon instructions.
- Ensure Patrick is comfortable, i.e. reposition, review risk assessment using appropriate tool, for example Waterlow (1998).
- Observations to be completed and recorded on dedicated postoperative chart with appropriate action as per hospital protocol:
  — TPR, SAO$_2$ (oxygen saturations), and BP
  — Neurovascular observations are imperative; Shields & Clarke (2011) suggest using Dykes' (1993) five Ps, where the nurse would assesses and document Patrick's pain, pulses, pallor, parasthesia and paralysis
  — Pain assessment score using the numerical scale 0–10
- Check Ilizarov frame (as above), neurovascular status of lower limb, pin sites for ooze, bleeding and signs of infection.
- Hospital protocol must be adhered to regarding care of cannula, i.e. patency and management of intravenous fluids (IV) fluids.
- Administer analgesia as ordered by anaesthetist. Patrick would most likely receive either a morphine-based PCA or an epidural infusion with a local anaesthetic. Both would be in conjunction with regular IV paracetamol. Nurse to observe for potential side effects of opioids. Analgesia can be used in conjunction with non-pharmacological methods, for example music.
- Monitor IV fluids (as per hospital protocol). Patrick may also tolerate sips of water later in the day. Also monitor output on fluid balance chart, reporting any concern to anaesthetist. Patrick may also have an indwelling urinary catheter and this often accompanies an epidural infusions (Wheetman 2006).
- Patrick to be reviewed by pain management team.
- Occupational therapist to review Patrick to make foot splint which aims to prevent neurovascular complication, i.e. dropped foot.
- Consider Patrick's altered body image and privacy needs of a young person.
- Patrick to be reviewed by Ilizarov team: orthopaedic consultant, anaesthetist, physiotherapist and specialist nurse.
- Administer IV prophylactic antibiotics as per hospital protocol.
- Complete check X-ray as per consultant's instruction.

Evaluate all nursing interventions and document.

Question 4. In an attempt to prevent pin site infection Patrick will be taught pin site management. Discuss the methods currently used within the UK.

The use of multiple pins has increased the risk of complications such as intractable pain, tethering and tenting of the surrounding skin, muscle spasm, swelling and soft tissue tension, and infection at the pin site, which is the main concern and can result in loosening of the pin, loss of fixation and osteomyelitis (Patterson 2005). In the UK the expert British nursing consensus group on pin site care (Lee-Smith *et al.* 2001) differentiate clearly between the terms 'reaction', 'colonisation' and 'infection' when discussing pin site care. Pin site care which is identified by Santy (2000) as requiring specialised nursing care is a psychomotor skill initially undertaken by the nurse and then executed by either the child or parent following appropriate education and a period of supervised practice. Clarke & Richardson (2008) address the evidence on how best to manage and care for pins and wires that fundamentally seek to reduce or prevent the aforementioned complications.

A review of the literature confirms that opinion differs on the most appropriate management of skeletal pin sites and that protocols are often based on doctor/nurse preference (Sims & Saleh 1996). There is little scientific evidence to support one technique over another (Gordon *et al.* 2000) and indeed the literature highlights the dearth of actual completed research studies on skeletal pin site care. Clarke & Richardson's study (2008) demonstrates both cleansing approaches, i.e. the lesser used 'traditional British' (Table 25.3) approach versus the contemporary 'Russian' method (Table 25.4). This information should be used in conjunction with local guidelines for wound care, infection control and following discussion and agreement with other relevant members of the healthcare team and reviewed on an ongoing basis.

Activity 25.1

Consider the impact on 'the family' when Patrick returns home with an Ilizarov frame on his leg for six months.

Question 5. How would the children's nurse prepare Patrick and his family for discharge, following application of an Ilizarov frame?

Activity of living: maintaining a safe environment.

- Commence discharge planning on admission: reflect upon Patrick's stage of development and identify individual needs *(assess)*.
- Early *planning*: ensure Patrick is eating and drinking normally in conjunction with a normal urinary output and bowel function.
- *Implementation*: establish communication pathways with MDT and refer to community health care, i.e. children's community nurse.
- Physiotherapy input regarding mobilisation, check if Patrick can complete stairs and educate on elevation of limb with crutches to aid mobility.
- Educate Patrick on a healthy balanced diet and effects of smoking (it can interfere with bone healing).
- Occupational therapy referral for potential housing aids, urinal, and wheelchair for distance, etc.
- Patrick to be taught and then demonstrate competence in undertaking 'Ilizarov turns' the osteogenesis component of the distraction process.

Table 25.3 'Traditional' pin site cleansing (Clarke & Richardson 2007).

Points	Action	Rationale
1.	Prepare patient: seek verbal consent, check patient's position or alternatively check if shower room vacant and record pain score.	Potential pain during pin site dressings – offer analgesia if appropriate.
	Collect the required equipment: Dressing pack Apron Sterile scissors Sterile gloves Non-sterile gloves Forceps (optional) Cleaning solution Tape 'Non-woven' gauze and *no* 'Q' tips (long cotton buds).	Day 1–2 post-surgery, reduce and renew dressings at bedside using aseptic technique as described in points 7–14 (no shower).

	'Q' tips (long cotton buds).	No fibres to be left at pin site.
2.	Wash and dry hands and put on plastic apron.	Prevent cross infection.
3.	Apply non-sterile gloves, remove existing dressings and discard in yellow clinical waste bag.	To expose pin sites.
4.	Inspect all pin sites.	Observe for signs of pin site reaction or infection.

| 5. | Wash hands. | Prevent cross infection. |
| 6. | Open all sterile dressings and equipment to be used. | In preparation for aseptic technique. |

continued

Table 25.3 (*Continued*)

Points	Action	Rationale
7.	Using a separate piece of non-woven gauze (gloved finger or forceps), clean each individual pin site with using a sweeping action.	In an attempt to prevent infection at pin site. Non-woven gauze will not shed; 'Q' tips produce shedding fibres.

| | Following 24–48 hour postoperative reduction and redressing of pin sites at bedside. Commence daily showering of pin sites, clean away exudate or dried blood away from skin using normal saline or chlorohexidine 2 mg/ml and attach required gauze rolls. Otherwise do not clean. | Example of shower chair (with pillow), to assist in the cleaning of pin sites. |

8.	Keep metal work socially clean Gently remove scabs and crusts around pin site.	In an attempt to prevent infection at pin site.
9.	Clean or dry rub surrounding skin with gauze. Do not massage.	To prevent skin tenting/tethering.
10.	Expose pin sites if non-symptomatic.	To prevent infection.
11.	Redress red or oozing pin site with gauze roll and secure with tape (alternatively at bedside on return from shower room).	To soak up exudate.
12.	Place solutions in secure cupboard, discard all dressings, gloves, and apron in clinical waste bag.	Health and safety. To prevent cross infection.
13.	Wash hands.	To prevent cross infection.
14.	Re-assess patient's pain score.	Review analgesia.

Table 25.3 (*Continued*)

Points	Action	Rationale
15.	Teach patient to shower at home and dry fixator with a clean towel used only for this purpose. Actively clean pin sites only if exudate present. Keep regime simple and provide instruction.	Tampering with pin sites excessively can lead to infection. Expect poor or non-compliance.
16.	Educate patient/family and community staff to look for signs of pin infection.	To identify problems early.
17.	Provide as much written and verbal information as possible with contact numbers. Provide opportunities to contact other patients and support groups.	To reduce anxiety, increase compliance and provide support.
18.	Provide psychosocial support.	Pins/wires amount to a major insult to self-image.

Adapted from Lee Smith *et al.* (2001).

Table 25.4   'Russian pin site cleansing' (Clarke and Richardson 2007)

Points	Action	Rationale
1.	Prepare patient: seek verbal consent, check patient's position and record pain score. Collect the required equipment: Dressing pack Sterile scissors Sterile gloves Bandages Non-sterile gloves Forceps (optional) Hydrex – pink chlorhexedine gluconate 0.5% w/v 70% v/v 'Non-woven' gauze squares	Potential pain during pin site dressings. Offer analgesia if appropriate. Day 2 post-surgery, reduce and renew dressings. Thereafter dressings will be changed at seven-day intervals (a shower can be taken prior to pin site care). No fibres to be left at pin site.
2.	Wash and dry hands then put on plastic apron.	Prevent cross infection.
3.	Pull back black rubber bungs (see below).	To provide access to existing dressings.
4.	Apply non-sterile gloves, remove existing bandages, dressings and discard in yellow clinical waste bag.	To expose pin sites.
5.	Inspect all pin sites.	Observe for signs of infection, etc.

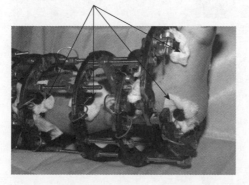

continued

Table 25.4 (*Continued*)

Points	Action	Rationale
6.	Wash hands.	Prevent cross infection.
7.	Open all sterile dressings and equipment to be used.	In preparation for aseptic technique.
8.	Apply sterile gloves.	To prevent cross infection.
9.	Prepare gauze squares by making slit in the gauze (keyhole dressing; see below).	To allow gauze to fit over wire at the pin site.
10.	Using a separate piece of gauze (gloved finger or forceps), clean each individual pin site with Hydrex- 0.5% w/v 70% v/v alcohol solution using a sweeping action.	In an attempt to prevent infection at pin site.

Rubber bung

11.	Do not remove crusts or scabs. Keep metal work socially clean.	In an attempt to prevent infection at pin site.
12.	Moisten all required gauze squares in Hydrex- 0.5% w/v 70% v/v alcohol solution and remove excess liquid from each gauze square.	In an attempt to prevent infection at pin site and reduce skin irritation.
13.	Apply the moistened keyhole gauze square dressing to each pin site.	Keyhole dressings of gauze, 2–3 layers thick moistened with Hydrex solution – alcoholic chlorohexidine. With excess liquid removed to prevent infection and skin irritation.

Key hole dressing

Table 25.4 (*Continued*)

Points	Action	Rationale
14.	Position the rubber bung onto each pre-soaked square gauze at each pin site (as demonstrated).	To secure gauze stays in position at pin site.

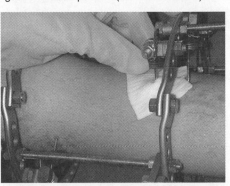

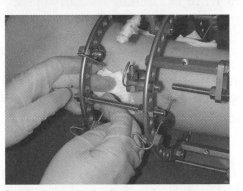

Points	Action	Rationale
15.	Bandaging each pin site.	Bandaging in figure of eight to secure dressings and ensure that the bungs do not lift.

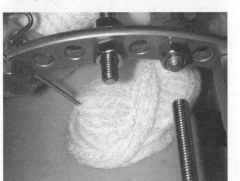

Points	Action	Rationale
16.	Place solutions in a secure cupboard and discard all dressings, gloves and apron in clinical waste bag/bin.	Health and safety. To prevent cross infection.
17.	Wash hands.	To prevent cross infection.
18.	Re-assess patient's pain score.	Review analgesia.
19.	Teach patient and family a similar regime. Keep regime simple and provide instruction.	Tampering with pin sites excessively can lead to infection. Expect poor or non compliance.

continued

Table 25.4 (*Continued*)

Points	Action	Rationale
20.	Educate patient/family and community staff to look for signs of pin infection. In some cases arrangements can be made to have the dressings completed by the Ilizarov nurse specialist.	To identify problems early.
21.	Provide verbal and written information with contact numbers. Provide opportunities to contact other patients and support groups.	To reduce anxiety, increase compliance and provide support.
22.	Provide psychosocial support.	Pins/wires amount to a major insult to self-image.

Adapted from Davies *et al.* (2005) and Lee Smith *et al.* (2001).

- Also teach and observe Patrick's competence in cleaning his pin sites as per hospital protocol in conjunction with the signs of infection (Clarke & Richardson 2008).

  An adapted 'Russian method' of pin site cleaning is currently used in Northern Ireland; variations of the traditional and Russian methods are used in the UK (Davies *et al.* 2005; Santy 2006).
- Provide contact numbers to enable troubleshooting with specialist/ward nurse regarding potential problems, for example pin site infection, neurovascular compromise (e.g. swelling, discoloured toes, cool to touch), pain, or early consolidation (fracture of new bone growth – it goes 'pop'), etc.
- Outpatient date to be given to review Patrick's progress.
- Check X-ray to be completed and viewed – discharge to be confirmed by orthopaedic consultant (*evaluation*).
- Doctor's letter for GP given to Patrick.
- Liaise with Patrick's school regarding returning to school or home tuition.
- Three-day supply of medication discussed, checked and given to Patrick with his parents; may include paracetamol and short-term codeine for pain. Discuss possibility of constipation due to restricted mobility and medication, may also be prescribed a stool softener.
- Discuss future admission and procedure to remove Ilizarov frame.
- Allow Patrick and his parents to ask questions.
- Document all care and discharge interventions.

References

Casey, A. (1988) A partnership with child and family. *Senior Nurse*, **8**(4), 8–9.

Clarke, S.E. (2003a) Orthopaedic paediatric practice: an impression pain assessment. *Journal of Orthopaedic Nursing*, **7**(3), 132–6.

Clarke, S.E. (2003b) Postoperative pain in children: a retrospective audit of continuous epidural analgesia in a paediatric orthopaedic ward. *Journal of Orthopaedic Nursing*, **7**(1), 4–9.

Clarke, S.E. & Richardson, O. (2007) Using intravenous paracetamol in children following surgery: a literature review. *Journal of Children's and Young People's Nursing*, **1**(6), 273–80.

Clarke, S.E. & Richardson, O. (2008) Skeletal pin site care, Chapter 42 In: Kelsey, J. & McEwing, G (eds). *Clinical Skills in Child Health Practice*. London: Churchill Livingstone Elsevier, 379–87.

Davies, R., Holt, N. & Nayagam, S. (2005) The care of pin sites with external fixation. *Journal of Bone and Joint Surgery*, **87B**, **5**, 716–19.

Dykes, C. (1993) Minding the five Ps of neurovascular assessment. *American Journal of Nursing*, **193**(6), 38–9.

Gordon, J.E., Kelly-Hahn, J., Carpenter, CJ. & Schoenecker, P.L. (2000) Pin site care during external fixation in children: results of a nihilistic approach. *Journal of Paediatric Orthopaedics*, **20**, 163–5.

Lee-Smith J., Santy, J., Davis, P., Jester, R. & Kneale, J. (2001) Pin site management. Towards a consensus: part 1. *Journal of Orthopaedic Nursing*, **5**, 37–42.

Patterson, M. (2005) Multicenter pin site study. *Orthopaedic Nursing*, **24**(5), 349–59.

Roper N., Logan W. & Tierney A. (1990) *The Elements of Nursing*, 3rd edn. London: Churchill Livingstone.

Santy, J. (2000) Nursing the patient with an external fixator. *Nursing Standard*, **14**(31), 47–52.

Santy, J. (2006) A survey of current practice in skeletal pin site management. *Journal of Orthopaedic Nursing*, **10**, 198–205.

Santy J., Vincent, M. & Duffield, B. (2009) The principles of caring for patients with Ilazarov external fixation. *Nursing Standard*, **23**(6), 50–55.

Shields, C. & Clarke, S (2011) Using neurovascular assessment tool within children's A&E *International Journal of Orthopaedic and Trauma Nursing*, **15**(1), 3–10.

Sims, M. & Saleh, M. (1996) Protocols for the care of external fixator pinsites. *Professional Nurse*, **11**, 261–4.

Waterlow, J. (1998) Pressure sores in children: risk assessment. *Paediatric Nursing*, **10**(4), 22–3.

Wheetman, A. (2006) Use of epidural analgesia in postoperative pain management. *Nursing Standard*, **20**(44), 54–64.

26

Developmental Dysplasia of the Hip

Sonya Clarke

Scenario

Wai-ki is a five-month-old baby girl who recently emigrated from China with her parents. During a routine visit to their GP concerns were raised regarding Wai-ki's lower limbs. A physical examination showed an uneven crease fold, leg length discrepancy, limited range of movement, with no evidence of pain. Both parents were present at the appointment with Dad interpreting (Mum has limited English). Wai-ki was referred to a paediatric orthopaedic consultant following her clinical examination.

A second physical examination in conjunction with an X-ray of Wai-ki's hips confirms developmental dysplasia of the right hip (DDH). The parents agree to an elective admission to a children's orthopaedic ward following an informed discussion with the paediatric orthopaedic consultant. Wai-ki is scheduled for a closed reduction of her right hip, adductor tenotomy and application of a hip spica cast (see Figures 26.1 and 26.2) under general anaesthetic.

Wai-ki undertakes the planned surgery (Dad was available to interpret) and returns to the ward in a double hip spica with no complications.

The proposed case history incorporates two nursing models for planning care, i.e. Roper *et al.* (2000) and Casey (1988). The author recommends the student undertakes additional reading around the specialist area of orthopaedics.

Care Planning in Children and Young People's Nursing, First Edition.
Edited by Doris Corkin, Sonya Clarke, Lorna Liggett.
© 2012 Blackwell Publishing Ltd. Published 2012 by Blackwell Publishing Ltd.

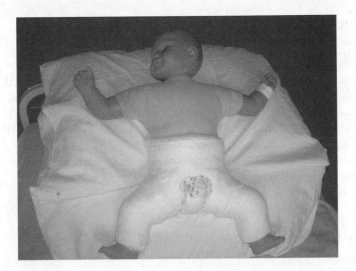

Figure 26.1 Child in hip spica cast. The nappy is effectively tucked into the hip spica.

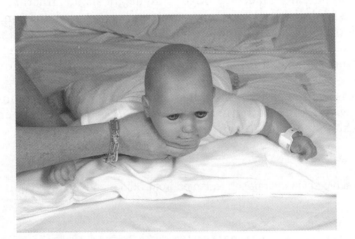

Figure 26.2 Child in hip spica cast, positioned prone with head supported.

 Questions

1. What is developmental dysplasia of the hip (DDH)?
2. What is a hip spica, and what does it do for Wai-ki?
3. How does the children's nurse plan the care for Wai-ki in relation to 'controlling body temperature'? (Use the adult-based Roper *et al.* (2000) model of care and Casey's model of nursing (1988), working in partnership with children and their families.)

Answers to questions

Question 1. What is developmental dysplasia of the hip (DDH)?

Clarke & Dowling (2003) described DDH as a spectrum of disorders related to abnormal development of the hip that may develop at any time during foetal life, infancy or childhood. A change in terminology from congenital hip dysplasia (CDH) to DDH more properly reflects the varying onset and types of hip abnormalities in which there is a shallow acetabulum, subluxation or dislocation (Kneale & Davis 2005). The cause of DDH is unknown, but certain factors such as gender, birth order, family history, intrauterine position, delivery type, joint laxity and post-natal positioning are believed to affect the risk of DDH (Kneale & Davis 2005).

Question 2. What is a hip spica, and what does it do for Wai-ki?

Young children (under the age of five years) who present with the condition DDH or fractured femur have traditionally been managed through body casting (Apley & Soloman 2008; Clarke & Dowling 2003; Cluett 2003). As no clear-cut term is used for body casting, confusion may arise for parent and health professional (i.e. body cast/hip spica/frog plaster/spica cast). The hip spica is composed of plaster of Paris or synthetic material. Variations in spica cast position are influenced through child diagnosis, i.e. fracture versus DDH. The spica cast presents with the leg(s) +/– full extension, +/– hip(s) abduction, +/– knee flexion and either long or partial leg in plaster, i.e. double or one and a half spica cast. For the child in spica cast, a brief stay in hospital is necessary to dry the plaster and prepare for discharge. Table 26.1 includes general management information in relation to hip spica management.

The hip spica cast demonstrated in Figures 26.1 and 26.2 aims to maintain abduction of the femoral head within the acetabulum of the hip joint, as containment encourages normal femoral head development within the pelvis.

Table 26.1   General hip spica information (adapted from Clarke and McKay 2006).

- Plaster of Paris is not waterproof.
- It will take at least 48 hours for the cast to dry.
- Special care must be taken to prevent damage to the cast during the first 48 hours.
- The child should be nursed on pillows and turned every two hours during the day and every four hours at night* until the cast is dry (*during hospitalisation as supervised by nurse as potential increased risk of cot death).
- Check circulation to the feet (neurovascular observations) (Shields & Clarke 2011).
- The cast should be firm and fit snugly.
- The edges will be padded, a bar may be fitted to stabilise the cast and MUST NEVER BE USED TO LIFT WITH.
- When dry, a reinforcing layer can be added to strengthen the hip spica.
- When the cast is dry, the child can be positioned on a blanket either on the floor, or on a beanbag.
- Always put toys within reach of the child.
- The child may crawl in a safe environment.
- Do not allow your child to insert small toys or objects under the cast.
- Your child can be nursed, not carried, do not hip nurse, as the added weight is harmful to the carer's spine and posture.
- Standing in cast is usually *not* advised.
- Care and attention needs to be given to the child regarding temperature control, to avoid a febrile convulsion while in hip spica.

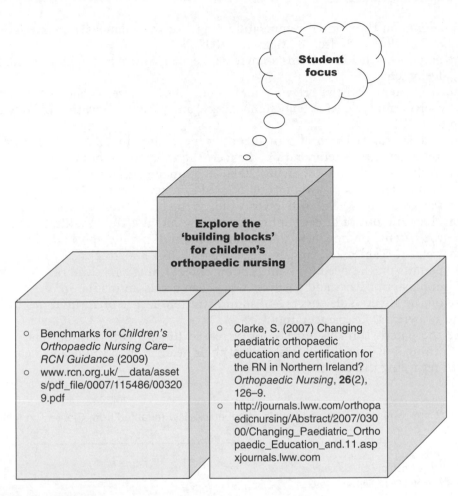

Figure 26.3 Student focus.

Care planning for child in hip spica: in-depth focus: see Figure 26.3.

Question 3. How does the children's nurse plan the care for Wai-ki in relation to 'controlling body temperature'? (Use the adult-based Roper *et al.* (2000) model of care and Casey's model of nursing (1988), working in partnership with children and their families.)

Activity of daily living: controlling body temperature.

Potential problem: Wai-ki is at risk of developing a pyrexia or febrile convulsion due to her age and application of a hip spica, i.e. legs, abdomen and lower chest covered by plaster of Paris, stockinet and padding.

Goal: to prevent or safely manage an elevated temperature, pyrexia or febrile episode.

Nursing intervention:

• Educate parents on the implications of their daughter's underdeveloped hypothalamus in relation to controlling body temperature and the potential for 'regular assessment'.

- Inform parents on the normal temperature range for their daughter at five months old, 36.6–37.8°C (Aylott in Kelsey & McEwing 2008).
- Educate parents on the 'basic signs' of pyrexia, i.e. baby warm to touch, flushed, irritable, crying, sleepy, etc.
- Educate the parents on the relevant terms, i.e. febrile (state of elevated temperature/ fever), hyperthermia (elevated body temperature) and pyrexia (elevation of body temperature up to 41°C).
- Educate and determine parental competence in the application of a suitable tool that can evaluate their daughter's temperature, the ideal thermometer should be accurate, reliable and safe. Aylott in Kelsey & McEwing (2008) recommend either the 'electronic thermometer' or 'tempa' dot in the axilla or the infrared tympani thermometer placed in the ear for children aged four weeks to five years old, as the oral route is unsafe.
- Position the child out of direct sunlight using safe moving and handling techniques.
- Educate the parents on how best to care for their child in a hip spica, washing, positioning, etc. (refer to Tables 26.1 and 26.2 plus Figures 26.1 and 26.2).
- Educate parents on the need for light bedding and clothing as a third of Wai-ki's body is covered in plaster of Paris and padding, which can act as an insulator.
- Educate on the effects/side effects and administration/dosage of antipyretics in the management of pyrexia, i.e. paracetamol.
- Educate the parents on the purpose of increased fluids (with caution) and removal of upper clothing. NB The child loses most of their heat through the head so care needs to be taken regarding the use of a hat.

Table 26.2 Care planning for the child in hip spica: quick view (adapted from Clarke and McKay 2006).

Washing and dressing
Problem: how do I wash my child's body and hair?
Goal: to safely wash child's hair and body.
Intervention:
1. No baths. Wash with flannel or sponge using soap (if applicable) and moisturise skin.
2. Wash hair over bath or basin: protect cast from water.
Useful notes
Wash child on bed turning from tummy to back.
For hair washing the parent can sit on a chair or bed edge and support child's head on a plastic covered parent's knee over a basin or bath – use jug or shower.
Rationale: to keep child clean and ensure good circulation.
Use two people for carer and child safety.
Check circulation – colour of skin should be pink and warm.
Evaluate: outcome of care.

Mobilisation/positioning
Problem: can my child be comfortable?
Goal: ensure child comfort.
Intervention:
1. Change position regularly (two hourly – on back/tummy/ position at 30 degree tilt).
2. Use pillows and wedge to change position.
3. Older children can turn themselves. Encourage turning, as it will make the child more comfortable.
4. Do not lift child by the arms but lift with hand supporting their bottom.
Rationale: prevents pressure sores.
Child at night should be on their back to reduce risk of 'cot death'.
Younger children should sleep on their backs and in their parents' room (use pillows and wedge in cot).
Evaluate: outcome of care.

Table 26.2 (*Continued*)

Elimination
Problem: how will my child go to the toilet?
Goal: to attend to child's elimination needs effectively.
Intervention:
1. If your child uses a nappy continue to do so. If not, use a bedpan or urinal. Child may regress during time in hip spica, i.e. may need to use nappy if recently potty trained.
2. Nappies, bedpan and urinal may be available and free of charge from your health visitor/children's nurse.
3. A child's nappy size may need to be reduced due to application of a hip spica (see Figure 26.1).
Rationale: to ensure safe toileting/prevent skin breakdown/reduce cast smelling from unpleasant odours and structure breakdown.
The ward nurse should address elimination needs prior to discharge.
Evaluate: outcome of care.

Working and playing
Problem: how can I occupy my child?
Goal: child is occupied, not bored or distressed.
Intervention:
1. Stimulating toys, TV, videos, reading, drawing, and computer (age appropriate).
2. School-home tuition may be an option (age appropriate).
3. Stimulation – good positioning of child so that they can see their surroundings, plus activities, will discourage bad behaviour.
Rationale: to prevent boredom and encourage child development.
Evaluate: outcome of care.

Maintaining a safe environment
Problem: how will I take my child shopping and secure them safely in the car?
Goal: ensure child safety at all times.
Intervention:
1. A suitable pram or special wheelchair may be available free or to rent prior to discharge.
2. For a younger child suitable car seats should be bought and fitted prior to discharge (see www.safetyfirst.com).
3. The ward staff can give full information on transport options. For the older child transport is problematic and an ambulance may be required.
4. Parents are advised to contact their car insurance broker.
Rationale: child safety, prevent prosecution – encourage social freedom.
Evaluate: outcome of care.

Eating and drinking
Problem: do I feed my child a normal diet?
Goal: ensure child receives age appropriate diet/fluids and adequate intake.
Intervention:
1. Yes, but smaller amounts – the cast is restrictive; also monitor weight as potential weight gain due to reduced mobility.
2. The child should be positioned at 45 degrees to aid digestion, comfort and reduce the risk of aspiration or choking.
Rationale: promote healing and prevent constipation. A balanced diet plus fluids.
Evaluate: outcome of care.

- Educate on the safety/implications of older practice, i.e. tepid sponging and fan therapy. A randomised controlled trial (RCT) by Thomas *et al.* (2009, p133) (N = 150) suggests 'apart from the initial rapid temperature reduction, addition of tepid sponging to antipyretic administration does not offer any more advantage in ultimate reduction of temperature; moreover it may result in additional discomfort'.
- Discuss future admission and procedure to remove hip spica.
- Allow parents to ask questions.
- Document all care and discharge interventions.

Evaluation: Wai-ki's body temperature remained within normal limits post-surgery (remember to document).

Activity 26.1

What is the evidence/effectiveness of tepid sponge and electric fan treatment for high fevers in children?
   Is there any harm in this treatment?

References

Apley, A.G. & Solomon, L. (2008) *Concise System of Orthopaedics and Fractures*. Oxford: Butterworth Heinman.

Aylott, M. (2008) Assessment temperature, pulse and respiration In: Kelsey, J. & McEwing, G. (2008). *Clinical Skills in Child Health Practice*. London: Churchill Livingstone Elsevier, 70–95.

Casey, A. (1988) The development and use of the partnership model of nursing care. In: Glasper, E.A & Tucker, A. (eds). (1993). *Advances in Child Health Nursing*. London: Scutari Press. pp83–93.

Clarke, S. (2007) Changing paediatric orthopaedic education and certification for the RN in Northern Ireland? *Orthopaedic Nursing*, **26**(2), 26–129.

Clarke, S.E. & Dowling, M. (2003) Spica cast guidelines for parents and health professionals. *Journal of Orthopaedic Nursing*, (**7**), 184–91.

Clarke, S.E. & McKay, M. (2006) Spica cast guidelines for parent and health professional: measure the effect of new evidenced based information using audit. *Journal of Orthopaedic Nursing*, **10**(3), 128–37.

Cluett, J. (2003) What you need to know about orthopaedics-hip spica. http://linkinghub.elsevier.com/retrieve/pii/S1361311106000422 (accessed 13 May 2011).

Kneale, J. & Davis, P. (2005) *Orthopaedic and Trauma Nursing*, 2nd edn. Edinburgh: Churchill Livingstone.

Newman, D.M.L. & Fawcett, J. (1995). Caring for a young child in a body cast: impact on the care giver. *Orthopaedic Nursing*, **14**(1), 41–6.

Roper, N., Logan, W.W. & Tierney, A.J. (2000) *The Roper-Logan-Tierney Model of Nursing: Based on Activities of Living*. Edinburgh: Elsevier Health Sciences.

Royal College of Nursing (2009) *Benchmarks for Children's Orthopaedic Nursing Care – RCN Guidance*. RCN.org

Shields, C. & Clarke, S (2011) Neurovascular observation and documentation for for children within Accident and Emergency: a critical review. *International Journal of Orthopaedic and Trauma Nursing*, **15**(1), 3–10.

Thomas, S.V., Vijaykumar, C., Naik, R., Moses, P.D. & Antonisamy, B. (2009) Comparative effectiveness of tepid sponging and antipyretic drug versus only antipyretic drug in the management of fever among children: a randomised controlled trial. *Indian Pediatrics*, **46**(17), 133–6.

Section 8

Care of the Gastro-intestinal Tract in Infants and Children

27

Gastro-oesophageal Reflux

Doris Corkin and Heather McKee

Scenario

Judith, now aged three months, was born at term weighing 3.7 kg and is in the sensorimotor stage of cognitive development (Bee & Boyd 2007). She is currently bottle feeding on casein based milk, demand fed every 3–4 hours and her weight is 5.0 kg.

Judith has been admitted to hospital with a two-week history of vomiting following feeds and according to her mother appears to be in pain, as she is irritable, clenching her fists and drawing up her knees. On admission to the ward the children's nurse advised Judith's mother to change Judith's casein-based milk back to whey, which is the preferred first choice.

Gastro-oesophageal reflux has been diagnosed after a few days, following a nursing and medical assessment and investigations. The doctor initially prescribed a trial period of infant Gaviscon and as it was unsuccessful then suggested thickening. Judith feeds with Carobel (Corkin 2008). However, Judith continues to vomit and is referred to the paediatric dietician who recommends an anti-reflux formula.

Judith is accompanied by her mother, a single mum, who is particularly anxious, and grandparents who are very supportive.

Care Planning in Children and Young People's Nursing, First Edition.
Edited by Doris Corkin, Sonya Clarke, Lorna Liggett.
© 2012 Blackwell Publishing Ltd. Published 2012 by Blackwell Publishing Ltd.

Activity 27.1

Plot Judith's weight on a centile chart. At birth Judith was assessed as within the 75th centile. At three months old Judith should now be between the 25th and 50th centile (see BMI chart in Chapter 17).

Questions

1. Discuss Judith's sensorimotor stage in cognitive development and possible characteristics.
2. Define gastro-oesophageal reflux.
3. What nursing and medical investigations are likely to have been undertaken?
4. How should gastro-oesophageal reflux be best treated and managed whilst being bottle fed?
5. Judith, three months old, weighing 5.0 kg has been prescribed oral omeprazole. When planning care what safety measures must the children's nurse consider prior to administration of medication?

Answers to questions

Question 1. Discuss Judith's sensorimotor stage in cognitive development and possible characteristics.

Jean Piaget (1896–1980) has been the most influential child development theorist, extensively observing children, including his own (www.piaget.org). The sensorimotor stage represents the first major stage of cognitive development and has been identified as the period extending from birth to about 18 months of age, where the child is essentially engaged in their environment (Bee & Boyd 2007). During this time Judith will develop increased muscle control and should have a strong attachment to her mother. After Judith was born, she began to learn to use her senses and can understand the world through motor and sensory activities. She can focus and follow moving objects, distinguish between pitch and volume of sound and see all colours. Now three months old, Judith can clearly recognise faces and respond to smiles and familiar sounds.

Question 2. Define gastro-oesophageal reflux.

Gastro-oesophageal reflux is the passage of gastric contents into the oesophagus, it is a very common gastro-intestinal disorder in infants and tends to resolve following the weaning period. This is caused by the immaturity of the lower oesophageal sphincter which allows frequent reflux of gastric contents into the oesophagus. Vomiting (which is neither projectile or bile-stained), can occur during or between feeds. Bleeding, however, may occur and appear as bright blood in the vomitus if oesophagitis is present. Commonly this may present as 'coffee ground' flecks of altered blood. Severe gastro-oesophageal reflux in some infants can lead to repeated episodes of aspiration and pneumonia and later present as faltering growth (Hutson *et al.* 1999). The diagnosis is established following a nursing assessment of the child's feeding pattern and a thorough physical examination by the medical team (Axton & Fugate 2009).

Question 3. What nursing and medical investigations are likely to have been undertaken?

Assessment: on admission to hospital the children's nurse would undertake a detailed nursing assessment and establish Judith's weight and feeding pattern and this would include a test feed. In order to establish diagnosis the medical team investigations will involve:

* A health/family history
* Physical examination from head to toe
* Diagnostic tests, such as barium swallow or pH probe monitoring which measures the oesophageal pH and percentage of time the pH falls below 4 in 24 hours

Question 4. How should gastro-oesophageal reflux be best treated and managed whilst being bottle fed?

Activity of living: eating and drinking as per Roper, Logan & Tierney model of care (Holland *et al.* 2008), see Chapter 1 for further reading.

 Plan: gastro-oesophageal reflux is a condition which nature will gradually resolve as Judith gets older. The children's nurse should aim to minimise the symptoms and keep Judith as comfortable as possible:

1. Thicken Judith's milk feed – following discussion with the medical team, this can be addressed by adding a thickener (Carobel) to the milk Judith is already receiving. The amount of Carobel can be increased, depending on the severity of the reflux. Alternatively, the paediatric dietician can be consulted and a formula tried, for example Enfamil AR or Staydown can be offered instead (Corkin & McDougall 2009).
2. It is important to highlight the need to calculate feeding requirements accurately based on Judith's weight and to educate her parent/grandparent regarding overfeeding, as it may be best to give Judith small frequent feeds initially until pain or discomfort eases.

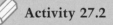 **Activity 27.2**

1. As Judith now weighs 5.0 kg, calculate her daily feeding requirements based on 150 ml per kg.
2. If Judith takes six bottle feeds in 24 hours how many millilitres would each one be?

---

3. Nurse Judith in a more upright position – infants benefit from being nursed in a suitable tilted bouncer/car chair or in buggy where their head is raised above the level of their

feet. This allows gravity to help keep Judith's milk feed in her stomach. Furthermore, the head of Judith's cot can also be raised by placing some folded towels *under* the cot mattress at the head end. Also, it is important to make sure that the cot is stable and Judith is safe at all times. Make Judith's mother aware of cot death prevention advice, such as the 'feet to foot' position, so that Judith's feet are at the end of the cot, thus preventing her from wriggling under her covers (Health Promotion Agency 2007).

4. Encourage nappy changing prior to feeding and ensure accurate recording of intake and output on fluid balance chart while in hospital.
5. Paediatrician may prescribe Judith some medication – in some cases the doctor may prescribe an acid-reducing preparation such as infant Gaviscon (reduces oesophagitis) or omeprazole, which can be administered in liquid form or alternatively ranitidine (BNFC 2010–2011). However, these medications should not be used in combination with Enfamil AR or SMA Staydown as these milks need stomach acids present to be effective. Medications will allow Judith to tolerate her feeds by either promoting gastric emptying or reducing the acidity of Judith's stomach contents. This medication is similar to those used by adults with heartburn or ulcers. Medication can help reduce the pain which Judith is experiencing when reflux does occur.
6. Surgery such as a fundoplication (see Chapter 11) may be performed in a minority of cases as a last resort (Daigneau 2003), especially those children with life-threatening conditions, for example a child with complex needs and a tracheostomy *in situ*.
7. Early weaning should be discouraged with Judith as the current government recommendation for starting weaning is six months (DH 2003) or at the very earliest 17 weeks of age after careful consideration.

Question 5. Judith, three months old, weighing 5.0 kg has been prescribed oral omeprazole. When planning care what safety measures must the children's nurse consider prior to administration of medication?

Administration of oral medication

Activity of living: maintaining a safe environment as per Roper, Logan & Tierney model of care (Holland *et al.* 2008).

 Implementation: the administration of oral medicines is an important, complex aspect within the multifaceted role of the children's nurse (see Table 27.1). Standards for medicine management are regulated by the Nursing and Midwifery Council (NMC 2008) and clearly highlight the nurse's responsibility to ensure safe practice when administrating medication. As medications can come in various forms for administration via multiple routes (Leathard 2001), it is essential for all nurses to have a working knowledge and understanding of these NMC standards as conventional drugs can have at least three names, for example:

Calpol – proprietary name

paracetamol – common (generic) name

acetaminophen – chemical name

Indeed, there are various omeprazole preparations available (BNFC 2010–2011). Many generic companies manufacture omeprazole in capsule and tablet form. However,

Table 27.1 Administration of oral medication.

Action: administration of oral medication	Reason
1. The children's nurse should be aware of Judith's plan of care and incorporate a family-centred approach (Casey 1988) in order to gain consent and parental co-operation.	To ensure clear communication pathway is implemented.
2. The children's nurse should be able to correctly refer to a paediatric prescribing textbook, for example *British National Formulary for Children* (BNFC 2010–2011).	To establish safe dose of medication, understand therapeutic effects and possible side effects.
3. Be aware of Judith's care plan, for example check for allergies, that prescription is valid, in keeping with Judith's age and weight and signed by doctor and dated.	To ensure safe practice and accurate calculation of dosage.
4. Children's nurses should wash their hands prior to and after procedure.	To prevent cross infection.
5. Safe administration of medication involves five 'c's/'r's (Griffith *et al.* 2003; Watt 2003b): • Correct/right dose • Correct/right medicine (check expiry date) • Correct infant/child (check unit number and details on hospital armband and records) • Correct route (e.g. oral, nasogastric, etc.) • Correct/right time Adhere to hospital policy, for example double checking by registered nurse/s involved at every stage of medicine administration process (NMC 2008).	Professional responsibility and accountability. To reduce risk.
6. The safe preparation, dispense and storage of medication must be adhered to as per ward policy and pharmacist.	Patient safety.
7. The children's nurse should accurately and immediately record medication (NMC 2010) after administration or if refused by Judith, ensuring signatures of both nurses are clearly written with date and time. Ensure disposal of equipment used to administer medicine, disposal of unused medicine and monitoring of effectiveness of drug action.	Ensuring safe practice and continuity of care.

AstraZeneca manufacture Losec Mups® (omeprazole tablets dispersible in water) and Losec capsules® (e.g. contents can be sprinkled directly onto spoonful of food).

As the NMC (2008) supports the administration of medicines by a carer, the majority of parents should be encouraged by the children's nurse to take part in the administration of medicines to their child in the paediatric setting, thus advocating a partnership approach to care (Casey 1988). Although the responsibility to ensure the medication is given remains with the children's nurse, age-appropriate considerations should always be taken into account and there should be negotiation with the parent regarding mixing of medication with food to disguise any unpleasant taste. Please note this is different to 'covert administration of medicines', which is regarded as deception without informed consent (advice@nmc-uk.org).

Formula for calculating drug dosage: this is calculated as shown here (Watt 2003a):

$$\frac{\text{what you require}}{\text{what you have}} \times \text{dilution} = \text{what you give}$$

A standardised formula can help reduce calculation/medicine errors, for example:

- 'What you require' is the prescribed dosage.
- 'What you have' is the concentration of drug in the medicine bottle.
- 'Dilution' is the amount of liquid in which the drug is dissolved.

Calculation of drugs

The administration of prescribed medication to infants and children must be viewed by the children's nurse as a key aspect of nursing care that requires sound knowledge of pharmacology, numeracy skills and the ability to communicate effectively with Judith and her family (Casey 1988).To ensure accurate dosing, body weight is used more frequently for ease of paediatric calculations. In order to calculate drug doses accurately the children's nurse must be able to demonstrate an understanding of child development theory, the units of drugs in current use and approved abbreviations, for example:

- Gram = g
- Milligram = mg
- Millilitre = ml
- Microgram = must be written in full

Student nurses should be involved in the procedure of drug calculation and administration as a learning tool. However, in order to meet legal, local trust and professional guidelines student nurses should *NEVER* single check oral medication and administer unsupervised. As nurses administer medications on a regular basis there is the potential for errors to occur (Griffith *et al.* 2003). According to Preston (2003) nurses' poor mathematical skills are an ongoing problem and use of calculators is acknowledged as part of the dose checking process. Reports regarding medication incidents with children have included wrong drug, wrong strength and wrong patient in 2008 (NPSA 2009). A recent study (Simons 2010) has identified computerised prescription systems as having been shown to reduce medication errors.

Storage and transportation of drugs

Safe storage of drugs involves both environmental and security factors, such as medicines trolley and refrigerator. Children's nurses must ensure all medicines are stored in accordance with the patient/drug information leaflet. According to the NMC (2008) registered nurses may transport medication to patients (including controlled drugs), where patients or their carers are unable to collect them, provided the registrant is conveying the medication to a patient for whom the drug product has been prescribed (e.g. from pharmacy to patient in community setting).

Acknowledgement

The authors thank Andrea McDougall, Paediatric Dietician, Royal Belfast Hospital for Sick Children (RBHSC), Northern Ireland, for her valuable comments.

References

advice@nmc-uk.org. *Covert Administration of Medicines: Disguising Medicines in Food and Drink* (accessed 6 August 2010).

Axton, S.E. & Fugate, T. (2009) *Paediatric Nursing Care Plans for the Hospitalized Child* (eds), 3rd edn. Upper Saddle River, New Jersey: Pearson Prentice Hall.

Bee, H. & Boyd, D. (2007) *The Developing Child*, 11th edn. London: Pearson.

British National Formulary for Children (BNFC) (2010–2011) *British Medical Journal*. London: PS Publishing.

Casey, A (1988) A partnership with child and family. *Senior Nurse*, **8**(4), 8–9.

Corkin, D. (2008) Artifical feeding, Chapter 14. In: Kelsey, J. & McEwing, G. (eds). *Clinical Skills in Child Health Practice*. Oxford: Churchill Livingstone, Elsevier.

Corkin, D. & McDougall, A (2009) Preparation of infant feeds, Chapter 27. In: Glasper, A., McEwing, G. & Richardson, J. (eds). *Foundation Skills for Caring*. Hampshire: Palgrave Macmillan.

Daigneau, C.V. (2003) The child with gastro-intestinal dysfunction, Chapter 33. In: Hockenberry, M.J., Wilson, D., Winkelstein, M.L. & Kline, N.E. (2003). *Wong's Nursing Care of Infants and Children*, 7th edn. London: Mosby.

Department of Health (DH) (2003) *Infant Feeding Recommendations*. London: DH.

Griffith, R., Griffith, H. & Jordan, S. (2003) Administration of medicines. Part 1: *Nursing Standard*, **18**(2), 47–53.

Health Promotion Agency (2007) *Birth to Five*. Belfast: Health Promotion Agency for Northern Ireland (permission from DH). www.healthpromotionagency.org.uk

Holland, K., Jenkins, J., Solomon, J. & Whittam, S. (2008) *Applying the Roper Logan Tierney. Model in Practice*, 2nd edn. Edinburgh: Churchill Livingstone.

Hutson, J.M., Woodward, A.A. & Beasley, S.W. (1999) *Jones' Clinical Paediatric Surgery*, 5th edn. Blackwell Science, Asia Pty.

Leathard, H.L. (2001) Understanding medicines: conceptual analysis of nurses' needs for knowledge and understanding of pharmacology (Part 1). *Nurse Education Today*, **21**, 266–71.

National Patient Safety Agency (NPSA) (2009) *Review of Patient Safety for Children and Young People*. London: NSPA.

Nursing and Midwifery Council (2008) *Guidelines on the Administration of Medicines*. London: NMC.

Nursing and Midwifery Council (2010) *Record keeping – Guidance for Nurses and Midwives*. London: NMC.

Preston, R.M. (2003) Drug errors and patient safety: the need for a change in practice. *British Journal of Nursing*, **13**(2), 72–8.

Simons, J. (2010) Identifying medication errors in surgical prescription charts. *Paediatric Nursing*, **22**(5), 20–24.

Watt, S. (2003a) Safe administration of medicines to children: Part 1. *Paediatric Nursing*, **15**(4), 40–43.

Watt, S. (2003b) Safe administration of medicines to children: Part 2. *Paediatric Nursing*, **15**(5), 40–44.

www.piaget.org Jean Piaget Society (accessed 30 July 2010).

Answers to Activity 27.2

1. $50 \times 5 = 750$ ml in 24 hours
2. $750 \div 6 = 125$ ml per feed

28

Cerebral Palsy and Nasogastric Tube Feeding
Gillian McEwing

Scenario

Colin is an eight-year-old boy who was diagnosed as having cerebral palsy at the age of nine months, after his parents had concerns regarding his slow development. As he grew older Colin was able to learn to walk, first with a frame and then independently. He can competently carry out the activities of daily living, such as dressing and feeding himself. However, Colin has some difficulties with fine motor tasks, he has left sided hemiparesis and has scoliosis.

Colin is cognitively intact, communicates verbally and has a good social life with friends and family. He had been experiencing an upper respiratory tract infection for nearly a week, his condition then deteriorated and Colin was admitted to hospital with pneumonia. He was treated with antibiotics at first intravenously but then progressed to oral administration. Fluid intake was initially maintained intravenously. Although Colin's condition is improving he is still unable to maintain his fluid and nutritional needs orally and requires enteral feeding.

Care Planning in Children and Young People's Nursing, First Edition.
Edited by Doris Corkin, Sonya Clarke, Lorna Liggett.
© 2012 Blackwell Publishing Ltd. Published 2012 by Blackwell Publishing Ltd.

Questions

1. What is cerebral palsy?
2. Discuss the rationale for enteral feeding.
3. What is enteral feeding?
4. Using the nursing process and a model of care, how would the children's nurse prepare Colin and his family for the insertion of a nasogastric tube?
5. Describe the procedure for passing a nasogastric tube.

Answers to questions

Question 1. What is cerebral palsy?

Cerebral palsy is an umbrella term used to describe a permanent non-progressive condition in which dysfunction of the brain affects movement, posture and co-ordination.

The condition can arise before, during or after birth. The severity and effects of the condition are wide ranging and less severe cases may not be detected until early childhood. Approximately 1800 children are diagnosed in the UK each year (SCOPE UK 2010) and the condition can affect individuals from any social background or ethnic group.

The damage to the brain may occur prenatally between conception and birth, during birth or during early childhood. Prenatal causes include: inefficient placenta, genetic disorders, infections, maternal high blood pressure or premature birth. Birth trauma may be due to prolonged labour, oxygen deficit or occasionally forceps delivery. Damage in the neonatal period may be caused by hypoglycaemia, respiratory problems, convulsions, blood group incompatibility or infection (Southcombe 2007).

There are four main classifications of cerebral palsy: *spastic*, when the child's movement is difficult or stiff; *ataxic*, where there is loss of depth perception and balance; *athetoid or dyskinetic*, where movement is uncontrolled or involuntary; or the condition may be a mixture of any or all of these. Half of children born with cerebral palsy have normal intelligence; others will have some learning difficulties. Many children with cerebral palsy have swallowing problems due to poor tongue control.

Question 2. Discuss the rationale for enteral feeding.

Poor nutrition is a complication of many childhood diseases which can affect the child's health by impairing immunity, delaying wound healing, reducing muscle strength and impairing psychological drive (Stroud *et al.* 2003). There are a number of reasons why illness may interfere with eating, digestion and absorption. The desire to eat can be affected by many things such as: lack of appetite, nausea, vomiting, dysphasia, pain on swallowing, altered taste due to medications and psychological factors. Ability to eat can be affected by impaired sucking, chewing and swallowing mechanisms and respiratory or cardiac conditions leading to breathlessness when feeding (Corkin & Chambers 2008). Digestion and absorption can be affected by altered pathophysiology of the gut, for example short-term conditions such as severe acute diarrhoea or long-term conditions including coeliac disease or short bowel syndrome.

When a child is at risk of suffering from under nutrition, enteral feeding can be considered, providing they have a functioning gastro-intestinal tract (Corkin & Chambers 2008).

There are four main groups of children that may require enteral feeding. These include children with:

- Neurological disorders, such as cerebral palsy (Parkes & Clarke 2010).
- Chronic conditions, such as cystic fibrosis, renal failure and bowel disorders.
- Short-term feeding problems, including prematurity, cancer and severe burns.
- Some miscellaneous conditions, such as anorexia nervosa (Corkin & Chambers 2008).

Box 28.1   Assessment of needs

Colin is unable to meet his nutritional needs orally as he has no desire to eat. His increased respiratory effort makes it difficult for Colin to swallow and breathe at the same time. He feels thirsty and hungry but is unable to eat or drink normally. Colin is only able to manage sips of fluid to make his mouth more comfortable. Following discussion with the dietician, medical staff, Colin and his parents, it has been decided that Colin will benefit from enteral feeding.

Question 3. What is enteral feeding?

Enteral feeding refers to the delivery of a nutritionally complete feed containing protein, carbohydrate, fat, water, minerals and vitamins directly into the stomach, duodenum or jejunum (NICE 2006).

Enteral feeding is an artificial method of providing nutrition to a child. There are three main routes for administration: orogastric, nasogastric and gastrostomy.

- *Orogastric* feeding involves a tube passing through the mouth and oral cavity down the back of the throat, into the oesophagus and then into the stomach.
- *Nasogastric* feeding is when a tube is passed through the nostril, down the back of the throat, into the oesophagus and then into the stomach.
- *Gastrostomy* feeding is performed through a tube surgically placed through the skin of the abdomen into the stomach.

Nasogastric feeding is usually considered for the child requiring short-term nutritional support and can be used for up to 4–6 weeks (Bowling 2004). Furthermore, it is suitable for those children unable to feed orally in acute or chronic illness. This is the most common method of enteral feeding, with nutrients being delivered directly into the gastrointestinal tract through a nasogastric tube.

> **Box 28.2**   Planning of care
>
> Colin has long-term needs resulting from his cerebral palsy and acute problems due to his respiratory infection. This has made it difficult for him to maintain his nutritional intake orally. With the use of antibiotics his condition should gradually improve and Colin will be able to eat and drink independently again. Therefore he only requires short-term assistance with meeting his nutritional needs and the nasogastric route would be the most suitable.

Question 4. Using the nursing process and a model of care, how would the children's nurse prepare Colin and his family for the insertion of a naso-gastric tube?

Activity of living: communication (Roper *et al.* 2000).

Best practice involves making sure Colin and his parents are fully informed regarding the benefits of inserting a nasogastric tube in order to meet Colin's nutritional needs. Information should be given verbally and when necessary supported by written information to meet the child and family's needs (NICE 2006). The individual's ability to understand must be considered when providing information with regard to language, culture, physical, sensory or learning disabilities. Effective communication will need to take into consideration Colin's age, cognitive ability, personality and coping skills. Misunderstandings can cause the child to become distressed; for a child there is no such thing as a minor procedure and often the severity of pain or discomfort does not correlate accurately with what the child feels they experience (Liossi 2002).

The procedure should be explained to both the Colin and his parents and they should be encouraged to ask questions.

Goal: Colin and his parents will understand the need to commence enteral feeding. They will be fully informed regarding the procedure for passing a nasogastric tube.

Implement and evaluate:

- The need for Colin to be fed for a short period using the nasogastric route will be discussed with Colin's parents.
- Care will be planned with the parents on how best to proceed with the procedure causing the least distress possible to Colin.
- The procedure will be explained to Colin at his level of understanding using his own language, avoiding misinterpretations and encouraging questions.
- Explore with Colin any fears he may have in relation to the procedure.

Activity of living: maintaining a safe environment (Roper *et al.* 2000).

Psychological preparation for an unpleasant procedure is essential (Holden *et al.* 1997; Penrod *et al.* 1999). This will help the child and parents to manage the procedure effectively and help ensure the procedure is completed as efficiently and safely as possible (Jonas 2007). Passing a nasogastric tube is an invasive procedure and it could cause anticipatory anxiety in Colin and his parents. Past experiences of unpleasant procedures must be taken into account. Providing information to children about the experience, encouraging emotional expression of concerns, and establishing a trusting relationship with the healthcare profes-sional will all help to reduce the stress of the procedure (O'Connor-Von 2000). Non-pharmacological interventions, such as parental presence, hugging and holding, distraction, deep breathing and guided imagery and relaxation can all help reduce Colin's anxiety. Increasing parental participation can be achieved by providing them with a role such as active coaching to help the child through procedure.

Goal: Colin and his parents will have given consent for the procedure. Colin will be calm and compliant throughout the procedure and aware of the boundaries of behaviour and how to communicate distress. His parents will understand their role during the procedure. Management of the procedure will involve good organisation and planning ahead.

Implement and evaluate:

- If possible, both Colin and his parents should give verbal consent for the procedure to take place.
- Discuss with Colin what is expected of him and the limits of acceptable behaviour throughout the procedure.
- The procedure will be explained to Colin's parents, and their role during the procedure should be agreed.
- Age-appropriate books or other visual aids can be used.
- The procedure will be planned. Delays will be avoided that may cause unnecessary dis-tress by preparing all the equipment beforehand and out of the child's sight unless the child specifically requests to see it.
- Step-by-step, honest, age-appropriate information will be provided to Colin and his parents to increase their sense of control (Jonas 2007).
- Throughout the procedure Colin will be allowed choices, if appropriate, such as which nostril will be used. This will increase co-operation and give Colin a sense of control and reduce feelings of helplessness.
- Following the procedure Colin will be praised, with emphasis on the positive aspects of the experience and age-appropriate reward stickers or certificates should be given.

Activity of living: eating and drinking (Roper *et al.* 2000).

A dietician will be involved to plan a feeding regime for Colin to ensure that he has the correct fluid and nutritional intake. Feeds can be given by gravity, as a bolus or by a pump continuously (Hanks & McEwing 2009). Feeds given continuously reduce the risk of gas-trointestinal symptoms but this does mean the child needs to be connected to the pump most of the time, which limits mobility. Feeds given as a bolus at meal times will help maintain normal body feeding patterns.

Goal: Colin will receive suitable enteral feeds to meet his physical and nutritional needs.
Implement and evaluate:

- When possible Colin will be fed at normal meal times.
- If Colin is able to take any food or fluid orally this should be given at the same time as the feed (Wiggins 2007).
- Enteral feeding should not be an unpleasant experience for Colin.

Question 5. Describe the procedure for passing a nasogastric tube.

See Table 28.1.

Table 28.1 The procedure for passing a nasogastric tube.

Action	Rationale and evidence
1. Collect the required equipment: Nasogastric tube Syringe pH indication paper Tape to secure Hydrocolloid dressing Oral fluid for older child Two gallipots Water or water-based lubricant Disposable gloves Scissors Plastic apron	When choosing a nasogastric feeding tube the size and material it is made from needs to be considered. There are two main types commonly used, polyvinylchloride (PVC) and polyurethane tubes. The PVC tubes quickly lose their flexibility when in contact with gastric secretions; these are therefore primarily used for short-term feeding as they need changing frequently according to the manufacturers' guidance (Hockenberry *et al.* 2003). The polyurethane tubes are more suitable for longer term feeding as they are softer and more flexible and can remain *in situ* for up to one month. Tubes are sized according to their internal lumen; 6, 8 and 10 French gauge (Fg) are usually used for children (Huband & Trigg 2000). It is essential to follow the manufacturers' guidelines regarding the size of the syringe used when aspirating the tube in order to prevent damage (Viasys 2000). When aspirating the tube the negative pressure created at the tip of the syringe is dependent on the size and type of syringe and the force exerted.
2. Wash and dry hands using recognised technique and put on plastic apron.	To prevent cross infection hands must be decontaminated immediately before each and every episode of direct patient contact or care (NICE 2003). Plastic aprons should be worn when required for a single episode of patient care and then discarded (NICE 2003).
3. Explain to the child and parent that you are going to pass the nasogastric tube, explain what the child should do if they wish you to stop.	Promote psychological support.
4. Clean work surface/trolley prior to placement of equipment.	Passing a nasogastric tube is a clean procedure.
5. Prepare a piece hydrocolloid dressing.	To prevent epidermal damage this should be three times the width of the tube and cover two-thirds of the child's cheek between the side of the nostril and the child's ear.
6. Cut adhesive tape and place within easy reach.	To secure adequately this should be wide enough to cover the nasogastric tube and overlap the sides sufficiently to hold it securely in place; however, it should not overlap the hydrocolloid dressing.
7. Wash and dry hands.	To prevent bacterial contamination of the tube.
8. Water/lubricant → gallipot.	To lubricate the tip of the tube.
9. Place strip of pH paper in second gallipot.	
10. Open syringe, place within easy reach.	
11. Put on disposable gloves.	To prevent bacterial contamination of the tube.
12. Remove nasogastric tube from packaging, ensure not damaged.	

continued

Table 28.1   (*Continued*)

Action	Rationale and evidence
13. Measure length of tube from nostril to ear, and then from ear to stomach, just past the xiphoid process. Note/ mark the point on the tube or hold the tube at the calculated point and keep between the fingers of your less dominant hand.	To determine the length of tube required. Traditionally the NEX measurement (length from nose to earlobe to the xiphoid process) is used to indicate the length of tube required. A study by Klasner *et al.* (2002) suggested that for paediatric gastric tube insertion, a graphic method based on height was a more accurate method for determining depth of tube insertion.

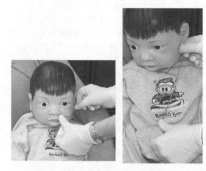

Action	Rationale and evidence
Ensure end cap of the tube is in place.	To prevent leakage of gastric contents.
14. Ask assistant (parent) to supportively hold child as appropriate to age and level of understanding.	To prevent the child moving during the procedure and provide comfort.

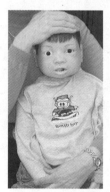

Older children may prefer to sit up with their head supported. Babies can be wrapped in a blanket and encouraged to suck a dummy through the procedure.

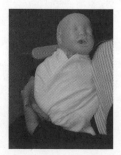

Table 28.1   (*Continued*)

Action	Rationale and evidence
15. Select clear nostril, older children can choose which nostril. Lubricate the tip of the tube using a water-based solution. Insert tip of tube into nostril. 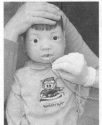 Angle tube slightly upwards and slide backwards along the floor of the nose into the pharynx.	Consider airway maintenance in infants who are obligatory nose breathers. Lubrication reduces the risk of friction and tissue damage. Follow manufacturers' guidelines regarding type of lubrication. Follows the normal contour of the nasal passage.
16. Continue to gently feed tube downwards. 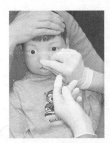 As the tube passes to the back of the nose, advise child to take sips of water (if appropriate) to help the tube go down or in the case of a baby offer them a dummy. A short pause may be necessary for the tube to pass through the cardiac sphincter into the stomach.	In the case of obstruction, pull tube back and turn it slightly and advance again. If obstruction is felt again try the other nostril. The tube should be gently inserted as the child swallows as this will assist with the movement of the tube and reduce any discomfort. If at any time during this procedure the child starts to cough or their colour deteriorates the procedure should be stopped immediately and the tube removed. The most common site for resistance when passing a nasogastric tube is at the laryngeal level at the arytenoid cartilages and piriform sinuses. Lateral neck pressure compresses the piriform sinuses and moves the arytenoid cartilages medially, relieving 85% of the incidences of impaction (Ozer & Benumof 1999).
17. Stop when the point marked on the tube reaches the outer edge of the child's nostril. 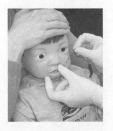	The tube should be in the stomach.

continued

Table 28.1   (*Continued*)

Action	Rationale and evidence
18. Ask person assisting to hold the tube in position. Check the nasogastric tube is in the child's stomach. Remove the end cap. Using syringe aspirate a small amount of gastric contents by gently pulling back on the plunger. Detach syringe, replace end cap. Test pH of fluid using pH indicator paper, readings should be less than 5.5. (NPSA 2005) Replace aspirate in infants at risk of electrolyte imbalance. If there is difficulty obtaining aspirate, lie the child on his/her left side and encourage to swallow a small amount of oral fluid if allowed.	When determining the position of nasogastric tubes insufflation and auscultation of air into the stomach is an unreliable method of checking tube position as it has been shown to give false positive results as bowel or chest sounds can be misinterpreted as evidence of gastric tube placement (Metheny *et al.* 1998). Placing the proximal end of the tube under water and observing for bubbles on expiration runs the risk of aspirating the water on inspiration, particularly when the child is ventilated (Thomas & Falcone 1998). Examining the colour of aspirate alone is not a safe indication of tube placement (Metheny *et al.* 1994). The use of blue litmus paper turning pink/red to indicate whether aspirate is acidic, is not safe as it does not indicate the degree of acidity present. This is crucial as bronchial secretions can be slightly acidic which will turn the litmus pink.
Attempt to push the tube away from the stomach wall by inserting 1–5 ml of air down the tube using a 20 or 50 ml syringe. Try advancing or retracting the tube slightly to alter the position in the stomach.	Testing the pH of aspirate is the recommended method. The NPSA 2005 recommends that feeding can commence if aspirate is below pH 5.5. However, care should be taken as the use of antacids, proton pump inhibitor drugs or H_2 receptor antagonists can elevate the pH of the gastric contents and limit the usefulness of this test in those children receiving these therapies. If any doubt exists on the correct placement of the nasogastric tube then consider re-passing the tube or checking position by X-ray.
19. Apply hydrocolloid dressing to child and secure tube using adhesive tape.	Most children benefit from using a barrier product such as hydrocolloid dressings and transparent films to protect the skin under strong adhesive tapes (Dollison & Beckstrand 1995; National Health Service Quality Improvement Scotland 2003).
20. Document nostril used, size, date and time of insertion. It is useful to make a note of the length of the tube extending from the nostril as this may help determine if the tube has been displaced (Best 2005).	PVC tubes lose their flexibility when in contact with gastric secretions and need changing frequently according to the manufacturer's guidance.

References

Best, C. (2005) Caring for the patient with a naso-gastric tube. *Nursing Standard*, **20**(3), 59–65.
Bowling, T. (2004) *Nutritional Support for Adults and Children.* Abingdon: Radcliffe Medical Press.
Corkin, D. & Chambers, J. (2008) Nutrition via enteral feeding devices. In: Kelsey, J., McEwing, G. (eds). *Clinical Skills in Child Health Practice.* Edinburgh: Elsevier. pp137–8.
Dolllison, E.J. & Beckstrand, J. (1995) Adhesive tape vs. pectin-based barrier use in pre-term infants. *Neonatal Network*, **14**(4), 35–9.
Hanks, C. & McEwing, G. (2009) Enteral feeding. In: Glasper, A., McEwing, G. & Richardson, J. (eds). *Foundation Skills for Caring Using a Student Centred Approach.* London: Palgrave Macmillan.
Hockenbury, M.J., Wilson, D., Winklestein, M.L. *et al.* (2003) *Wong's Nursing Care of Infants and Children,.* 7th edn. St Louis: Mosby.

Holden, C., Sexton, E. & Lesley, P. (1997) Enteral nutrition for children. *Nursing Standard*, **11**(32), 49–54.

Huband, S. & Trigg, E. (2000) *Practices in Children's Nursing: Guidelines for Hospital and Community*. Edinburgh: Churchill Livingstone.

Jonas, D.A. (2007) Management of procedural pain. In: Glasper, A., McEwing, G. & Richardson, J. (eds). *Oxford Handbook of Children's and Young People's Nursing*. Oxford: Oxford University Press.

Klasner, A.E., Luke, D.A. & Scalzo, A.J. (2002) Pediatric orogastric and nasogastric tubes: a new formula evaluated. *Annals of Emergency Medicine*, **39**, 268–72.

Liossi, C. (2002) *Procedure Related Cancer Pain in Children*. Abingdon: Radcliffe Medical Press.

Metheny, N.A, Reed, L, Berglund, B. & Wehrle, M.A. (1994) Visual characteristics of aspirates from feeding tubes as a method of predicting feeding tube placement. *Nursing Research*, **43**(5), 282–7.

Metheny, N.A., Whrie, M.A., Wiersama, L. & Clark, J. (1998) Testing feeding tube placement: ausculatation vs. pH method. *American Journal of Nursing*, **98**(5), 37–43.

National Health Service Quality Improvement Scotland (2003) *Nasogastric and Gastronomy Feeding for Children Being Cared for in the Community. Best Practice Statement*. Edinburgh: Nursing and Midwifery Practice Development Unit.

National Institute of Clinical Excellence (2003) *Infection Control: Prevention of Healthcare-associated Infection in Primary and Community Care*. London: NICE.

National Institute of Clinical Excellence (2006) *Nutritional Support in Adults*. London: NICE.

National Patient Safety Agency (NPSA) (2005) Reducing the harm caused by misplaced naso-gastric feeding tubes. *Interim Advice for Healthcare Staff*. London: NHS.

O'Conner-Von S (2000) Preparing children for surgery: an integrative research review. *AORN*, **71**(2), 334–43.

Ozer, S. & Benumof, J. (1999) Oro- and naso-gastric tube passage in intubated patients: fiberoptic description of where they go at the laryngeal level and how to make them enter the esophagus. *Anesthesiology*, **91**(1), 137–43.

Parkes, J. & Clarke, S. (2010) Children with complex motor disability. In: Glasper, E.A and Richardson, J. (eds). *A Textbook of Children's and Young People's Nursing*, 2nd edn. Edinburgh: Churchill Livingstone, Elsevier.

Penrod, J., Morse, J.M. & Wilson, S. (1999) Comforting strategies used during nasogastric tube insertion. *Journal of Clinical Nursing*, **8**(1), 31–8.

Roper, N., Logan W.W. & Tierney, A.J. (2000) *The Roper-Logan-Tierney Model of Nursing: Based on the Activities of Living*. Edinburgh: Elsevier Health Sciences.

SCOPE. www.scope.org.uk/help-and-information/cerebral-palsy-and-associated-impairments/introduction-cerebral-palsy

Southcombe, B. (2007) Cerebral palsy. In: Glasper, A., McEwing, G. & Richardson, J. (eds). *Oxford Handbook of Children's and Young People's Nursing*. Oxford: Oxford University Press.

Stroud, M., Duncan, H. & Nightingale, J. (2003) Guidelines for enteral feeding in adult hospital patients: Gut. *An International Journal of Gastroenterology and Hepatology*, **52**(7), 1.

Thomas, B.W. & Falcone, R.E. (1998) Confirmation of naso-gastric tube placement by colourimetric indicator detection of carbon dioxide: a preliminary report. *Journal of the American College of Nutrition*, **17**(2), 195–7.

Viasys (2000) *Effect of Syringe Pressure on Viasys Feeding Tubes*, protocol 170. Viasys, Conshohocken.

Wiggins, S. (2007) Feeding via a naso-gastric tube. In: Glasper, A., McEwing, G. & Richardson, J. (eds). *Oxford Handbook of Children's and Young People's Nursing*. Oxford: Oxford University Press.

29

Enteral Feeding – Gastrostomy Care
Catherine Paxton

Scenario

Jane is a two-year-old girl who was born prematurely at 28 weeks gestation and suffered a grade IV intraventricular haemorrhage. This has left her with an evolving cerebral palsy. 'Cerebral palsy is a disorder of posture, movement and tone due to a static encephalopathy acquired during brain growth in fetal life, infancy or early childhood' (McKinlay 2008, p888). Jane lives with her parents, Lynne and Paul, and twin brother John who is meeting his developmental milestones and suffered no health problems as a result of his prematurity. Her maternal grandparents are involved with Jane's care on a daily basis.

Jane has had feeding problems since her birth, with her family devoting large parts of each day to feeding, each meal taking up to two hours to finish. This leaves them with little time to spend on other family activities. Jane was fed via a nasogastric tube for a period of time but she kept pulling this out and the family found it increasingly stressful to repass the nasogastric tube. Many of these feeding issues have been highlighted in the literature. Craig *et al.* (2003) carried out interviews with parents and one of the themes that came out was their experience of feeding. Some mothers reported that mealtimes lasted between five and eight hours a day. Within their book, Sullivan (2009) further explore the complexities and practicalities of nutritional support in children with neurodisabilities.

Jane has always been smaller than her brother, with her weight and length tracking along the 0.4th centile on her UK-WHO growth chart (Wright *et al.* 2010). Following a recent viral illness her weight has drifted below the 0.4th centile and her oral feeding skills have deteriorated, meaning it is becoming increasingly difficult to feed Jane. She has been referred to her local children's hospital so Jane's family can discuss the possibility of her having a gastrostomy tube inserted.

At this appointment, Jane's family met the surgeon, who discussed the procedure and the nutrition nurse, who showed them a gastrostomy tube, gave them literature to take home and answered any questions the family had. They also met the dietitian to discuss possible feeding methods once the tube is inserted. The feeds can be given as a daytime bolus or as an overnight feed via a feeding pump.

The decision to proceed and allow Jane to have a gastrostomy tube inserted was a difficult one for the family to make. The decision to go ahead with insertion of a gastrostomy tube was helped by meeting the parents of a couple of other children who had had a gastrostomy tube inserted. Gunton-Bunn & McNee (2009) carried out a review of the literature looking at the psychosocial impact of gastrostomy placement and highlighted a number of issues that are important for children's nurses to consider. These issues included the quality of information they were given at time of discussing gastrostomy tubes, what helped them to make the decision and how the gastrostomy tube impacted on life after placement.

 Questions

1. What is a gastrostomy tube and name the different types of gastrostomy tubes?
2. Discuss the nursing care of Jane in relation to the first 48 hours following insertion of her gastrostomy tube.
3. How would the children's nurse prepare Jane and her family for discharge following insertion of a gastrostomy tube?

Answers to questions

Question 1. What is a gastrostomy tube and name the different types of gastrostomy tubes?

A gastrostomy tube is a feeding tube that connects the stomach with the surface of the abdominal wall. It is usually placed in children who require medium to long-term nutrition support.

In 1980, Gauderer *et al.* reported a technique to insert a feeding tube that did not require a laparotomy – the percutaneous endoscopic gastrostomy (PEG), which uses an endoscope to insert a gastrostomy tube. Under general anaesthetic, the endoscope is passed through the mouth, down the oesophagus and into the stomach. A light at the end of the endoscope, along with finger indentation is used to identify a suitable position in the stomach to place the tube (Figure 29.1a). The skin is cleaned and a small incision is made in the skin, a wide-bore needle is passed through the incision into the stomach. A guide wire is passed through the needle; this is grasped by a forcep which is passed through the end of the endoscope (Figure 29.1b). The endoscope and guide wire are pulled up the oesophagus and out through the mouth. The PEG tube is attached to the guide wire at the mouth, the guide wire is then pulled out through the abdominal wall pulling the PEG tube into the stomach, and an endoscope is then passed to check tube position (Figure 29.1c). See also Figure 29.2.

This PEG tube needs to remains *in situ* until the stoma tract has healed, usually 6–8 weeks, and can then be replaced. It can be replaced with a G-tube or low-profile skin level

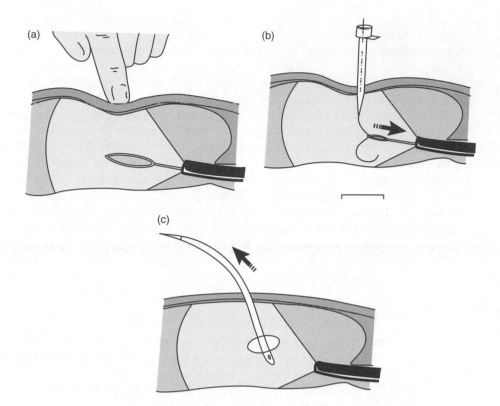

Figure 29.1   Percutaneous endoscopic gastrostomy tube placement (Cotton & Williams 1996). Reproduced with kind permission.

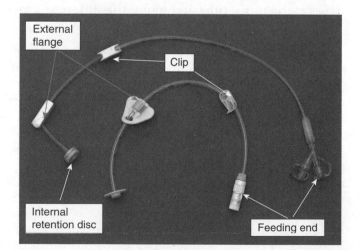

Figure 29.2   Percutaneous endoscopic gastrostomy (PEG) tubes and component parts.

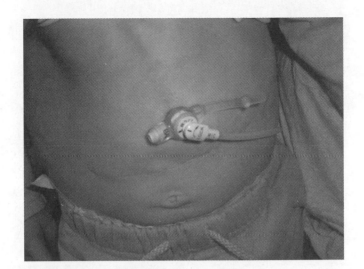

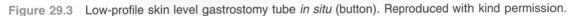

Figure 29.3 Low-profile skin level gastrostomy tube *in situ* (button). Reproduced with kind permission.

feeding tube more commonly called a button (see Figure 29.3). Both of these gastrostomy tubes are held in the stomach by a water filled balloon (see Figure 29.4). According to Khair (2003) these button devices are designed to sit flush to the skin, making them more cosmetically acceptable to some children and their families.

All planned care should adopt an appropriate model of nursing, for example Casey (1988) and Roper *et al.* (2000). Casey's model looks at working in partnership with families and it is important to work with Jane's family as they will be providing her ongoing care following discharge. Coleman *et al.* (2003) further explore the concept of family and carer participation by looking at a practice continuum tool. This highlights an important concept in children's nursing, identifying that there will be times of Jane's care where it will be appropriate for it to be all nurse led, for example in the immediate postoperative period, moving through to times where it is all parent or family led, for example just prior to discharge home having completed training for home enteral tube feeding. Although Roper *et al.* (2000) address 12 activities of daily living (see Chapter 1) this chapter will only address maintaining a safe environment, personal cleansing and dressing and eating and drinking in relation to postoperative care and discharge planning.

Question 2. Discuss the nursing care of Jane in relation to the first 48 hours following insertion of her gastrostomy tube.

Activity of living: maintaining a safe environment.
  Assess and plan postoperative interventions:

- Family-centred partnership approach to care; involve the parents when collecting Jane from recovery and return Jane to her prepared bed space. Jane's parents and grandparents to be involved in all aspects of care.
  Implement postoperative interventions:
- In order to be able to manage any postoperative airway problems that may arise ensure that the bed space has working oxygen and suction for Jane's return from theatre.

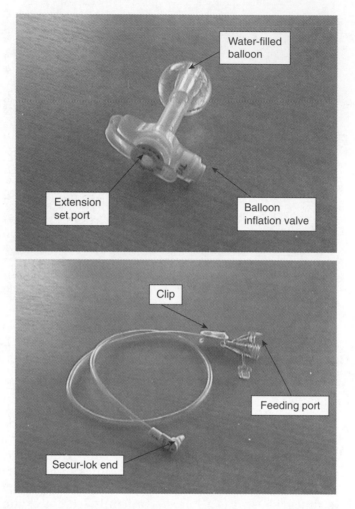

Figure 29.4 Low-profile button and extension set (Lothian Enteral Tube Feeding, Best Practice 2007). Reproduced with kind permission.

- Attach Jane to appropriate monitoring and infusion equipment as per hospital policy.
- Read medical and nursing notes, adhering to anaesthetist and surgeon's instructions.
- Record observations, TPR, SAO₂ (oxygen saturations), and BP on appropriate postoperative documentation. Frequency of monitoring as per hospital protocol.
- Using an appropriate pain assessment tool for children with a neurodevelopmental disorder, assess and record pain score. Swiggum *et al.* (2010) identify a range of assesment tools that might be used for children with cerebral palsy (see also Appendix 3, RCN 2010 pain guidelines).
- Administer analgesia as required in accordance with medical prescription. Note, although insertion of a gastrostomy is a relatively simple procedure, children can experience high levels of post-procedure pain requiring regular paracetamol, non-steroidal and occasionally opiate based medications.
- Observe gastrostomy stoma site for redness, leakage and swelling. Adjust external fixator (see Figure 29.2) on gastrostomy tube if it appears tight.

- Hospital policy may be to attach the gastrostomy tube to a drainage bag and leave on free drainage in the immediate postoperative period to allow for drainage of gastric contents and stomach decompression.
- Provide ongoing support to Jane's family and provide explanations for all interventions.

Activity of living: eating and drinking.
Assess and plan postoperative interventions:

- To assess Jane's nutritional status using a nutrition screening tool, for example Paediatric Yorkhill Malnutrition Score (PYMS) (Gerasimidis *et al.* 2010). Plan how to meet Jane's nutritional requirements following insertion of her gastrostomy tube.
- To monitor and maintain Jane's hydration.

Implement postoperative interventions:

- Nil by mouth/feeding tube for first 12–24 hours post-gastrostomy tube insertion (Lee *et al.* 2003). This practice can vary depending on hospital policy and it may be the surgeon's practice to use the gastrostomy tube a few hours after insertion.
- Administer intravenous fluids as per prescription, adhering to local hospital intravenous policy on monitoring of intravenous cannula site and infusion pump pressures.
- Commence enteral feeds according to dietician plan once medical staff have advised feeding can commence.
- Wash hands, put on gloves and apron before handling feed or setting up feed pump (see Figure 29.5). Best (2008) highlights importance of food hygiene when setting up enteral feed pumps.

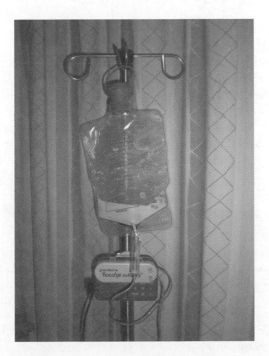

Figure 29.5 An enteral feed pump.

Activity of living: personal cleansing and dressing.
Assess and plan postoperative interventions:

- Assess Jane's personal cleansing and dressing requirements in partnership with her parents.
- Ensure that all equipment required to carry out Jane's personal hygiene has been collected and is close to hand.

Implement postoperative interventions:

- Maintain oral hygiene, especially while nil by mouth.
- Always wash and dry hands before handling the PEG tube.
- Put on gloves and an apron.
- Clean the PEG stoma site using gauze and sterile water or saline, this should be demonstrated to Jane's family and they should then be supervised carrying out the procedure.
- The gastrostomy stoma site should be cleaned and dried once a day.
- Avoid using any creams or talcum powder around the gastrostomy stoma site.

Evaluate all nursing interventions and document
   Activity: did you do what you aimed to do and what was the outcome to reduce risk of infection?

Question 3. How would the children's nurse prepare Jane and her family for discharge following insertion of a gastrostomy tube?

Assess and plan for a safe discharge:

- Discharge planning should ideally begin on admission. Jane is *assess*ed as clinically fit for discharge home: apyrexial, tolerating oral and gastrostomy feeds, gastrostomy site is satisfactory. Jane's family are educated and confident they can carry out Jane's ongoing care at home.
- Identify those members of the multidisciplinary team in the community that need to be contacted and any equipment the family will require to provide ongoing care for Jane at home. Corkin & Chambers (2008) highlight the information that should be provided for families in preparation for discharge home.

Activity of living: maintaining a safe environment:
Implementation of discharge plan:

- Ensure local hospital training checklist is completed and signed, such as that found in NHS Quality Improvement Scotland Best Practice Statement *Caring for Children and Young People in the Community Receiving Enteral Tube Feeding* (2007, p29).
- All equipment (feed pump and stand, giving sets and syringes) required for discharge home is supplied.
- Jane is registered with a homecare company for ongoing feed and equipment supplies.
- Referral to children's community nurse for support and advice at home and to arrange training on use of the gastrostomy tube for staff at Jane's nursery.

- Discharge medication checked as per hospital policy, given and administration instructions explained to the family. Paracetamol and ibuprofen for pain relief, meprazole and domperidone for gastroesophageal reflux as per doctor's advice.
- Doctor's letter for GP is given to Jane's family.
- Outpatient appointment arranged and given to the parents.

Activity of living: eating and drinking:

- Parents are educated and able to use the enteral feeding pump and administer bolus feeds.
- Jane is tolerating her feeds as per the dietician's feed plan. No or minimal vomiting, bowels are moving regularly without any difficulty.
- Parents know what to watch for in terms of Jane not tolerating feeds, for example vomiting, loose stools or constipation.
- Referral to speech and language therapist for ongoing input with oral feeding skills.
- Parents have a copy of the dietician's feed plan and a contact number for their dietician.

Activity of living: personal cleansing and dressing:

- Parents are advised to dress Jane in vests with popper fasteners to keep her gastrostomy tube tucked underneath her clothing and prevent it from getting caught when being lifted.
- For the first two weeks following gastrostomy tube insertion showers are preferable to immersion baths. Jane has a bathing chair and can be sat in this to be showered.
- Parents demonstrate competent cleaning and drying of the stoma site: turning the gastrostomy tube through 360 degrees and adjustment of external fixator as required. Once home a clean cloth, unscented soap and water should be used to clean the stoma site.
- No swimming or hydrotherapy for six weeks post-gastrostomy tube insertion.
- Contact nutritional nurse specialist for advice on any gastrostomy tube related complications. Common complications include leakage, blockage, overgranulation (see Figure 29.6) and infection (Crawley-Coha 2004).

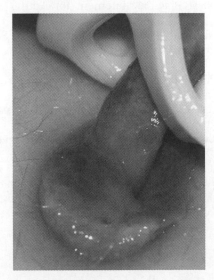

Figure 29.6 Overgranulated tissue at stoma site.

Evaluate all nursing interventions and document
Activity: did you do what you aimed to do and what was the outcome?

References

Best, C. (2008) Enteral tube feeding and infection control: how safe is our practice? *British Journal of Nursing*, **17**(16), 1036–41.

Casey, A. (1988) A partnership with child and family. *Senior Nurse*, **8**(4), 8–9.

Coleman, V., Smith, L. & Bradshaw, M. (2003) Enhancing consumer participation using the practice continuum tool for family-centred care. *Paediatric Nursing*, **15**(8), 28–31.

Corkin, D.A.P. & Chambers, J.A. (2008) Nutrition via enteral feeding devices, Chapter 15A. In: Kelsey, J. & McEwing, G. (eds). *Clinical Skills in Child Health Practice*. Edinburgh: Churchill Livingstone, Elsevier.

Cotton, P. & Williams, C. (1996) *Practical Gastrointestinal Endoscopy*, 4th edn. Oxford: Wiley-Blackwell.

Craig, G.M., Scambler, G. & Spitz, L. (2003) Why parents of children with neurodevelopmental disabilities requiring gastrostomy feeding need more support. *Developmental Medicine & Child Neurology*, **45**,183–8.

Crawley-Coha, T. (2004). A practical guide for the management of pediatric gastrostomy tubes based on 14 years of experience. *Journal of Wound, Ostomy and Continence Nursing*, **31**(4), 193–200.

Gauderer, M.W.L., Ponsky, J.L. & Izant, R.J. Jr (1980) Gastrostomy without laparotomy: a percutaneous endoscopic technique. *Journal of Pediatric Surgery*, **15**, 872–5.

Gerasimidis, K., Keane, O., Macleod, I., Flynn, D.M. & Wright, C.M. (2010) A four-stage evaluation of the Paediatric Yorkhill Malnutrition Score in a tertiary paediatric hospital and a district general hospital. *British Journal of Nutrition*, **104**(5), 751–6.

Gunton-Bunn, C. & McNee, P. (2009) Psychosocial implications of gastrostomy placement. *Paediatric Nursing*, **21**(7), 28–31.

Khair, J. (2003) Managing home enteral tube feeding for children. *British Journal of Community Nursing*, **8**(3),116–26.

Lee, A.C.H., Carter, H.P. & Crabbe, D. (2003) Percutaneous endoscopic gastrostomy. Procedure in practice. *British Journal of Perioperative Nursing*, **13**(7), 298–99, 301–2, 305.

Lothian Enteral Tube Feeding Best Practice Statement for Adults and Children (2007) Edinburgh (unpublished).

McKinlay, I. (2008) Cerebral palsy. In: McIntosh, N., Helms, P.J., Smyth, R.L. & Logan, S. (2008) *Forfar & Arneil's, Textbook of Pediatrics*, 7th edn. Edinburgh: Churchill Livingstone, Elsevier, 888–97.

NHS QIS Best Practice Statement (2007) *Caring for Children and Young People in the Community Receiving Enteral Tube Feeding*. Edinburgh: NHS QIS.

Roper N., Logan W.W. & Tierney A.J. (2000) *The Roper-Logan-Tierney Model of Nursing: Based on Activities of Living*. Edinburgh: Elsevier Health Sciences.

Sullivan, P.B. (2009) *Feeding and Nutrition in Children with Neurodevelopmental Disability*. London: MacKeith Press.

Swiggum, M., Hamilton, M.L., Gleeson, P. & Roddey, T. (2010) Pain in children with cerebral palsy: implications for pediatric physical therapy. *Pediatric Physical Therapy*, **22**, 86–92.

Wright, C.M., Williams, A.F., Elliman, D., *et al.* (2010). Using the new UK-WHO growth charts. *British Medical Journal*, **340**, c1140, 647–50.

Section 9

Care of Children and Young Persons with Endocrine Disorders

30

Nephrotic Syndrome

Janet Kelsey

Scenario

Gary, aged four years, has recently started to wake up with puffy eyes and tiredness. His abdomen is now swollen and his urine has become frothy and reduced in amount. Gary went to his GP with both his parents where he was found to have ++++ of protein in his urine. Gary was referred to the local children's assessment unit where he was assessed and admitted to the children's ward.

 Questions

1. What is nephrotic syndrome (NS)?
2. Discuss specific NS nursing care of Gary, especially during the first three days since admission to hospital.
3. Explain the normal mechanism for maintaining tissue fluid balance.
4. Describe pharmaceutical management of NS.

Care Planning in Children and Young People's Nursing, First Edition.
Edited by Doris Corkin, Sonya Clarke, Lorna Liggett.
© 2012 Blackwell Publishing Ltd. Published 2012 by Blackwell Publishing Ltd.

Answers to questions

Question 1. What is nephrotic syndrome (NS)?

Nephrotic syndrome is a condition marked by oedema, decreased serum albumin and albuminuria. A syndrome is a group of signs and/or symptoms which occur together, the cause of which is not always obvious. The disease is characterised by degenerative lesions in the kidney (nephrosis). There is increased permeability of the glomeruli and consequently a high loss of plasma protein in the urine (albuminuria). Nephrotic syndrome is defined as the combination of 'significant' proteinuria (protein: creatine ratio greater than 200 mg/mmol), hypoalbuminemia (less than 25 g/L) and generalised oedema. The cause is not fully understood. However, it is thought that there may be an immune pathogenic response (Lane 2008).

Proteinuria is definitive of nephrosis; it occurs because of changes to capillary endothelial cells, the glomerular basement membrane, or podocytes, which normally filter serum protein selectively by size and 'charge'. The result is urinary loss of macromolecular proteins, primarily albumin, but also opsonins, immunoglobulins, erythropoietin, transferring, hormone-binding proteins and antithrombin III in conditions that cause non-selective proteinuria (McMillan 2010).

As the plasma protein concentration falls so does the colloid osmotic pressure that it exerts; therefore fluid moves out of the capillaries and accumulates in the tissue spaces to cause oedema. The resulting fall in the blood flow through the kidneys causes them to secrete renin, an enzyme which stimulates the production of aldosterone by the adrenal cortex. This causes an increase in the re-absorption of water and salt through the kidney tubules. This re-absorption exacerbates the generalised oedema (Dolan & Gill 2008).

Children presenting with NS are likely to be lethargic, irritable and have poor appetite; they may also have diarrhoea and abdominal pain and an upper respiratory tract infection. Blood pressure is usually normal or low. Persistent hypertension is rare in minimal change disease (MCD) or focal segmental glomerulosclerosis (FSGS), and should raise suspicion of some other form of glomerular disease such as membranoproliferative disease (Dolan & Gill 2008).

Approximately 80% of cases of childhood NS have MCD, the commonest glomerular disease of childhood, with a median age at presentation of four years, which is more common in males than females (ratio 3:2). Over 90% of cases with MCD will respond to steroid therapy, but 70% of these will develop a relapsing course (Hodson *et al.* 2009). Steroid responsiveness is the most important determining factor in the long-term prognosis of NS. Conditions such as FSGS and mesangiocapillary glomerulosclerosis (MCGN) account for the remaining 20% of cases of NS. These conditions tend to present in the older child and the majority do not respond to oral steroid therapy (Dolan & Gill 2008).

Question 2. Discuss specific NS nursing care of Gary, especially during the first three days since admission to hospital.

Children presenting with their first episode of NS are admitted to hospital for diagnostic assessment, nursing and medical management, and parental education. Therefore, the initial nursing assessment should be in partnership with child and family (Casey 1988), and include the following specific to NS: observation of the level of oedema – weight on admission is taken as a baseline observation. Note any swelling around the eyes, ankles and other dependent parts and record the level of pitting – in Gary's case the scrotal area should be observed for swelling, irritation or redness and the skin should be inspected for any evidence of breakdown. Ask Gary and his mother about his appetite, urinary output and signs of tiredness or irritability. Assess vital signs, including blood pressure, and ask about recent infections. Carry out urinalysis to identify protein loss and specific gravity.

It is likely that the following problems will be identified specific to his NS:

- An excess fluid volume
- Risk of imbalanced nutrition
- Risk of impaired skin integrity
- Risk of tiredness and/or irritability
- Risk of infection
- Lack of understanding of the disease process and care planning

The NS specific goals of Gary's nursing care are therefore to relieve oedema and return fluid balance to within normal parameters, improve his nutrition, maintain skin integrity, to conserve Gary's energy, to prevent infection, and for Gary and his family to learn about the disease and the care required both in immediate future and long term. Gary will also require venepuncture as part of the investigations into his NS and should be prepared for this procedure and it should be carried out as for any child.

Activity of living: eating and drinking (Roper *et al.* 2000)
Assess
Goals:

- Gary's oedema will be reduced and this will be evidenced by appropriate weight loss and reduced abdominal girth.
- Gary will not become hypovolaemic.
- Gary will have an adequate nutritional intake to meet his normal growth needs, evidenced by him eating 80% of his meals.

Implement and evaluate:

- Daily weighing to determine increase or decrease in weight as a result of either retention of fluid or successful diuresis.
- Recording of oral/parenteral input and measurement of output to help calculate fluid requirements and to provide a visual means of determining the degree of diuresis.
- Observation of level of oedema. To identify the presence of oedema digital pressure is applied to the swollen area; removal of digital pressure leaves a characteristic indentation or pitting of the tissues.
- If Gary has mild oedema he does not require fluid restriction.
- Test all urine for protein losses and measurement of specific gravity.
- Observation for signs of hypovolaemia to include cool peripheries, capillary refill time >2 seconds, a core-peripheral temperature gap of >2°C, tachycardia and dizziness. Although hypotension is a late sign of hypovolaemia, blood pressure should be monitored regularly.
- Any signs of hypovolaemia should be reported immediately.
- A no-added-salt diet whilst there is >++ proteinuria, this is dependent on the level of oedema and changed as appropriate.
- Offer a balanced diet which appeals to Gary.

(Bagga 2008; Dolan & Gill 2008; Gipson *et al.* 2009).

Activity of living: maintaining a safe environment.
Assess
Goals:

- Gary will be free from signs of infection, as evidenced by normal vital signs with no respiratory symptoms.
- Skin integrity will be maintained, as evidenced by his skin remaining free from breakdown with no evidence of redness or irritation.

Implement and evaluate:

- Temperature, pulse and respiration are measured and recorded four hourly. A rise in temperature, pulse and respiration rates might indicate an underlying infection. The breathing rate, rhythm and depth should be observed to identify the accumulation of fluid in the pleural cavity (pleural effusion).
- Any symptoms of respiratory distress should be reported immediately.
- Protect Gary from anyone with an infection; this includes children, staff, family and visitors. Prevention of cross infection is important for all patients, but children with NS are at increased risk of bacterial infection, most commonly with *Streptococcus pneumoniae*. This increased susceptibility is due to urinary loss of immunoglobulins and complement components. It is therefore desirable to provide some isolation initially to prevent cross infection, though many units do not advocate such measures except where the child is on immunosuppressive drug therapy.
- Administer prophylactic antibiotics if prescribed.
- Inspect all skin surfaces regularly for breakdown; ensure Gary changes his position at a minimum of two hourly. Bathe and dry skin carefully especially in skin folds.
- Offer a scrotal support if Gary's scrotum is swollen.

Activity of living: working and playing.
Assess
Goal: Gary will conserve energy and play appropriately, as evidenced by him resting as needed and engaging in a level of play he is comfortable with.
Implement and evaluate:

- Encourage Gary to rest when he is tired. Bed rest is not encouraged as there is an increased risk of thrombosis due to the loss of proteins such as anti thrombin 111; this might be exacerbated by hypovolaemia (Renal Clinicians Group 2005).
- Assist Gary to mobilise when he is feeling more able.
- Provide play activities appropriate to age.
- Play with Gary at his pace.

Activity of living: communication.
Assess
Goal:

- Gary and his family will verbalise an understanding of the disease and his care needs.

Implement and evaluate:

- Ascertain current level of knowledge and understanding.
- Involve family in planning care.
- Provide a written plan of care.
- Teach the family about the use of steroids.
- Teach family about how to keep Gary in optimum health; this should include recognising signs of infection, how to respond to increasing weight either due to oedema or the potential to become overweight following steroid therapy, how to respond to increasing proteinuria and advice regarding vaccinations.

Question 3. Explain the normal mechanism for maintaining tissue fluid balance.

Tissue fluid balance is maintained by the counteraction of two pressures: blood pressure and the osmotic pressure of plasma protein. This is achieved by the following processes:

1. At the arterial end of the capillaries the blood pressure is greater than the osmotic pressure. As a result fluid is forced through the capillary walls into the tissue spaces.
2. At the venous end the osmotic pressure is greater than the blood pressure and fluid is therefore drawn into the capillary.

Normally these two opposing factors keep a steady balance of fluid in the tissues. Any factor which disturbs this equilibrium may lead to oedema.

Oedema is said to be present when there is excess fluid in the interstitial spaces. For example, sodium and water retention leads to increased blood pressure and loss of protein in the urine (proteinuria). This leads to a decrease in plasma protein (hypoproteinaemia) and therefore decreases osmotic pressure. Fluid then collects and stagnates in the interstitial space.

Question 4. Describe pharmaceutical management of NS.

Corticosteroids

Hodson *et al.* (2007) recommend that prednisolone therapy should be for a minimum of 12 weeks and that alternate day therapy is not stopped abruptly but tapered over the next 2–4 months. However, Gipson *et al.* (2009) recommend daily prednisone for six weeks, followed by alternate days for six weeks and no steroid taper. All children should be issued with a steroid warning card and advised that the medicine should be taken with food to reduce the gastrointestinal side effects.

Corticosteroids are both anti-inflammatory and immunosuppressive. The objectives of steroid therapy are to induce and maintain remission and to minimise side effects (Box 30.1). Diuresis generally occurs one to two weeks after therapy starts. This is followed by a reduction in the oedema. Prolonged steroid therapy may be associated with side effects.

Box 30.1   Corticosteroid side effects

Behavioural problems
Increased appetite
Weight gain/obesity
Acne
Hirsutism
Increased susceptibility to infection
Posterior subcapsular cataracts
Hypertension
Growth suppression
Pubertal delay
Adrenal suppression
Acute pancreatitis
Osteoporosis
Impaired glucose metabolism

Box 30.2   Side-effects of cyclophosphamide (Dolan & Gill 2008)

Bone marrow suppression
Reversible hair loss
Gastro-intestinal upset
Haemorrhagic cystitis
Impaired fertility
Malignancy

Children who are not responding to steroids are given alternative immunomodulatory agent drugs. Cyclophosphamide is usually used (Bagga 2008; Gipson *et al.* 2009). It has been shown to induce a two-year, relapse-free period in approximately 70% of children with steroid sensitive NS and 25% of children with steroid dependent NS. Cyclophosphamide is also used as a cytotoxic drug. It interferes with normal division and development of cells by binding to the DNA, stopping cell division.

Levamisole may be used in children who have occasional relapses. However, it is considered less useful for children who are steroid dependent (Renal Clinicians Group 2005). The chief side effect is leucopenia: flu-like symptoms, liver toxicity, convulsions and skin rashes are rare (Bagga *et al.* 2008).

Cyclosporin may be given as a steroid sparing agent, but BP and renal function must be monitored. Side effects include hypertension, hirsutism, gum hypertrophy, nephrotoxicity, hypercholesterolemia and elevated transaminases (Bagga *et al.* 2008; Renal Clinicans Group 2005).

Antibiotics

Prophylactic penicillin may be beneficial whilst the child is oedematous and has proteinuria, but this is usually discontinued when the child goes into remission. Suspected infections should be treated promptly (Renal Clinicians Group 2005).

Albumin

The clinical indications for albumin are clinical hypovolaemia and severe symptomatic oedema. However, children should be monitored closely during administration due to the possibility of intravascular overload (Dolan & Gill 2008; Renal Clinicians Group 2005).

Diuretics

Diuretics may be used to control oedema until remission begins, but close observation for hypovolaemia is essential and the child's electrolytes should be checked regularly (Dolan & Gill 2008).

Immunisation

Live vaccines should not be given to immunosuppressed children; all children with nephrotic syndrome should be vaccinated against pneumococcal infections. Varicella vaccination may be offered when the child is in remission and not immunocompromised (Bagga 2008; Renal Clinicians Group 2005).

References

Bagga, A. (2008) Revised guidelines for the management of steroid-sensitive nephrotic syndrome. *Indian Journal of Nephrology*, **18**, 1.

Casey, A. (1988) A partnership with child and family. *Senior Nurse*, **8**(4), 8–9.

Dolan, M. & Gill, D. (2008) Management of nephritic syndrome. *Paediatrics and Child Health*, **18**(8), 369–74.

Gipson, D.S., Massengill, S.F., Yao, L., *et al.* (2009) Management of childhood onset nephrotic syndrome. *Pediatrics*, **124**, 747–57.

Hodson, E.M., Willis, N.S. & Craig, J.C. (2007) Corticosteroid therapy for nepphrotic syndrome in children. *Cochrane Database Syst Rev*, 20007: CD001533.

Hodson, E.M., Willis, N.S. & Craig, J.C. (2009) Corticosteroid therapy for nephrotic syndrome in children (Review) *The Cochrane Library*, Issue 1. www.thecochranelibrary.com (accessed 2 September 2009).

Lane, J. (2008) Nephrotic syndrome. E-medicine nephrology. http://emedicine.medscape.com/ (accessed 13 March 2009).

MCMillan, J. (2010) Nephrotic syndrome Merck manuals on line medical library. www.merck.com/ mmpe/sec17/ch235/ch235c.html#BABDDJGD (accessed 28 September 2010).

Renal Clinicians Group (2005) *Guidelines for the Management of Nephritic Syndrome*. Renal Unit Royal Hospital for Sick Children, Galsgow: Yorkhill Division.

Roper, N., Logan, W. & Tierney, A.J. (2000) *The Roper-Logan-Tierney Model of Nursing: Based on Activities of Living*. London: Elsevier.

www.clinicalguidelines.scot.nhs.uk/Renal%20Unit%20Guidelines/Nephrotic%20Syndrome%20. pdf (accessed 2 September 2009).

31

Newly Diagnosed Diabetic

Pauline Cardwell and Doris Corkin

Scenario

Miley, a six-year-old girl who is in the pre-operational stage of cognitive development (Bee & Boyd 2010), has become 'out of sorts' recently. She lives at home with her parents and her twin brothers who are 18 months old. Her parents describe Miley as normally a very energetic child, and recently as being too tired to play and more impatient than usual. They also notice that her breath is 'smelly' and she woke during the night complaining of 'a sore tummy'.

Whilst at the GP surgery, Miley has her urine tested and it is quickly identified that the sample contains glucose and ketones. Additionally, the practice nurse carries out a blood glucose test which reveals a sugar level of 22.5 mmol/L (normal range 4–8 mmol/L, Diabetes UK 2008a). Dr Good, her GP, advises Miley's parents that it is likely she has diabetes and that she needs to go to hospital for further investigations and management of her condition.

Miley is referred to the children's medical ward by her GP with a provisional diagnosis of diabetes mellitus (DM). On admission to the ward Miley's parents appear anxious, distressed and demanding answers to questions. According to Miley's parents, she has been drinking excessive amounts of fluids, passing urine frequently (polyuria), losing weight and generally feeling unwell, over the last 2–3 weeks. Following further investigations in the children's ward, Miley's diagnosis of diabetes mellitus type 1 (DMT1) is confirmed with an HbA1c (12.3%) blood test that measures long-term blood glucose (normal non-diabetic HbA1c is 3.5–5.5%). In diabetes <7.5% is target (www.medweb.bham.ac.uk), so treatment and management of disease need to be established.

What is diabetes mellitus?

This is a chronic disease which is characterised by a raised blood glucose level, resulting from a lack of the hormone insulin or a resistance to insulin in the body. The disease is categorised into two main types: type 1 and type 2, which will impact on the ongoing management of the condition.

 Questions

1. Explain the pathophysiology of diabetes mellitus type 1.
2. Discuss the impact of this condition for Miley and her family.
3. Outline how to monitor blood glucose levels and administer insulin.
4. Describe the information that Miley and her parents will require to manage her condition safely after discharge from hospital in relation to managing hypoglycaemia and hyperglycaemia attacks.

The proposed answer plans offer 'lists of potential responses' with limited rationale, it is therefore recommended for the individual student/healthcare professional to explore the issues through further reading. Answers are not meant to be definitive or restrictive and may be amended to facilitate changing circumstances at any time.

Answers to questions

Question 1. Explain the pathophysiology of diabetes mellitus type 1.

Diabetes mellitus type 1 (DMT1) is the most common endocrine disorder in children, which can occur at any stage of development during childhood, even during infancy, with an increasing incidence in the UK (Faulkner & Clark 1998; Burns *et al.* 2010). Literature would suggest that the aetiology of DMT1 is not completely understood, but may be triggered by genetical or environmental factors (Morrow 2006). The condition is characterised by the failure to produce insulin in the beta cells within the islets of Langerhans in the pancreas.

DMT1 relates to a deficiency of insulin production, which requires a well balanced, healthy diet, glucose monitoring, insulin injections and exercise (Lowes & Lyne 1999; Faulkner & Chang 2007). A lack of insulin within the body inhibits the metabolism of carbohydrates, proteins and fats. Insulin is required to facilitate the uptake of glucose, which is the primary energy of body cells (Axton & Fugate 2009). If the body is not able to access glucose it then metabolises fat and proteins, which causes an increase in food intake and weight loss.

Diabetes mellitus type 2 (DMT2) is a combination of insulin deficiency and insulin resistance and is linked to obesity or family history of DMT2, with increasing incidence in children (Axton & Fugate 2009; Moules & Ramsay 2008). Treatment is mainly focused on diet and exercise, although oral medication may be required.

Characteristics of DMT1 include:

- Polyuria
- Polyphagia
- Polydipsia
- Acetone breath
- Weight loss
- Abdominal pain
- Ketonuria
- Glucosuria
- Hyperglyceamia
- Lethargy
- Enuresis in toilet trained children

✎ Activity 31.1

Explore the above medical terms and reflect upon your clinical experience of caring for a newly diagnosed diabetic child.

Question 2. Discuss the impact of this condition for Miley and her family.

Activity of living: communication and dying, as per Roper, Logan & Tierney model of care (Holland *et al.* 2008).

This is an overwhelming and daunting diagnosis for Miley and her family. Learning that Miley has diabetes will be difficult for her parents to come to terms with, as they may feel shock, denial, anger, fear, sadness, guilty or responsible for their child's chronic condition (Morrow 2006). Adapting to and managing diabetes will no doubt disrupt the normal routine within the family home and place a great strain on the family unit. The fact that DMT1 is a life-long condition which can have long-term complications, for example damage to eyes, heart and kidneys, can be devastating for Miley's parents (Diabetes UK 2008a). Whilst this can be a stressful time for Miley and her parents their concerns should be clearly recorded and addressed as appropriate in her care plan. Service Delivery and Organisation (SDO 2010) identify in their recommendations the importance of recording and communicating effectively care plans, by methods which are quality assured and effective in meeting patient education and self-care needs. Should problems arise around compliance with treatment of DMT1 serious life-threatening consequences may occur, such as admission to intensive care for life-saving interventions or indeed early mortality in severe cases.

Miley's parents will require ongoing education and support from the children's diabetes care team which will include the consultant paediatrician, paediatric diabetes nurse specialist, paediatric dietitian and other professionals as required, with access to contact details. Information will be provided in verbal and written forms in a timely manner, to suit Miley and her parents' needs and they should be given the opportunity to ask questions and clarify information provided (NICE 2010). Parents should also be made aware of charities, for example Diabetes UK, as they have many valuable age-appropriate resources to help inform Miley and themselves about her condition.

Question 3. Outline how to monitor blood glucose levels and administer insulin.

Activity of living: maintaining a safe environment as per Roper, Logan & Tierney model of care (Holland *et al.* 2008).

Blood glucose monitoring is a central aspect of care for Miley and her parents, to ensure treatments are ongoing and responsive to needs. This allows Miley's parents to appreciate the changes in her glucose levels in response to growth and development, illness, exercise and changes in her lifestyle. Miley's parents must be confident in performing blood glucose monitoring and recording accurately, to assist in developing a log of Miley's response to care delivered and changes in her management regime. See plan in Box 31.1.

Administration of insulin injection

The administration of insulin injections is a complex aspect of care delivery within the multifaceted role of the children's nurse. Standards for medicine management are regulated by the Nursing and Midwifery Council (NMC 2008) and clearly highlight the nurse's responsibility to ensure safe practice when administrating medication. Abdomen, thigh and upper arms are the most commonly used injection sites for insulin administration, which is administered at a 90 degree angle using the appropriate delivery device. These sites need to be rotated in order to prevent lipoatrophy, which will inhibit the absorption of insulin, thus leading to instability in overall condition. Ensure all equipment used to deliver insulin is used and disposed of as per manufacturer's guidelines/hospital policy.

As the NMC (2008) supports the administration of medicines by a carer, the parents should be encouraged by the children's nurse to become competent in the administration of insulin injections to Miley in the paediatric setting, thus supporting a partnership approach to care (Casey 1988). Although the responsibility to ensure the insulin is administered remains with the children's nurse in the hospital setting, the nurse also needs to ensure the parents are educated and confident to deliver insulin injections as prescribed. In most cases the insulin will be delivered by a syringe, pen device or a pump. Insulin is administered in units and in the initial period of management the units administered may be adjusted by the doctor or diabetes nurse specialist, to achieve adequate control that gives blood glucose results pre-meals of 4–8 mmol/L. Considerations appropriate to Miley's age and stage of development should always be taken into account, with clear negotiation and support for the parents regarding Miley's ongoing care needs, for example when Miley refuses her insulin injection. The use of play therapy or distraction techniques can be a useful aid to the children's nurse in engaging Miley in her ongoing care needs.

Types of insulin

Insulin is a protein which is used to treat DMT1 and is delivered via subcutaneous injection or pump infusion. Regimes are determined on an individual basis, requiring up

---

Box 31.1   Care plan

Action: how to monitor blood sugars	Reason
1. The children's nurse should be aware of Miley's plan of care and incorporate a family-centred approach (Casey 1988) in order to gain consent, parental co-operation and involvement.	To ensure clear communication pathway is implemented.
2. The children's nurse should collect all equipment, such as electronic blood glucose meter and reagent test strip (check expiry date and ensure test strip code is compatible with glucose meter code), lancet (finger-pricking device), sharps disposing box and tissue to wipe site after obtaining blood sample.	To ensure safe practice and accurate blood glucose testing.
3. Be aware of Miley's care plan, for example check blood glucose 20–30 minutes before meals (aim for 4–8 mmol/L), at bedtime or at other times as indicated.	To monitor condition and record findings.
4. The children's nurse and Miley should wash their hands (warm water to increase capillary blood flow) and dry prior to and after procedure. Then nurse should apply gloves prior to carrying out procedure (Morrow 2006).	To prevent cross infection.
5. Ensure test strip is inserted into glucose meter and is ready to receive blood sample.	Prevent nerve damage and ensure rotation of sites.
Blood glucose testing involves pricking the side of Miley's finger (either second or third) using appropriate finger pricking device, to obtain small drop of blood.	Ensuring adequate sample for analysis.
Bring the reagent strip to the pricked finger and touch it to the droplet of blood as per manufacturer's guidelines. Apply gentle pressure with tissue to sample site to remove excess blood.	
6. Dispose of finger- pricking device or component as appropriate in sharps box as per hospital policy.	Nurse and patient safety.
Ensure blood glucose meter is cleaned between patient use.	
7. The children's nurse should accurately and immediately record the blood sugar result in Miley's diary and nursing care plan (NMC 2005). Ensure doctor is informed of latest result.	Ensuring safe practice and supporting continuity of care.
8. Praise Miley for her co-operation and participation throughout the procedure and reward as appropriate, for example a badge or bravery certificate.	To promote Miley's involvement in ongoing care needs.
Discuss with parents the use of reward charts in the home to support compliance with ongoing monitoring.	Parental education.

to four injections per day. There are four different categories of insulin (BNFC 2010–2011; NICE 2010):

- Rapid-acting – onset of action 15 minutes
- Short-acting – onset of action 30–60 minutes

- Intermediate-acting – onset of action approximately 1–2 hours
- Long-acting – once-daily dose to produce a constant level of insulin

Selection of insulin used is usually based on needs of child and made by the consultant in charge of care.

Calculation of insulin dose

The administration of prescribed medications to children must be viewed by the children's nurse as a key aspect of nursing care that requires sound knowledge of pharmacology, numeracy skills and the ability to communicate effectively with Miley and her family (Casey 1988; Smith & Coleman 2009). To ensure accurate dosing, body weight is used more frequently for ease of paediatric calculations. In order to calculate drug doses accurately the children's nurse must be able to demonstrate an understanding of child development theory, the units of drugs in current use and approved abbreviations.

Student nurses should be involved in the procedure of drug calculation and administration as a learning tool. However, in order to meet legal, trust and professional guidelines student nurses should *NEVER* single check an insulin injection and administer unsupervised. As nurses administer medications on a regular basis there is the potential for errors to occur (Griffith *et al.* 2003; NPSA 2010).

Storage of drugs

Safe storage of drugs involves both environmental and security factors, such as a lockable medicines trolley and refrigerator. Children's nurses must ensure all medicines are stored in accordance with the patient /drug information leaflet. Parents need to ensure that they have an adequate supply of insulin to meet Miley's needs and it should be stored in a refrigerator until required. Once the insulin vial/penfill is in use it can be stored at room temperature and must be discarded after one month (Sadik 2001). As with all medicines they must be stored safely and out of the reach of children, including Miley and her twin brothers.

When in the school environment, Miley's medicines and monitoring equipment must be stored safely and appropriately to ensure continuity of care whilst in school (Diabetes UK 2011), which is supported by an individual care plan.

Question 4. Describe the information that Miley and her parents will require to manage her condition safely after discharge from hospital, in relation to managing hypoglycaemia and hyperglycaemia attacks.

Discharge plan: in order for Miley's parents to manage her condition safely after discharge from hospital it is essential to discuss, amongst other aspects of care, the management of low and high blood sugars to prevent the possibility of long-term complications and life-threatening events occurring.

Hypoglycaemia, often referred to as a 'hypo', is when the blood sugar level is low (below 4mmol/L). These hypos can have a rapid onset and are caused by (Diabetes UK 2009):

- A delayed/missed meal or snack
- Not enough food – especially carbohydrates
- Too much insulin has been given
- Increased activity levels

Box 31.2   Hypoglycaemia

Symptoms of hypoglycaemia

- Hunger
- Sweating
- Shaking/trembling
- Irritability
- Palpitations
- Lack of concentration
- Glazed eyes
- Mood changes – anger/aggressive behaviour
- Drowsiness
- Vagueness

Treating hypoglycaemia

- Immediately give a sugary drink or food such as, lucozade or coke, glucose tablets, sweets, teaspoonfuls of sugar or glucogel.
- Follow this with other long-acting carbohydrates, for example sandwiches, fruit, cereal bar, biscuits or a meal if due.
- Seek further guidance from diabetes care team.

Box 31.3   Hyperglycaemia

Symptoms of hyperglycaemia

- Urinary frequency
- Thirst – increased
- Tiredness/lethargy
- Weight loss
- Visual disturbances – blurring

Treatment of hyperglycaemia

- Can have a quick onset and may lead to diabetic ketoacidosis (DKA), which can be life threatening in severe cases and require hospitalisation.
- Close monitoring of blood glucose levels and recording of same (up to four times per day).
- Good adherence to dietary regime and support from diabetic care team.
- Review of insulin regime and injection technique.

Nursing alert!
If the child is unconscious do not give anything to eat or drink, call for medical assistance immediately and stay with the child until help arrives.

Hyperglyceamia is when the blood glucose level is high (>15 mmol/L) and is linked to poor control of the condition. Causes for the high glucose levels include: missing doses of insulin/oral treatments, poor injection technique or eating a high carbohydrate diet. Physical stress can initiate extra glucose production by the body, leading to hyperglycaemia (www.diabetes.co.uk).

Children with diabetes in school

Whilst education is an important aspect of life for children and young people, care for the child with diabetes in school must be appropriate to their needs, parallel with optimising their academic performance. Schools must adopt positive attitudes towards children with diabetes and adopt a child-centred policy which offers children and their parents support in the school environment from appropriately trained staff (Diabetes UK 2008b).

References

Axton, S.E. & Fugate, T. (2009) *Paediatric Nursing Care Plans for the Hospitalized Child*, 3rd edn. Upper Saddle River, NJ: Pearson Prentice Hall.

Bee, H. & Boyd, D. (2009) *The Developing Child*, 12th edn. London: Pearson.

British National Formulary for Children (BNFC) (2010–2011) *British Medical Journal*. London: PS Publishing.

Burns, M.R., Bodansky, H.,J. & Parslow, R.C. (2010) Paediatric intensive care admissions for acute diabetes complications. *Diabetic Medicine* **27**, 705–708.

Casey, A. (1988) A partnership with child and family. *Senior Nurse*, **8**(4), 8–9.

Diabetes UK (2008a) *When Your Child Has Diabetes – What You Can Expect*. London: Diabetes UK.

Diabetes UK (2008b) *Making All Children Matter: Support for Children with Diabetes in Schools*. London: Diabetes UK.

Diabetes UK (2009) *Children With Diabetes at School – What all Staff Need to Know*. London: Diabetes UK.

Diabetes UK (2011) Diabetes week 2011 – Lets talk Type I diabetes in schools. www.diabetes.org.uk/In_Your_Area/N_Ireland/Public-meetings/ (accessed 22 June 2011).

Faulkner, M.S. & Chang Lu.I. (2007) Family influence on self care, quality of life and metabolic control in school-age children and adolescents with type I diabetes. *Journal of Paediatric Nursing* **22**, 59–68.

Faulkner, M.S., & Clark, F.S. (1998) Quality of life for parents of children and adolescence with type 1 diabetes. *Diabetes Educator*, **24**, 721–7.

Griffith, R. Griffith, H. & Jordan, S. (2003) Administration of medicines. Part 1: *Nursing Standard*, **18**(2), 47–53.

Holland, K., Jenkins, J., Solomon, J. & Whittam, S. (2008) *Applying the Roper. Logan. Tierney. Model in Practice*, 2nd edn. Edinburgh: Churchill Livingstone.

http://medweb.bham.ac.uk/easdec/prevention/what_is_the_hba1c.htm (accessed 13 August 2010).

Lowes, L. & Lyne, P. (1999) A normal life-style: parental stress and coping in childhood diabetes. *British Journal of Nursing*, **6**(28), 30–33.

Morrow, P. (2006) Caring for children with diabetes and other endocrine disorders, Chapter 34. In: Glasper, A. & Richardson, J (eds). *A Textbook of Children's and Young People's Nursing*. London: Churchill Livingstone, Elsevier.

Moules, T. & Ramsay, J. (2008) *The Textbook of Children's and Young People's Nursing*, 2nd edn. Oxford: Blackwell Publishing.

National Institute for Health and Clinical Excellence (2004, updated 2010) *Type 1 Diabetes: Diagnosis and Management of Type 1 Diabetes in Children, Young People and Adults*. Clinical guideline 15. London: NICE.

NHS National Patient Safety Agency (2010) Rapid Response Report. Safer Administration of Insulin. NPSA/2010/RRR013.

Nursing and Midwifery Council (2008) *Guidelines on the Administration of Medicines*. London: NMC.

Nursing and Midwifery Council (NMC, 2005) *Guidelines for Records and Record Keeping*. London: NMC.

Sadik, R. (2001) Case 12. Gareth Jones: three-year old with diabetes. In: Sadik, R. & Campbell, G. (eds). *Client Profiles in Nursing, Child Health*. London: Greenwich Medical Media Limited.

Service Delivery and Organisation (2010) *The Organisation and Delivery of Diabetes Services in the UK: a Scoping Exercise*. www.sdo.nihr.ac.uk/files/project/249-final-report.pdf (accessed 13 August 2010).

Smith, L. & Coleman, V. (2009) *Child and Family-Centred Healthcare*, 2nd ed. London: Palgrave Macmillan.

www.diabetes.co.uk/Diabetes-and-Hyperglyceamia.htlm (accessed 12 August 2010).

32

Acute Renal Failure/Kidney Injury

Hazel Gibson, Gloria Hook and Rosi Simpson

This scenario aims to give insight into how recognition, assessment and early intervention of predisposing factors can prevent and influence outcomes of acute renal failure (ARF) and acute kidney injury (AKI). Plotz *et al.* (2008) observed a high incidence of significant AKI in the at-risk paediatric population.

Scenario

Twelve-year-old Jack, who lives with his mother and two siblings, was admitted to his local general hospital with abdominal pain. He had an appendicectomy (see Chapter 24) for a perforated appendix.

Postoperatively his abdominal pain, nausea and vomiting persisted. An abdominal CT scan (computed tomography) showed a pelvic collection and intravenous antibiotics were commenced.

Jack's nausea and vomiting continued despite regular anti-emetics. On day 7 postoperatively he had an episode of *frank haematuria*. Following this he became *anuric* and it was noted that his intake and output record was incomplete. Bloods taken at this time showed elevated levels of *urea* and *creatinine* (see Table 32.1).

A medical decision was made to transfer Jack to the regional children's hospital for further management and treatment. On admission his serum creatinine and urea levels had increased further, his serum CO_2 level was reduced, his CRP was raised, and he had become hypertensive and remained anuric (see Table 32.1). A diagnosis of acute renal failure was made secondary to dehydration.

Care Planning in Children and Young People's Nursing, First Edition.
Edited by Doris Corkin, Sonya Clarke, Lorna Liggett.
© 2012 Blackwell Publishing Ltd. Published 2012 by Blackwell Publishing Ltd.

Table 32.1 Definitions.

Frank haematuria: the passage of blood in the urine that is visible to the naked eye.
Anuric: the failure of the kidneys to produce urine.
Urea: the main breakdown product of protein metabolism, the product that unrequired nitrogen is excreted by the body in urine.
Creatinine: a product of protein metabolism found in muscle.
CO_2: serum CO_2 indicator of respiratory/metabolic acidosis.
CRP (C reactive protein): a protein whose plasma concentrations are raised in infection and inflammatory states and in the presence of tissue damage or necrosis.

Questions

1. Define acute renal failure/kidney injury.
2. With reference to a model of care, identify the immediate problems when planning Jack's care.
3. Continuing with the nursing process and model of care, discuss in further detail the immediate problems identified in Jack's care plan.
4. What would indicate that Jack may require renal replacement therapy (RRT)?
5. Using the information provided give rationale for the dialysis modality chosen for Jack.
6. How would you assess if Jack is recovering his renal function?

Answers to questions

Question 1. Define acute renal failure/kidney injury.

Acute renal failure (ARF) was the traditional way of describing and defining damage to the kidneys (Davies 2009). It is a sudden, potentially reversible inability of the kidney to maintain normal body chemistry and fluid balance and is usually accompanied by oliguria (urine output <0.5 ml/kg/hour or <1 ml/kg/hour in a neonate), but polyuric ARF can also occur (Rees *et al.* 2007). In 2005 a group of experts proposed the term 'acute kidney injury' as a new system of classifying renal damage (Mehta *et al.* 2007).

Along with the new terminology it was felt that acute kidney injury (AKI) should be diagnosed as an abrupt (within 48 hours) reduction in kidney function, defined as an a increase in serum creatinine or a percentage increase ≥50%, or a reduction of urine output from a known baseline (Mehta *et al.* 2007). A new modified staging system was proposed to classify the cause of renal disease in children. The stages were to reflect the increasing severity of AKI and used serum creatinine and urine output as markers.

Paediatric – modified RIFLE (pRIFLE)

R	Risk
I	Injury
F	Failure
L	Loss – need for renal replacement therapy (RRT) >4 weeks
E	End-stage renal disease (ESRF), requiring dialysis >3 months

(Bellomo *et al.* 2004)

Paediatric – modified RIFLE (pRIFLE)

Stage	Estimated CCL	Urine output criteria
1. Risk	eCCl<25%	<0.5 mls/kg/hour for >8 hours
2. Injury	eCCl <50%	<0.5 mls/kg/hour for >16 hours
3. Failure	eCCl <75%	<0.5 mls/kg/hour for >24 hours
or	eCCl <35 ml/min/1.73 m²	anuric for 12 hours

CCl = creatinine clearance

(Akcan-Arikan *et al.* 2007)

Ricci *et al.* (2008), have shown that this classification is a good predictor of outcome, showing that mortality increased with worsening Rifle class. It is hoped that these new guidelines will standardise and improve diagnoses and outcomes for renal patients. Currently no studies have been able to determine exactly at what point 'renal replacement therapy' (RRT) should be initiated. This can differ widely between units and even individual practitioners.

Activity 32.1

For further reading into acute renal failure/kidney injury, causes and classification:
www.gosh.nhs.uk/gosh_families/information_sheets_acute_renal_failure
UK Renal Association (2008) *Acute Kidney Injury, Clinical Practice Guidelines*, 4th edn.
  Accessed online 10 May 2011 at: www.renal.org/guidelines

Question 2. With reference to a model of care, identify the immediate problems when planning Jack's care.

'Nursing prevention strategies for ARF depend on nurse's knowledge of pathophysiology, toxicity of pharmacological agents and therapeutic clinical measures that can precipate ARF in children'.
Activity of living: elimination (Roper *et al.* 1990).
Assess: Jack is anuric.
Activity of living: eating and drinking.
Assess: Jack has continued nausea and vomiting leading to dehydration. This could lead to potential problems of:

• Over hydration – if IV fluids erected, inability to adhere to 24 hour fluid allowance.
• Catabolism – due to reduced calorie intake and inability to tolerate oral nutrition.
• May require dietetic involvement, for example nasogastric feed, supplements/enteral feeds.

Activity of living: maintaining a safe environment.

Assess: Jack has the potential problem of fluid excess related to anuria, excessive fluid administration and sodium and water retention.

Potential electrolyte imbalance due to:

↓ renal potassium excretion (hyperkalaemia)
↓renal sodium excretion (hypernatraemia)

Activity of living: breathing and circulation.

Assess: Jack has the potential problem of pulmonary oedema due to fluid overload, and fluid retention. He has the potential problem of hypertension due to fluid overload.

Activity of living: controlling body temperature.

Assess: Jack has the potential problem of infection due to compromised nutritional status.

Activity of living: communication (Casey 1988).

Assess: Jack and his family are anxious due to the suddenness, severity of his illness, the potential for long-term kidney damage. Jack is almost a teenager with the potential problem of compliance/concordance.

Question 3. Continuing with the nursing process and model of care, discuss in further detail the immediate problems identified in Jack's care plan.

Activity of living: elimination.
Plan:

- To find cause of anuria and if possible restore renal function
- To prevent fluid overload

Implement:

- Weigh twice daily – morning and evening.
- Ensure blood is retained daily – increase frequency if indicated – assist with same.
- Record minimum four hourly vital signs – heart rate (HR), blood pressure (BP), respiratory rate (RR). Paediatric vital signs are individualised specific to age, size and underlying medical condition:
  — Assess fluid status from results
  Decreased BP, increased HR continued dehydration
  Increased BP fluid overload
  Increased RR pulmonary oedema
- Calculate individual fluid requirement and ensure accurate record completion.

Activity of living: eating and drinking.
Plan:

- To ensure required nutritional and fluid intake and prevent a catabolic state
- To reduce uraemia
- To minimise nausea and vomiting

Implement:

- Record a minimum daily weight.
- Give IV fluids as prescribed – adhere to local hospital policies and procedures for administration of intravenous fluids.
- Assist with venepuncture to retain daily bloods or more frequently as indicated.
- Liaise with dietician for daily dietetic assessment.
- Give prescribed anti-emetics as per local hospital policy for administration of medicines and monitor effect.
- Record accurate hourly intake and output to account for insensible loss ($300\,ml/m^2$) + previous 24 hours' output and other losses.
- Offer small amounts of high calorie, low salt, low potassium, calculated protein foods – take into account personal likes and dislikes.
- Consider the need for supplementary/enteral feeding if oral nutrition cannot be tolerated.
- Provide parent and child information and explanation of dietary needs.
- Consider parental or child involvement in recording diet and oral intake.

Activity of living: maintaining a safe environment.
Plan: monitor serum potassium and reduce to a safe level.
Implement:

- Assist with the collection of a minimum of daily bloods – increase frequency if clinically indicated.
- Liaise with dietician and ensure dietary potassium restriction is adhered to in diet.
- Give prescribed medications as per hospital policy and monitor effects/side effects, for example sodium bicarbonate drives potassium from blood into the cells.
- Consider the need for ECG monitoring, depending upon serum electrolyte levels.
- Provide parental and child information on diet and potassium containing foods.
- If potassium remains elevated give explanation and information in preparation for dialysis.

Activity of living: breathing and circulation.
Plan: to reduce BP to a safe level.
Implement:

- Record a minimum of four hourly BP and HR (increase frequency if condition indicates).
- Give anti-hypertensives as prescribed as per local hospital policy and monitor effects/side effects.
- Ensure parents and child are aware of their fluid allowance and the importance of compliance.
- Consider child and parents' involvement in the recording of oral fluid intake
- Weigh to assess hydration status, i.e. fluid overload may contribute to increased BP.
- If BP remains elevated provide parents and child with information and explanation if dialysis is considered. Consider age appropriate and developmental needs when providing written and verbal information.
- Involve play therapist – distraction.

NB when administering prescribed medications, the frequency and/or dose may need adjusted due to the child's reduced renal function.

Activity 32.2

Familiarise yourself with normal paediatric biochemistry/haematology parameters, for example local laboratory parameters:
  www.scarborough.nhs.uk/BiochemistryReferenceRanges
  www.scarborough.nhs.uk/TestReferenceRanges

Evaluation: evaluate all nursing procedures and complete relevant documentation.
Activity: did you achieve what you set out to achieve?

Question 4. What would indicate that Jack may require renal replacement therapy (RRT)?

Blood indicators

- Increased creatinine as a result of reduced excretion of waste products of metabolism.
- Decreased CO_2 indicating metabolic acidosis due to excessive loss of bicarbonate.
- Hyperkalaemia (increased serum potassium level) due to reduced excretion.
- Uraemia (increased serum urea level) due to retention of nitrogenous waste.
- Falling haemoglobin level due to reduced production of hormone erythropoietin.

Clinical/physical observations

- Anuria – fluid accumulates as kidneys fail to excrete excess body water weight increases.
- Positive/negative oedema – peripheral/ pulmonary oedema due to accumulation of fluid in extravascular space which has moved from intravascular to extravascular space.
- Hypertension (blood pressure above 95th centile for height/weight) (Pediatric Hypertension Association 2006).
- Reduced appetite, nausea +/- vomiting

Jack's bloods are continually monitored, together with an accurate intake and output chart and regular observations. Unfortunately Jack's blood pressure remains elevated and despite the importance of adhering to a fluid allowance, Jack sneaks extra oral fluids.

This results in his continued hypertension and oedema, which develops into the more serious condition of pulmonary oedema.

See Figures 32.1 and 32.2.

Box 32.1 Types of dialysis

Peritoneal dialysis (PD)
- Neonates – adults
- Initially small fill volumes to reduce risk of leakage, respiratory compromise
- Hospital and home based
- Contra-indicated in abdominal surgery, anatomical problems, social situations
- Uses a large surface area
- Avoids sudden fluid and solute shifts
- Burden of care for parent/carer

Haemodialysis (HD)
- Immediate use
- Hospital based at specialist centre
- Disruption to family life
- Demand vascular access via double lumen central venous catheter or arteriovenous (AV) fistula
- Increase fluid and dietary restrictions

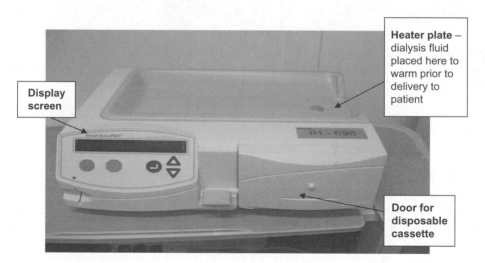

Figure 32.1 Home choice peritoneal dialysis machine.

Question 5. Using the information provided give rationale for the dialysis modality chosen for Jack.

Haemodialysis was the modality of choice due to:

- Recent abdominal surgery
- Urgent normalisation of serum potassium
- Urgent removal of fluid due to pulmonary oedema and hypertension
- Allows nutritional supplements to be given during treatment

Jack receives haemodialysis three times per week for three weeks.

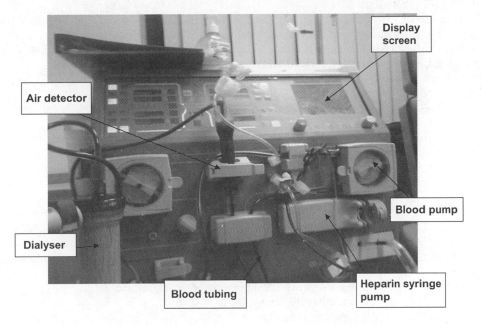

Figure 32.2   Haemodialysis machine.

Question 6. How would you assess if Jack is recovering his renal function?

Blood indicators

- Decreased serum creatinine – improved excretion of waste products of metabolism
- Decreased serum urea levels – improved excretion of nitrogenous waste
- Increased CO_2 – correction of acidosis
- Normalising level of potassium – excretion of electrolytes

Physical indicators

- Increased urinary output – reduced need for fluid removal by dialysis and fluid restriction
- Daily weight reduces
- Normalising BP – reduced need for antihypertensives
- Decreased serum urea level – increased appetite
- Ability to tolerate diet and fluids

Jack's general wellbeing improves, with increased energy levels, normalisation of BP (appropriate for age, height and weight), and blood results returning to within normal parameters.

Preparation is made for discharge and follow-up.

References

Akcan-Arikan, A., Zappitelli, M., Loftis, M.M., Washburn, K.K., Jefferson, L.S. & Goldstein, S.L. (2007) Modified RIFLE criteria in critically ill children with acute kidney injury. *Kidney International*, **71**, 1028–35.

Bellomo, R., Ronco, C., Kellum, J.A., *et al.* (2004) Acute renal failure – definition, outcome measures, animal models, fluid therapy and information technology needs: the Second International Consensus Conference of the Acute Dialysis Quality Initiative (ADQI) Group. *Critical Care*, **8**(4), R204–12.

Casey, A. (1988) A partnership with child and family. *Senior Nurse*, **8**(4), 8–9.

Davenport, A. & Stevens, P. (2008) *UK Renal Association Acute Kidney Injury, Clinical Practice Guidelines*, 4th edn. www.renal.org/guidelines (accessed 10 May 2011).

Davies, A. (2009) Diagnosing and classifying acute kidney injury. *Journal of Renal Nursing*, **1**(1), 9–12.

Mehta, R., Kellum, J.A., Shah, S.V., *et al.* (2007) Acute Kidney Injury Network: report of an initiative to improve outcomes in acute kidney injury. *Critical Care*, **11**(2), R31.

Plotz, F.B., Bouma, A.B., van Wijk, J.A., Kneyber, M.C. & Bokenkamp, A. (2008) Pediatric acute kidney injury in the ICU: an independent evaluation of pRIFLE criteria. *Intensive Care Medicine*, **34**(9), 1713–17.

Rees, L., Webb, N. & Brogan, P.A. (2007) *Paediatric Nephrology*. Oxford: Oxford University Press.

Ricci, Z., Cruz, D. & Ronco, D. (2008) The RIFLE criteria and mortality in acute kidney injury: a systematic review. *Kidney International*, **73**(5), 538–46.

Roper, N., Logan, W. & Tierney, A. (1990) *The Elements of Nursing*, 3rd. edn. London: Churchill Livingstone.

www.gosh.nhs.uk/gosh_families/information_sheets_acute_renal_failure

www.scarborough.nhs.uk/BiochemistryReferenceRanges

www.scarborough.nhs.uk/TestReferenceRanges

Further reading

Andreoli, S.P. (2009) Acute kidney injury in children. *Paediatric Nephrology*, **24**(2), 253–63.

Department of Health (2004) *The National Service Framework for Renal Services*. London: DH.

Goldstein, S.L. (2006) Pediatric acute kidney injury: it's time for real progress. *Pediatric Nephrology*, **21**, 891–5.

Hewson, D. (2003) What I tell families about haemodialysis in children. *British Journal of Renal Medicine*, Autumn 13–16.

Kiessling, S.G., Goebel, J. & Somers, M.J.G. (2009) *Pediatric Nephrology in the ICU*. Verlag Berlin Heidelberg, Germany: Springer.

Moghal, N.E., Brocklebank, J.T. & Meadow, S.R. (1988) A review of acute renal failure in children: incidence, etiology and outcome. *Clinical Nephrology*, **49**, 91–5.

National High BP Education Programme Working Group (2004) High BP in children and adolescents. The fourth report on the diagnosis, evaluation and treatment of high BP in children and adolescents. *Pediatrics*, **114**(2 supp 4th report), 555–76.

Nursing Care Plan Management (2009) *Nursing Care Plan for Acute Renal Failure*. www.nursing-management.blogspot.com (accessed 19 March 2010).

Peacock, P. & Sinert, R.H. (2009) *Acute Renal Failure*. http//:e-medicine.medscape.com (accessed 10 June 2010).

Pediatric Hypertension Association (2006). www.pediatrichypertension.org/BPLimitsChart.pdf (accessed 10 May 2011).

Redmond, A., McDevitt, M. & Barnes, S. (2004) Acute renal failure: recognition and treatment in ward patients. *Nursing Standard*, **18**(22), 46–53.

Resuscitation Council (UK) (2008) *Paediatric Immediate Life Support*, 1st edn. London: Resuscitation Council (UK).

Royal College of Nursing (2000) *Paediatric Nephrology Nursing, Guidance for Nurses*. London: RCN.

Shaheen, I.S., Watson, A.R. & Harvey, B. (2006) Acute renal failure in children: etiology, treatment and outcome. *Saudi Journal of Kidney Diseases and Transplantation* (serial online), **17**, 153–8.

Strazdins, V., Watson, A. & Harvey, B. & European Pediatric Peritoneal Dialysis Working Group (2004) Renal replacement therapy for acute renal failure in children: European Guidelines. *Paediatric Nephrology*, **19**(2), 199–207.

Uchino, S., Bellomo, R., Goldsmith, D., Bates, S. & Ronco, C. (2006) An assessment of the RIFLE criteria for acute renal failure in hospitalised patients. *Critical Care Medicine*, **34**, 1913.

UK Renal Association (2008) *Acute Kidney Injury, Clinical Practice Guidelines*, 4th edn. www.renal.org/guidelines (accessed 10 May 2011).

Williams, D.M., Sreedhar, S.S., Mickell, J.J. & Chan, J.C. (2002) Acute kidney failure: a pediatric experience over 20 years. *Archive of Paediatric Adolescent Medicine*, **136**(9), 893–900.

Section 10

Care of Infants and Young Persons with Skin Conditions

33

Infant with Infected Eczema
Gilli Lewis and Debbie Rickard

Scenario

Henry is a ten-month-old infant who has been admitted to the children's ward for treatment of his infected eczema. Henry has three siblings, two of which also have eczema. Henry's father had mild eczema as a child. The family of six live in a small two- bedroom, council-owned house.

Henry is covered in lesions; he has a weeping, crusting, staphylococcal infection. He appears irritated and itchy and is crying on assessment. This is his third admission to hospital; he has previously been admitted for treatment of bronchiolitis and exacerbated eczema. Apart from his eczema, Henry is now physically well. He is afebrile, feeding normally, but his sleep has been affected. Henry has been bottle fed infant formula milk since birth, and he commenced solid food at six months of age; no allergic responses have been noted to date.

Care Planning in Children and Young People's Nursing, First Edition.
Edited by Doris Corkin, Sonya Clarke, Lorna Liggett.
© 2012 Blackwell Publishing Ltd. Published 2012 by Blackwell Publishing Ltd.

Questions

1. What is eczema?
2. On Henry's admission to the ward, the children's nurse will need to complete a nursing assessment, from which a nursing plan of care may be developed. Describe how the nurse would carry out this assessment.
3. Identify the key healthcare deficits/issues/problems Henry and his mother, Sharon, present with and using an appropriate model of nursing plan goals of nursing care in relation to these problems.
4. Henry has been admitted with infected eczema. Describe the nursing care plan which the children's nurse should follow to ensure Henry receives appropriate evidence-based skin care.

Answers to questions

Question 1. What is eczema?

Eczema is a common inflammatory skin condition, affecting one in five children in the UK (NICE 2007). Eczema has a higher incidence in infancy and childhood but can affect individuals throughout life and is typically an episodic disease of exacerbation and remissions. Effective therapy improves quality of life for children with atopic eczema and their parents and carers. It is known that a lack of education and support about therapy leads to poor adherence, and consequently to treatment failure (NICE 2007; Smith *et al*. 2010).

Eczema often has a genetic component that leads to the breakdown of the skin barrier. This makes the skin susceptible to trigger factors, including irritants and allergens, which can make the eczema worse. Many cases of eczema clear or improve during childhood, but some persist into adulthood. Some children who have eczema will go on to develop asthma and/or allergic rhinitis; this sequence of events is sometimes referred to as the 'atopic march' (Weinberg 2005).

Eczema is usually characterised by epidermal changes, pruritus (itch), and lesions with indistinct borders. These lesions can appear as erythema, papules, or scales; they can present in an acute, subacute or chronic phase. Oedema, serous discharge and crusting occur with continued irritation and scratching. In chronic cases, the skin may become thickened and leathery and hyperpigmented from recurrent irritation and scratching. This is called lichenification. The location of eczema may depend on the underlying cause. There is an association with personal or family history of atopy (atopic eczema, allergic rhinitis and/ or asthma).

Affected sites vary with age (see Figure 33.1). Infantile eczema commonly affects the face, sparing around the mouth, and later the hands, feet and elsewhere (Halkjoer *et al*. 2006).

Eczema is sometimes referred to as atopic dermatitis (AD). Although termed atopic, up to 60% of children with characteristic eczema symptoms and history do not have demonstrable IgE-mediated sensitivity to allergens (Flohr 2004), an observation that led the World Allergy Organisation to propose a revised nomenclature (Johansson *et al*. 2004). Approximately 70% of cases of atopic dermatitis start in children under five years of age (Williams & Wüthrich 2000). In addition, asthma develops in approximately 30% of children with atopic dermatitis, and in 35% with allergic rhinitis (Gold & Kemp 2005).

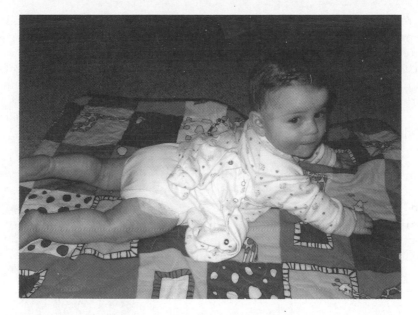

Figure 33.1 Eczema on child's face, back of legs and feet.

When an individual has eczema there is an impaired barrier function (Bieber 2008). This genetically determined skin barrier defect leads to a loss of water from the skin (Proksch & Lachapelle 2005). When the skin barrier is impaired from dryness (xerosis) of the skin and/or excoriated (in response to the pruritis from the skin xerosis) this allows bacteria, viruses and allergens to penetrate the skin (Bieber 2008; Brown & Butcher 2005; Cork *et al.* 2006; Proksch *et al.* 2006). As expressed by Leung *et al.*(2004), 'the skin represents the interface between the body and the surrounding environment' (p654).

Historically, it would appear that eczema has been poorly understood and frequently under treated (Cork *et al.* 2006; Grillo *et al.* 2006). There is no curative therapy and emphasis is on effective management and increasingly prophylaxis (Bieber 2008; Eichenfield 2004; Lester *et al.* 2001; Threstrup-Peterson 2002; Williams 2000). With the increasing prevalence of eczema it is no longer dismissed as a trivial disorder; indeed, the impact of this chronic condition on the individual, families and the community is increasingly being recognised (Grillo *et al.* 2006; Kemp 1999; Moore *et al.* 2006).

Question 2. On Henry's admission to the ward, the children's nurse will need to complete a nursing assessment, from which a nursing plan of care may be developed. Describe how the nurse would carry out this assessment.

Assessment

The initial assessment will be carried out during a family interview, in which the nurse may ask questions relevant to the care of the child. During the family interview it is important to be aware that caregivers of children with eczema are often frustrated and exhausted. If possible, hospitalisation of the child should be avoided as these children are highly susceptible to infections. However, admission may sometimes be the only answer to provide intensive therapy or to relieve an exhausted caregiver.

In this interview it is important to cover the history of Henry's condition, including treatments that have been tried and any identified or known allergens or triggers. It is useful to include a review of the home environment and daily routine. The nurse should evaluate Henry's mother's knowledge of eczema.

To aid management of eczema in children, the children's nurse should take detailed clinical and drug histories that include questions about:

* Time of onset, pattern and severity of the eczema
* Response to previous and current treatments
* Understanding of treatments and how these are used/implemented
* Possible trigger factors (irritant and allergic)
* The impact of the eczema on Henry and his parents
* Dietary history including any dietary manipulation
* Growth and development
* Personal and family history of atopic diseases

In addition to the interview, data collection about Henry must include obtaining vital signs, observing general nutritional state and a complete examination of all body parts, with careful documentation of the eruptions and their location and size. It is helpful to touch the skin to assess skin integrity; rough skin is an indicator of skin dryness. Unaffected areas, as well as those that are weeping and crusted, should be indicated. Henry's current height and weight should be measured and recorded.

It may be necessary to reassess when Henry is physically better, and Sharon is not so exhausted (physically and/or emotionally).

Question 3. Identify the key healthcare deficits/issues/problems Henry and his mother, Sharon, present with and using an appropriate model of nursing plan goals of nursing care in relation to these problems.

Identified problems

* Impaired skin integrity related to lesions and inflammatory process
* Risk of serious infection related to broken skin and lesions
* Acute pain related to intense itching, irritation and broken skin
* Disturbed sleep pattern related to itching and discomfort
* Deficient knowledge of caregivers related to disease condition and treatment

Model of nursing

Anne Casey's model of nursing (Casey 1993) guides nurses to work in partnership with children and their families. The philosophy behind the model is that the best people to care for the child are the family, with help from various professional staff. After all, following discharge from hospital, it is the family who will provide the ongoing care at home.

However, forming a partnership of care is not simple, and requires skill and sensitivity. Negotiating care is discussed by Anne Casey in her model. The ability to negotiate care is an underestimated skill, which is essential if nurses are to come alongside families/ caregivers in true partnership when planning care for children.

The nurse, in this case, will need to discuss the identified problems and possible goals of nursing care with Sharon.

Goals for Henry:

1. Improving and maintaining skin integrity; minimising flares
2. Preventing infection of skin lesions
3. Maintaining comfort, relief of itch
4. Improving sleep patterns
5. Enabling normal growth and development

Goals for Sharon/other caregivers:

1. Increasing knowledge about disease process
2. Increasing knowledge about management of the disease and its rationale
3. Improving confidence and competence in providing skin care; caring for Henry well

Question 4. Henry has been admitted with infected eczema. Describe the nursing care plan which the children's nurse should follow to ensure Henry receives appropriate evidence-based skin care.

The nursing care plan will be based on the problems identified during assessment, and the goals as discussed with Sharon and stated above.

Improving and maintaining Henry's skin integrity, minimising flares

1. The ultimate aim of treatment is to maintain skin integrity and minimise flares by replacing moisture and reducing inflammation. The key to helping maintain skin integrity is to moisturise.
2. Henry needs a daily skin care routine which should be incorporated into his usual daily routine. Discuss Henry's current skin care routine with Sharon.

Using emollient
- Emollients should form the basis of eczema management (Cork *et al.* 2006; Noorman *et al.* 2005), and generally should always be used, even when the eczema is clear. However, this is dependent on the severity of eczema and the flares.
- Emollients are moisturisers, which have emulsifiers and/or humectants, which affect the permeability barrier function of normal and diseased skin (Duval *et al.* 2003; Rajka 1997).
- Clinical experience has shown that the amount of emollient used is important in bringing about an improvement in eczema (Cork *et al.* 2003a; Marks 1997; Taieb 1998). Emollients should be used in larger amounts and more often than other treatments. Other treatments such as topical steroids do not replace emollients; they must always be used in conjunction with emollients unless condition is mild. (The emollient should be applied on top of the other treatments.) Emollients should be used in response to symptoms and prophylactically in response to known triggers.

- The nurse needs to ascertain that Sharon understands the use of emollients, as part of Henry's skin care routine. Any misunderstandings and gaps in knowledge can then be discussed.
- The nurse should show Sharon how to apply emollients, including how to smooth emollients onto the skin rather than rubbing them in. Sharon should be advised that regular application of emollients is a way that she can help her child and relieve his symptoms.
- Proven improved clinical response to effective emollient use motivates individuals, families and health professionals to continue with emollient use in eczema management (Cork *et al.* 2003b).

Topical corticosteroids, such as hydrocortisone

- Henry is likely to require some topical corticosteroid treatment.
- The nurse should inform Sharon that they should apply topical corticosteroids to areas of active eczema, which may include areas of broken skin. For the older child, a more potent steroid may be used 1–2 times weekly for maintenance in conjunction with emollient therapy.
- Topical steroids should be applied only to the red areas, including the face, as prescribed. This helps to reduce redness and inflammation. If the skin is still itchy despite being well hydrated this may indicate the need for a topical steroid as there may be an inflammatory response in the skin not visible to the eye.
- The prescribed topical steroid should be applied daily after bathing to all inflamed areas of skin. The steroid application may be prescribed more or less frequently, depending on potency of the steroid used.
- The nurse should discuss the benefits and harms of treatment with topical corticosteroids with Sharon, emphasising that the benefit outweighs possible harm when they are applied correctly. The appropriate use of steroids, such as hydrocortisone, have been shown to be perfectly safe (Charman *et al.* 2000). It is important for parents to know the potency of the topical steroid that is used. Hydrocortisone is extremely mild and there are likely to be little or no side effects from use. Poor adherence to therapy is usually the cause of exacerbations of eczema, rather than simply severity of disease. Poor adherence to therapy can occur for several reasons, including misunderstanding of topical preparations, such as topical steroids, and their use and potential side effects (Charman *et al.* 2000; Smith *et al.* 2010). Poorly managed eczema can damage the skin as much as overuse of topical steroids.
- Potent topical corticosteroids should not be used in children aged less than 12 months of age without specialist paediatric or dermatological supervision.

Topical calcineurin inhibitors

Topical tacrolimus and pimecrolimus are not recommended for the treatment of mild atopic eczema or as first-line treatments for eczema of any severity; topical tacrolimus and pimecrolimus are also not recommended for children under two years of age.

Wet wrap therapy (WWT)

- Henry may benefit from the use of WWT. If Sharon is not familiar with this treatment, the nurse would need to explain its use and demonstrate its application. Then later, the nurse could watch Sharon apply the wet wraps and evaluate if Sharon needs more instruction, information or encouragement to enable her to provide this therapy when Henry is discharged home.

- Wet wrap therapy involves the application of wet elasticated viscose tubular bandages as occlusive dressings, either to the whole body (limbs and trunk) – 'wet wrapped', or only to the worst affected areas (e.g. two limbs). An emollient is applied thickly to the skin with two bandages applied, the first wet after being soaked in water, the second dry. The water in the dressings helps to rehydrate the skin, and when it evaporates, it has a cooling effect. It is usually well tolerated due to the gradual cooling effect on the skin, and the rapid improvement in skin inflammation (Oranje *et al.* 2006). It is suspected that the constant hydration and reduction in inflammation reduces the itching. Wet wrap therapy has been particularly effective when the eczema is hard to control and there is intolerable itching (pruritus) (Devillers & Oranje 2006). Wet wraps also create a mechanical barrier against scratching, which allows improved healing of excoriated lesions and some protection against infection and environmental allergens. The absorption of topical medications is increased by the hydration and occlusion provided by the wet wraps. However, eczema which is severely infected may worsen with wet wraps (Oranje *et al.* 2006).

Preventing infection of skin lesions

- Sharon should be advised that eczema is frequently complicated by minor bacterial superinfections (Hoeger *et al.* 2000). Moreover, *Staphylococcus aureus* colonisation/ infection is commonly associated with disease severity in children with eczema (Hon *et al.* 2005, 2008), and is now well recognised as a trigger for exacerbating eczema (Bieber 2008).
- Sharon should be taught how to recognise the signs and symptoms of bacterial infection with staphylococcus and/or streptococcus (weeping, pustules, crusting). Eczema failing to respond to therapy, or rapidly worsening eczema (fever and malaise), indicates the need to seek prompt medical attention. Recognition of early signs and symptoms may prevent exacerbations and/or recurrent infections.
- Sharon should obtain new supplies of topical eczema medications after treatment for infected eczema because products in open containers can become contaminated with microorganisms and act as a source of infection.
- Systemic antibiotics that are active against *Staphylococcus aureus* and streptococcus will be administered to treat widespread bacterial infections of eczema.
- Antiseptics such as triclosan or chlorhexidine may be prescribed, at appropriate dilutions, as adjunct therapy to decrease bacterial load in children who have recurrent infected or exacerbated eczema. Long-term use should be avoided. There is also evidence that dilute bleach baths as a cheap antimicrobial may reduce bacterial colonisation. However, as bleach is a drying agent, it should not be used daily.

Preventing re-infection

- The nurse will admit Henry and family into an isolation room/ward to prevent cross infection in hospital. It should be explained to Sharon that this is for Henry's protection, as he is susceptible to infections. (It is also for the protection of other children who may be at risk of infection from Henry.)
- The nurse will administer oral or intravenous antibiotics to Henry as prescribed.
- If there are open lesions, the nurse must use aseptic techniques to prevent infection. Ideally the use of gloves is minimal as touch is a form of communication and ongoing use of gloves can increase risk of allergy development.

Maintaining comfort, relief of itch

- The nurse should plan soothing baths (see below) before nap/bedtime.
- Itch is often due to skin dryness; regular use of emollient usually will relieve this.
- Emollient should be applied whenever the skin is dry, red or itchy.
- Oral antihistamines are frequently prescribed for children with eczema to eliminate itch. The rationale is that this treatment acts on the H1 receptor to decrease histamine release and therefore eliminates itch (this is not the cause of itch in eczema unless it is an allergic response). In addition, the older antihistamines may have a sedative effect, which may assist with sleep in the short term (clinicians are moving away from this due to the ongoing side effects). However, there are no good quality studies demonstrating the efficacy of antihistamines in reducing symptoms of itch in children with atopic eczema (Dimson & Nanayakkara 2003).
- Cotton, loose fitting, 'all-in-one' clothing is recommended to cause least irritation.
- Henry's nails should be cut short and filed, to minimise damage from scratching.
- Distraction – ensure both Henry and Sharon have toys and books or magazines to entertain them. This will help to prevent Henry from continually scratching, and ease the loneliness and boredom from being in isolation in hospital.

Bathing
- Daily baths are regarded as the mainstay for infants and young children.
- Tepid baths are no longer recommended. There is no evidence to support their use. In fact, it is suggested that the vasodilation created by a warm bath only aids absorption of emollient in the water.
- Henry should be placed into a warm bath, with a soap substitute like emulsifying ointment melted in hot water first. As there is a staphylococcal infection present, antiseptic bath oil (like Oilatum Plus or QV Flare Up) should be added to the water *in addition* to the emollient.
- After the bath, Henry should be patted dry, not rubbed.
- Apply creams and ointments immediately after the bath to maximise absorption.

For Sharon, the nursing plan goals are:

- Increasing knowledge about disease process.
- Increasing knowledge about management of the disease and its rationale.
- Improving confidence and competence in providing skin care.

Education
- This is a key part of the nursing care plan for Henry. The aim here is to provide Sharon with enough information and confidence so that she will be able to provide good skin care herself. The aim is to transfer the power of knowledge from the nurse to the parent.
- Following a discussion with Sharon, in which an appraisal of her knowledge may be gleaned, the nurse should spend time educating Sharon about eczema and its treatment. She/he should provide information in verbal and written forms, with practical demonstrations.
- The nurse will need to assess Sharon's ability to take in this information, i.e. it may need to be done in short episodes with demonstrations of care and an arrangement to complete

education by the end of hospitalisation, follow-up by paediatric community nurses following discharge or following attendance to a nurse eczema clinic, if available.

• When discussing treatment options with Sharon the nurse should tailor the information they provide to suit Henry and Sharon's cultural practices relating to skin care and the way they bathe.

• The nurse should at all times be positive and supportive in their education. If Sharon is willing, the nurse should encourage her to provide the skin care for Henry, as discussed, under supervision initially and then on a daily basis. This should increase Sharon's confidence and competence in providing appropriate skin care for Henry.

• Assess Sharon's energy levels: is she sleep deprived? Does she need a break, assistance with Henry's care or even time to spend with his siblings? Encourage involvement of Sharon's partner and other family or social supports in Henry's care, so that the responsibility does not rest solely with Sharon.

• Encourage Sharon to ask questions particularly if she does not see the expected improvement.

• Nurses are increasingly recognised as the health professional to enable effective management of eczema (Cork *et al.* 2003b; Lawton 2004; Moore *et al.* 2006, Schuttelaar *et al.* 2009). The key to effective management of eczema is education and support which provides an individual plan that empowers the individual and/or family to successfully self care (Beattie & Lewis-Jones 2003; Cork *et al.* 2003a; Grillo *et al.* 2006).

Evaluation

Finally, it will be important for the nurse to evaluate all planned care for Henry and his mum, Sharon, and then re-plan care to address any remaining or ongoing healthcare or knowledge deficits.

References

Beattie, P.E. & Lewis-Jones, M.S. (2003) Parental knowledge of topical therapies in the treatment of childhood atopic dermatitis. *Clinical and Experimental Dermatology*, **28**, 549–53.
Bieber, T. (2008) Mechanisms of disease atopic eczema. *The New England Journal of Medicine*, **358**(14), 1483–94.
Brown, A. & Butcher, M. (2005) A guide to emollient therapy. *Nursing Standard*, **19**(24), 68–75.
Casey, A. (1993) The development and use of the partnership model of nursing care. In: Glasper, E.A. & Tucker, A. (eds). *Advances in Child Health Nursing*. London: Scutari Press.
Charman, C.R., Morris, A.D. & Williams, H.C. (2000) Topical corticosteroid phobia in patients with atopic eczema. *British Journal of Dermatology*, **142**, 931–6.
Cork, M.J., Timmins, J., Holden, C., et al. (2003a) An audit of adverse drug reactions to aqueous cream in children with atopic eczema. *The Pharmaceutical Journal*, **271**, 747–8.
Cork, M.J., Britton, J., Butler, L., Young, S., Murphy, R. & Keohane, S.G. (2003b) Comparison of parent knowledge, therapy utilization and severity of atopic eczema before and after explanation and demonstration of topical therapies by a specialist dermatology nurse. *British Journal of Dermatology*, **149**, 582–9.
Cork, M.J., Robinson, D., Vasilopoulos, Y., et al. (2006) Improving the treatment of atopic eczema through understanding of gene-environment interactions. *Exchange (quarterly journal of the National Eczema Society)*, **121**, 7–13.

Devillers, A. & Oranje, A.P. (2006) Efficacy and safety of wet-wrap dressings in the treatment of children with atopic dermatitis: a review of the literature. *British Journal of Dermatology*, **154**, 579–85.

Dimson, S. & Nanayakkara, C. (2003) Do oral antihistamines stop the itch of atopic dermatitis? *Arch. Dis. Child*, **88**, 832–3.

Duval, C., Lindberg, M., Boman, A., Johnsson, S., Edlund, F. & Loden, M. (2003) Differences among moisturisers in affecting skin susceptibility to hexyl nicotinate, measured as time to increase skin blood flow. *Skin Research and Technology*, **9**, 59–63.

Eichenfield, L.F. (2004) Consensus guidelines in diagnosis and treatment of atopic dermatitis. *Allergy*, **59**, Suppl.78, 86–92.

Flohr, C., Johansson, S.G.O., Wahlgren, C.F. & Williams, H.C. (2004) How atopic is atopic dermatitis? *J Allergy Clin Immunol*, **114**, 150–8.

Gold, M.S. & Kemp. A.S. (2005) Atopic disease in childhood. *Med J Aust. 21*, **182**(6), 298–304.

Grillo, M., Gassner, L., Marshman, G., Dunn, S. & Hudson, P. (2006) Pediatric atopic eczema: the impact of an educational intervention. *Pediatric Dermatology*, **23**(5), 428–36.

Halkjoer, L.B., Loland, L., Buchvald, F.F., *et al.* (2006) Development of atopic dermatitis during the first three years of life. *Arch Dermatol*, **142**, 561–6.

Hoeger, P.H., Ganschow, R. & Finger, G. (2000) Staphylococcal septicemia in children with atopic dermatitis. *Pediatric Dermatology*, **17**, 111–4.

Hon, K.L., Lam, M.C., Leung, T.F., *et al.* (2005) Clinical features associated with nasal *Staphylococcus aureus* colonisation in Chinese children with moderate-to-severe atopic dermatitis. *Annals of the Academy of Medicine, Singapore*, **34**, 602–5.

Hon, K.L., Leung, A.K., Kong, A.Y., Leung, T.F. & Ip, M. (2008) Atopic dermatitis complicated by methicillin-resistant *Staphylococcus aureus* infection. *Journal of the National Medical Association*, **100**, 797–800.

Johansson, S.G., Bieber, T., Dahl, R., *et al.* (2004) Revised nomenclature for allergy for global use: Report of the Nomenclature Review Committee of the World Allergy Organization. *J Allergy Clin Immunol*, **113**, 832–6.

Kemp, A. (1999) Atopic eczema. *Journal of Paediatrics: Child Health*, **35**, 229–31.

Lawton, S. (2004. Nurse-led care: the role of nurses in eczema clinics. *Nurse Prescribing*, **2**, 239–43.

Lester, S., Goodwin, P. & Watkins, J. (2001) Atopic eczema: the benefits of specialist nursing. *Paediatric Nursing*, **13**, 14–17.

Leung, D.Y.M., Boguniewicz, M., Howell, M.D., Nomura, I. & Hamid, Q.A. (2004) New insights into atopic eczema. *The Journal of Clinical Investigation*, **113**, 651–6.

Marks, R. (1997) How to measure the effects of emollients. *Journal of Dermatological Treatment*, **8**, S15–S18.

Moore, E., Williams, A., Manias, E. & Varigos, G. (2006) Nurse-led clinics reduce severity of childhood atopic eczema: a review of the literature. *British Journal of Dermatology*, **155**, 1242–8.

NICE (2007) *Atopic Eczema in Children – Management of Atopic Eczema in Children from Birth up to the Age of 12 Years.* Clinical Guideline produced by the National Collaborating Centre for Women's and Children's Health Commissioned by the National Institute for Health and Clinical Excellence (NICE). London: NICE.

Noorman, G., Tomicic, S., Bottcher, M., Oldaeus, G., Stromberg, L. & Falth-Magnusson, K. (2005) Significant improvement of eczema with skin care and food elimination in small children. *Acta Paediatrica*, **94**, 1384–8.

Oranje, A.P., Devillers, A.C.A., Kunz, B., *et al.* (2006) Treatment of patients with atopic dermatitis using wet-wrap dressings with diluted steroids and/or emollients. An expert panel's opinion and review of the literature. *Journal of European Academy of Dermatology and Venereology*, **20**, 1277–86.

Proksch, E. & Lachapelle, J.M. (2005) The management of dry skin with topical emollients – recent perspectives. *JDDG*, 768–74.

Proksch, E., Folster-Holst, R. & Jenson, J.M. (2006) Skin barrier function, epidermal proliferation and differentiation in eczema. *Journal of Dermatological Science*, **43**, 159–69.

Rajka, G. (1997) Emollient therapy in atopic dermatitis. *Journal of Dermatological Treatment*, **8**, S19–S21.

Schuttalaar, M.L., Vermeulen, K.M., Drukker, N. & Coenraads, P.J. (2009) A randomized controlled trail in children with eczema: nurse practitioner vs. dermatologist. *British Journal of Dermatology*, **162**, 162–70.

Smith, S.D., Hong, E., Fearns, S., Blaszczynski, A. & Fischer, G. (2010) Corticosteroid phobia and other confounders in the treatment of childhood atopic dermatitis explored using parent focus groups. *Australasian Journal of Dermatology*, no. doi: 10.1111/j.1440-0960.2010.00636.x

Taieb, A. (1998) Emollient therapy in atopic dermatitis: rediscovering the benefits of emollient therapy in eczema. *Journal of Dermatological Treatment*, **9**, S7–11.

Threstrup-Peterson, K. (2002) Treatment principles of atopic dermatitis. *European Academy of Dermatology and Venereology*, **16**, 1–9.

Weinberg, E. (2005) Atopic march. *Current Allergy & Clinical Immunology*, **18**, 4–5.

Williams, H.C. (2000) Epidemiology of atopic dermatitis. *Clinical & Experimental Immunology*, **25**, 522–9.

Williams, H.C. & Wüthrich, B. (2000) The natural history of atopic dermatitis. In: Williams, H.C. (ed.). *Atopic Dermatitis: the Epidemiology, Causes, and Prevention of Atopic Eczema*. Cambridge: Cambridge University Press.

34

Burns Injury

Idy Fu

Scenario

Ka Man, a 13-year-old girl, emigrated from China five years ago with her parents and a younger brother Ka Wai, aged 8. She was studying form 1 in a local secondary school 2 km from home. The family lived in a small rented apartment in one of the crowded districts on Hong Kong Island. Ka Man had sustained superficial and deep partial-thickness burns to her right lower leg and right foot respectively, from a tilted pot of boiled soup while she was helping her mother carry the pot to the dining room where she tripped over. She was sent to the nearby A&E department immediately, accompanied by her mother. She remained conscious and orientated but was very restless and complaining of severe pain over her right leg.

When Ka Man arrived at the hospital, her temperature was 35.8°C, blood pressure: 80/50 mmHg, pulse: 128 beats/min, respiration rate: 36 breaths/min and SpO_2: 90%. Her right lower leg was swollen and large blisters were found. She was put on oxygen therapy at 6 L/min via a face mask and intravenous fluid infusion was commenced. Ka Man was also given a dose of IV morphine to relieve her pain. Blood sample was taken for laboratory studies – complete blood count, renal and liver function tests, and blood gas analysis. After a thorough assessment by the A&E physician, Ka Man was transferred to the burns unit for close observation and further management.

Three days after admission, Ka Man was gradually recovering from the burn injury, with stable haemodynamics and satisfactory urine output. The oedema had subsided over her right lower leg and epithelialisation started to take place. However, the right foot remained pale and some necrotic tissues were found at the wound surface. After being reassessed by the surgeon, Ka Man was scheduled for debridement and grafting surgery of her right foot with split-thickness skin grafts harvested from her left anterior thigh.

Care Planning in Children and Young People's Nursing, First Edition.
Edited by Doris Corkin, Sonya Clarke, Lorna Liggett.
© 2012 Blackwell Publishing Ltd. Published 2012 by Blackwell Publishing Ltd.

> ## Questions
>
> 1. How should burn injuries be classified in children?
> 2. Discuss the immediate nursing assessments for Ka Man in relation to her burn injury.
> 3. Develop a nursing care plan for Ka Man during the resuscitation phase (first 24–48 hours) of a burn injury.
> 4. Explain the specific nursing care for managing the grafted and donor wounds of Ka Man postoperatively.

Answers to questions

Question 1. How should burn injuries be classified in children?

The severity of a burn injury is assessed by the percentage of surface area affected (the extent of injury) and the degree of involvement of the epidermis, dermis and underlying structures (the depth of injury). Indeed, the deeper the injury the greater the number of layers that are damaged. The seriousness of the injury is also determined by other important factors such as the age of the child, the location of the wound, the general health of the child, and the presence of respiratory involvement or any associated conditions. A burn injury that accounts for 10% of the total body surface area (TBSA) can be life threatening in small children with any delayed or inappropriate treatment.

Superficial (first-degree) burns involve damage of the epidermis. The protective functions of skin remain intact and therefore systemic infections are rare. The injury often results in redness of skin, with pain as the predominant symptom, and the wound usually heals in 5–10 days without scarring.

Partial-thickness (second-degree) burns are injuries to the second layer of skin, the dermis. The seriousness of a partial-thickness burn depends on how much of the dermis has been injured. These wounds are painful and extremely sensitive to temperature changes, exposure to air, and light touch because the nerve endings remain intact. Superficial partial-thickness wounds appear moist and mottled, pink or red, and blanch when pressure is applied. There are usually blisters present (see Box 34.1). Deep partial-thickness wounds appear dry and whitish in colour but do not blanch. A superficial partial-thickness wound usually heals spontaneously in approximately 14 days with varying degree of scarring, whereas a deep and large partial thickness burn is generally best treated with excision and grafting to reduce risk of hypertrophic scarring and contracture.

Full-thickness (third-degree) burns are serious injuries involving the entire epidermis and dermis and extending into the subcutaneous tissue. Wound colour varies from red to tan, waxy white, brown or black, with a dry, leathery appearance. These wounds are rarely painful because the nerve endings are damaged as well as the sweat glands and hair follicles. However, a partial-thickness burn is often present at the periphery of a full-thickness wound; therefore the child is not pain free. As the epidermis and entire dermis are destroyed, re-epithelialisation is not possible; thus surgical excision and grafting are required for wound healing.

Box 34.1   Care of blisters

Taken from *Clinical Practice Guidelines on Burns*, the Royal Children's Hospital Melbourne (2010).

The care of blisters depends on their size and location. Blisters are usually left alone if they are not large and not obstructing the dressing. If large bulbous blisters are present that are obstructing a dressing or causing restriction to local circulation, the blisters should be punctured and fluid aspirated for better dressing application.

If the fluid inside the blisters become opaque and infection is suspected, the blister epidermis should be removed completely. Loose epidermis from broken blisters may be debrided with caution as bleeding can occur when part of the blister remains attached to the skin.

Full-thickness (fourth-degree) burns are injuries involving underlying structures such as muscle, fascia, tendon and bone. These wounds have the same characteristics as third-degree burns.

Question 2. Discuss the immediate nursing assessments for Ka Man in relation to her burn injury.

In partial thickness burns water, plasma proteins and electrolytes are lost through the damaged tissues. The release of inflammatory and vasoactive mediators activated by the burn injury increases the capillary permeability, causing shifting of fluid from the vascular compartment to the interstitial space, resulting in further fluid loss. When intravascular volume continues to decrease without correction, hypovolaemic shock develops. The nurse therefore needs to assess Ka Man's blood pressure, pulse rate, and capillary refill every 30–60 minutes in order to detect hypovolaemic shock promptly. Urinary function should also be monitored hourly to ensure fluid resuscitation is adequate for tissue perfusion, which is indicated by maintaining a urine output of 1.0–1.5 ml/kg/hour (Pham *et al.* 2008). As the thermoregulatory function of the skin is impaired and body heat is lost from the burnt surfaces, the nurse should monitor Ka Man's temperature for hypothermia every hour until stable.

The conscious level of Ka Man should be assessed regularly to identify possible neurological complications resulting from altered electrolyte balance, in which the child may present with confusion, weakness and seizures. Neurovascular assessment of the affected limb must be performed hourly to rule out circulatory obstruction caused by compartment syndrome, particularly in circumferential burns, which is characterised by changes in colour and/or temperature, absence of distal pulse, loss of sensation, and deep throbbing pain.

Furthermore, the extent of injury should be assessed and the percentage of burnt areas estimated using the Lund & Browder Chart (Table 34.1) as a baseline to gauge wound healing process. The Rule of Nines method (Table 34.2) is not recommended for small

Table 34.1 The Lund and Browder method for assessing percentage of burn injury in children.

Surface area (anterior and posterior)	Age				
	0–12 month	1–4 year	5–9 year	10–15 year	>15 year
Head	19%	17%	13%	11%	9%
R & L thighs	5.5% × 2	6.5% × 2	8% × 2	8.5% × 2	9% × 2
R & L lower legs	5% × 2	5% × 2	5.5% × 2	6% × 2	6.5% × 2
Neck	2%				
Trunk	26%				
R & L upper arms	4% × 2				
R & L lower arms	3% × 2				
R & L hands	2.5% × 2				
R & L buttocks	2.5% × 2				
R & L feet	3.5% × 2				
Genitalia	1%				

R = right-sided; L = left-sided.

Table 34.2 The Rule of Nines method for assessing percentage of burn injury in adults.

Surface area	Anterior	Posterior
Head & neck	4.5%	4.5%
Torso	18%	18%
R & L legs	9% × 2	9% x 2
R & L arms	4.5% × 2	4.5% x 2
Genitalia	1%	—
Total	100%	

R = right-sided; L = left-sided.

children as the rates of growth in the head, thigh and lower leg vary across different age groups (Orgill 2009). However, it is useful as a rough estimate until the Lund & Browder chart can be used.

The nurse should assess the pain intensity of Ka Man regularly and monitor the effectiveness of analgesics given. Hyperventilation may develop as a result of severe pain and anxiety in the burnt child; therefore respiration rate and pattern should be assessed hourly to observe for respiratory complications. Changes in respiratory function and gas exchange are characterised by restlessness, irritability, increased work of breathing and alterations in blood gas values. In addition, the nurse needs to assess the tetanus status and allergy history of the child.

Question 3. Develop a nursing care plan for Ka Man during the resuscitation phase (first 24–48 hours) of a burn injury.

See Table 34.3.

Table 34.3 Nursing care plan for Ka Man with burn injury.

Nursing diagnosis (see Chapter 1)	Expected outcome	Nursing interventions/rationales
Fluid volume deficit related to fluid loss from damaged skin and increased capillary permeability.	Ka Man will maintain adequate fluid hydration status with stable haemodynamic parameters.	1. Monitor Ka Man's vital signs, urine output, mental state, skin turgor and moisture of mucous membrane *to determine adequacy of fluid replacement*. 2. Administer intravenous fluids as ordered by doctor, and check for patency of IV line *to ensure adequate replacement for fluid loss*. 3. Weight Ka Man daily at the same time *to rule out urinary retention or excessive diuresis*. 4. Monitor laboratory results (e.g. potassium, sodium, haemoglobin, haematocrit) *to detect fluid and electrolyte imbalance*. 5. Keep an accurate record of Ka Man's intake and output daily *to monitor for fluid balance*.
Risk for altered tissue perfusion related to oedema of the affected limb.	Ka Man will have optimal circulation to the affected limb without neurovascular complications.	1. Check distal pulse and sensation of the affected limb and monitor closely for signs and symptoms of circulatory obstruction *to observe for development of compartment syndrome*. 2. Elevate the affected limb 20 to 30 degrees *to promote venous return and reduce leg swelling*. 3. Remove restrictive clothing on the affected limb *to prevent circulatory obstruction*. 4. Avoid applying restrictive or pressure dressings over inured limb *to prevent obstruction of blood flow*. 5. Perform Doppler examination if diminished distal pulse is noticed *to detect circulatory obstruction early*. 6. Teach Ka Man to report any abnormal feelings in the affected limb *to allow early detection of neurovascular complications*.
Acute pain related to tissue destruction and exposed nerve endings at the skin surface.	Ka Man will report decreased level of pain with more restful periods.	1. Assess Ka Man's pain level every hour using age-appropriate assessment tool *to determine the need for pain medication*. 2. Administer pain medication at regular intervals when indicated *to achieve better pain control and prevent occurrence of severe pain*. 3. Determine the best route for administering analgesics and assess for effectiveness *to ensure maximal absorption and adequate pain relief*. 4. Monitor Ka Man's vital signs, emotional state, appetite, activity level, and sleep pattern *to collect data regarding level of pain she is experiencing*. 5. Offer breakthrough analgesics as necessary prior to wound dressing changes *to reduce discomfort*. 6. Use a bed cradle *to avoid bed linen from pressing on the affected limb*. 7. Handle the injured limb carefully and gently *to minimise discomfort and prevent unnecessary injuries*. 8. Explain all procedures beforehand *to reduce anxiety-associated pain*. 9. Employ age-appropriate, non-pharmacological pain relief strategies, for example music, television, games *to distract Ka Man from pain*. 10. Allow Ka Man to participate in self-care activities as appropriate, for example bathing, removing dressing *to promote a sense of control in pain management*. 11. Encourage parents to visit and stay with Ka Man as needed *to help comfort and support her recovery*. 12. Teach Ka Man to touch/stroke the unaffected areas *to provide physical contact and promote comfort*. 13. Educate Ka Man and her family on the characteristics of pain from a burn wound and their role in pain management *to promote family-centered care and effective coping*.

Impaired skin integrity related to thermal injury.

Ka Man will demonstrate no signs of wound infection and reduction in the size of burn wounds.

1. Implement standard precautions vigilantly when caring for Ka Man *to prevent cross infections.*
2. Cleanse all burnt surfaces thoroughly and regularly with normal saline, and debride devitalised skin as necessary *to decrease risk of infection and promote healing.*
3. Employ aseptic technique when performing dressing changes *to prevent infection.*
4. Use appropriate wound dressing materials *to reduce dressing change and unnecessary disturbance to wounds.*
5. Handle wound dressing with care during removal *to prevent damaging the newly-formed tissues.*
6. Apply topical antimicrobial preparation as ordered by doctor (e.g. silver sulfadiazine) *to decrease risk of infection.*
7. Start hydrotherapy treatment when haemodynamics are stable, using disinfected bathing equipments *to promote removal of devitalised tissues and colonised micro-organisms.*
8. Administer prophylactic antibiotics as prescribed by doctor if indicated and observe for side effects of medication *to reduce the risk of infection.*
9. Consider the use of temporary skin substitute *to protect the wounds, promote healing and reduce pain.*
10. Monitor for signs and symptoms of wound infection (fever, changes in amount, colour, or odour of drainage) and educate Ka Man to report any abnormalities promptly *to allow early recognition and treatment.*
11. Offer high-protein, high-calorie meals to Ka Man as tolerated or commence enteral (N/G) feeding if indicated *to augment nutritional requirements for wound healing.*
12. Administer supplementary vitamins and minerals as ordered by doctor *to facilitate tissue regeneration.*
13. Collect wound swabs for culture if symptomatic *to monitor the course of infection.*

Ineffective thermoregulation related to damaged skin barrier and increased body heat loss through evaporation from burnt surfaces.

Ka Man will maintain a normal body temperature of 37 ± 0.5°C.

1. Monitor Ka Man's temperature hourly until stable, then every 2–4 hourly *to ensure early detection and treatment of hypothermia.*
2. Observe for any chills or shivering *to identify signs of hypothermia.*
3. Maintain a warm environment and avoid unnecessary exposures of the body *to prevent excessive heat loss.*
4. Warm the IV fluids prior to administration if indicated, *to offset expected heat loss.*
5. Keep the water temperature for hydrotherapy at 36.7°C and limit the procedure time to 20 minutes *to prevent excessive heat loss and reduce stress.*
6. Use a thermal insulating blanket with a bed cradle over the injured limb if necessary *to reduce radiant heat loss and increase body temperature.*

continued

Table 34.3 (*Continued*)

Nursing diagnosis (see Chapter 1)	Expected outcome	Nursing interventions/rationales
Impaired physical mobility related to pain and impaired joint movement.	Ka Man will achieve optimal physical functioning with minimal complications.	1. Keep the right foot at 90 degrees with the use of assistive devices (e.g. splint, foot board) *to maintain a functional position and minimise deformity.* 2. Perform ROM exercises every four hours for 15 minutes or as tolerated with adequate analgesic cover *to increase muscle tone and prevent joint stiffness.* 3. Use appropriate wound care method (refer to Box 34.2) and avoid tight bandaging over the affected limb *to reduce restriction in joint movement.* 4. Assist Ka Man to change position regularly and use pressure-relieving devices to support bony areas *to prevent pressure sore formation.* 5. Teach Ka Man to perform active ROM exercises to unaffected extremities and ambulate as soon as feasible *to maintain optimal joint and muscle functions.* 6. Encourage participation in self-care activities *to increase mobility and improve morale.* 7. Administer analgesics before any strenuous activities *to reduce pain and increase activity tolerance.* 8. Consider early physiotherapy consultation for rehabilitation planning *to minimise level of disability.*
Disturbed body image related to alteration in appearance and mobility.	Ka Man will express her concerns on altered physical appearance and demonstrate acceptance to the burn injury.	1. Observe Ka Man for significant behavioural and/or emotional changes *to identify depressive symptoms for early interventions.* 2. Provide opportunities for Ka Man and her family to discuss the possible outcomes of injury *to allay fear and increase coping.* 3. Be honest with Ka Man and her family, providing relevant information on the recovery process *to build a trusting relationship.* 4. Encourage Ka Man to participate in wound care *to improve acceptance of the altered physical appearance.* 5. Convey positive attitude and offer appropriate coping strategies *to enhance acceptance of the injury.* 6. Promote independence in self-care activities as much as condition allows *to increase sense of control and improve self-esteem.*

Axton & Fugate 2009; Hockenberry *et al.* 2005; Sadik & Campbell 2001; Severe Burn Injury Service Model of Care, NSW Department of Health (2004); Speer 1999.

> **Box 34.2** The 'closed (occlusive) method' for burn wound (Smeltzer *et al.* 2008)
>
> 1. All dressing changes need to be carried out aseptically with adequate pain relief prior to the procedure.
> 2. The burn wounds should be covered with sterile non-adherent dressing, then gently wrapped with bandage circumferentially in a distal-to-proximal manner.
> 3. Do not allow any two burnt surfaces to come in contact (e.g. between digits, skin folds) to promote webbing of digits and prevent contractures.
> 4. The dressing that covers a burn wound must be about 2 cm thick to be effective for absorbing exudates and preventing it from reaching the surface where it can become infected.
> 5. The amount of wound exudate determines the frequency for dressing change.

Question 4. Explain the specific nursing care for managing the grafted and donor wounds of Ka Man postoperatively.

All wounds should be kept clean and dry postoperatively. The children's nurse should assess both wound sites regularly for excessive bleeding as haemorrhage is one of the most important complications after grafting surgery (Kagan *et al.* 2009; Orgill 2009). A sterile non-adherent dressing is used to cover the skin donor site, which is often kept intact for 3–5 days if no complications develop. A split-thickness skin graft harvest involves the epidermis and superficial (papillary) dermis, thus the donor wound at the left thigh normally heals spontaneously within 7–14 days.

For the grafted (recipient) site, small sutures may be used to secure the graft to the excised wound bed. The wound is covered with occlusive non-adherent dressing (often impregnated with antibiotic ointment to reduce bacterial proliferation) which may be removed on the fourth or fifth postoperative day, depending on the surgeon's practice. Graft detachment may result if there is haematoma formation or bacterial contamination at the wound site. The nurse should monitor the grafted area closely for any abnormalities.

Other factors that may cause graft failure include peripheral oedema and mechanical shearing forces (Kagan *et al.* 2009). Therefore Ka Man must be advised to stay in bed for 7–10 days with her right foot splinted and leg elevated to maintain functional positioning, reduce the risk of graft loss due to movement and facilitate adhesion of graft to the wound bed. The children's nurse should handle Ka Man's operated leg with care and protect the grafted site from any pressure or trauma. Ka Man should also be informed not to perform any exercise or activity that stretches the graft or puts it at risk for trauma for 3–4 weeks. The nurse should monitor Ka Man's pain level more closely after surgery and provide additional analgesics to her if needed to achieve effective pain control.

References

Axton, S. & Fugate, T. (2009) *Pediatric Nursing Care Plans for the Hospitalized Child*, 3rd edn. Upper Saddle River, NJ: Pearson Prentice Hall.

Hockenberry, M.J., Wilson, D. & Winkelstein, M.L. (2005) *Wong's Essentials of Paediatric Nursing*, 7th edn. St Louis: Mosby.

Kagan, R.J., Peck, M.D., Ahrenholz, D.H., *et al.* (2009) *Surgical Management of the Burn Wound and use of Skin Substitutes*. Chicago: American Burn Association.

NSW Department of Health (2004) *NSW Severe Burn Injury Service – Model of Care*. www.health.nsw.gov.au/pubs/2004/burninjurymoc.html.

Orgill, D.P. (2009) Excision and skin grafting of thermal burns. *The New England Journal of Medicine*, **360**(9), 893–901.

Pham, T.N., Cancio, L.C. & Gibran, N.S. (2008) American Burn Association practice guidelines burn shock resuscitation. *Journal of Burn Care and Research*, **29**(1), 257–66.

Royal Children's Hospital Melbourne (2010) *Clinical Practice Guidelines on Burns* http://www.rch.org.au/clinicalguide/cpg.cfm?doc_id=5158.

Sadik, R. & Campbell, G. (2001) *Client Profiles in Nursing: Child Health*. London: Greenwich Medical Media.

Smeltzer, S.C., Bare, B.G., Hinkle J.L. & Cheever K.H. (2008) *Brunner & Suddarth's Textbook of Medical-Surgical Nursing*, 11th edn. Philadelphia: Lippincott Williams & Wilkins.

Speer, K.M. (1999) *Pediatric Care Planning*, 3rd edn. Springhouse, PA: Springhouse Corporation.

Section 11

Care of Children and Young Persons with Life-Limiting Conditions

35

Young Person with Spinal Muscular Atrophy
Doris Corkin and Julie Chambers

Scenario

At eight months old, Michaela was diagnosed with spinal muscular atrophy (SMA) type 2, a degenerative muscle wasting disease (Hockenberry *et al*. 2003). Marie and Michael, her parents, were very aware of the signs of this life-limiting disease as their older daughter Martina had the same condition and died when she was 14 years old. This situation has brought a major upheaval into the lives of the whole family and has lead to a long-standing relationship with healthcare professionals, which at times has caused the parents great frustration, especially when trying to articulate the care they need.

Spinal muscular atrophy can cause the chest muscles to become paralysed; therefore a huge amount of effort is required to breathe. Michaela now 18 years old, has a portacath *in situ* (see Chapter 19) and currently uses non-invasive ventilation (BiPAP) overnight and sometimes has oxygen during the day, particularly if she has a chest infection. Spinal muscular atrophy means that Michaela is totally dependent and requires 24-hour care and assistance with all aspects of activities of living, especially personal cleansing and dressing. She has also had rods inserted into her spine to help manage the effects of her scoliosis.

Parents Marie and Michael have now been full-time carers for their daughters for over 20 years, taking on the responsibility of providing care, with the support of their community children's nursing team since it was established in 2000; prior to this it was the district nursing service.

Care Planning in Children and Young People's Nursing, First Edition.
Edited by Doris Corkin, Sonya Clarke, Lorna Liggett.
© 2012 Blackwell Publishing Ltd. Published 2012 by Blackwell Publishing Ltd.

🖉 **Activity 35.1**

Please see http://www.patient.co.uk/doctor/Spinal-Muscular-Atrophy.htm for further information.

Questions

1. What is spinal muscular atrophy (SMA) and how is it diagnosed?
2. Why do SMA patients have difficulty breathing?
3. Explain: (a) Non-invasive ventilation.
   (b) Use of a BiPAP machine in the home.
4. Discuss the importance of communication by healthcare professionals when caring for Michaela, a young person with a life-limiting condition, in the community setting.
5. Using the Roper, Logan & Tierney model in practice devise a care plan to address Michaela's personal cleansing and dressing.

Answers to questions

Question 1. What is spinal muscular atrophy (SMA) and how is it diagnosed?

Spinal muscular atrophy is a genetic disorder that affects the nerve cells in the anterior horn area of the spinal cord, breaking the link between brain and muscles, therefore muscles cannot be used and become wasted (Hockenberry *et al.* 2003). This can lead to problems with breathing as well as motor activities such as walking and feeding, because SMA causes weakness of the voluntary muscles in the arms and legs.

Individuals normally have two genes (inherited from parents); with SMA a gene is mutated or missing. It is primarily diagnosed through a blood test, along with suggestive history and physical examination, although the doctor may request a muscle biopsy or electromyography (EMG) testing, which measures the muscle's electrical activity (www.fsma.org). There are four types of SMA (see Figure 35.1), which are inherited diseases.

Reflect upon scenario: apply Roper, Logan & Tierney (1996) model of care.

Question 2. Why do SMA patients have difficulty breathing?

Activity of living: breathing.
Children and young people with a life-limited condition such as SMA type 2 will have symptoms that are difficult for families and health professionals to manage. Michaela tends to have great difficulty with her breathing and production of secretions. Two main functions of the respiratory system are:

- To provide a large area for gas exchange between air and circulating blood.
- To move air to and from gas-exchange surfaces of the lungs.

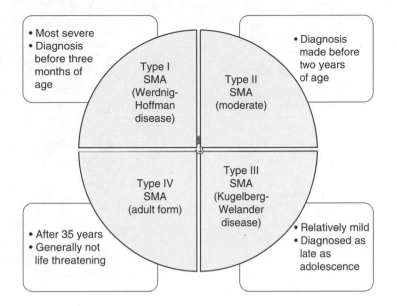

Figure 35.1   Spinal muscular atrophy (SMA) I, II, III and IV.

The two lungs are different: the right has three lobes and the left has two lobes, while the diaphragm acts as the floor of the thoracic cavity. When breathing, the respiratory muscles contract and the air inhaled passes through the upper airways, nose, trachea and bronchus to alveoli in the lungs, where gas exchange takes place (see Figure 35.2) – carbon dioxide (CO_2) is eliminated and replaced with oxygen (O_2).

Bronchus obstruction and muscle (intercostal and accessory) weakness are the two main causes of breathing difficulties in SMA patients, affecting the respiratory system. Regarding bronchus obstruction – carbon dioxide stays within the alveoli causing breathlessness and frequent coughing (Respironics 2008).

Question 3. (a) Explain non-invasive ventilation.

Activity of living: breathing (Roper *et al.* 1996).

Non-invasive ventilation is the term used to describe how a ventilator delivers air to the person's lungs under pressure. The ventilator assists in keeping the small airways and air sacs inflated in the lungs. When the person breathes in the airflow is strongest, so that as much air as possible is taken in. When the person breathes out the airflow is reduced but the pressure remains positive. This is known as bi-level positive airway pressure (BiPAP) and is prescribed by a doctor to help keep the airways open, allowing more air to enter and leave the lungs (Air Products 2009). This type of ventilation assists the person when breathing, working with them and not against. The 'non-invasive' term means that the ventilation process is achieved using a mask. The mask can either fit over both mouth and nose (Michaela's is this type) or just the nose. Non-invasive ventilation reduces the effort of breathing and enables the person's respiratory requirements to be maintained.

In summary, non-invasive ventilation therapy can improve lung function, increase oxygen intake, on expiration ensures more efficient flushing out of carbon dioxide, improve overall wellbeing and can reduce hospital readmissions.

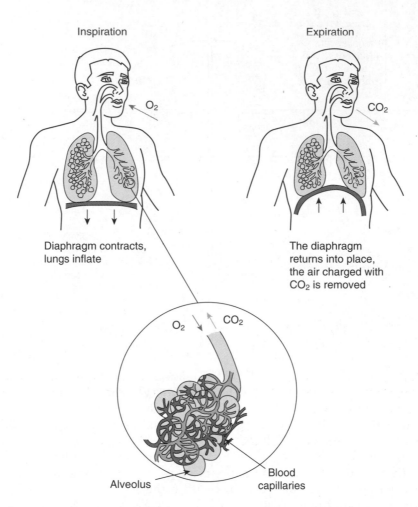

Inspiration

Expiration

O$_2$

CO$_2$

Diaphragm contracts, lungs inflate

The diaphragm returns into place, the air charged with CO$_2$ is removed

O$_2$ CO$_2$

Alveolus

Blood capillaries

Figure 35.2   Gas exchange within the lungs. Reproduced with kind permission of Philips Respironics.

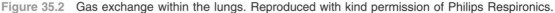

Question 3. (b) Explain the use of a BiPAP machine in the home.

Activity of living: Maintaining a safe environment (Roper *et al.* 1996).
As with all medical devices, equipment should be treated with care and damp dusted weekly. Do not store equipment on the floor, and unplug prior to cleaning (see Figure 35.3). A BiPAP machine should be serviced at least yearly.

Care of mask and headgear

Always wash the patient's face prior to putting the mask on to minimise build up of grease from facial pores. The mask should then be cleaned daily with a damp cloth. Remove mask shell or cushion pad weekly and wash in warm soapy water, rinse in clear water and allow to air dry. The mask should be renewed yearly. Hand wash headgear every week and replace when there appears to be loss of tension, remembering not to tumble dry.

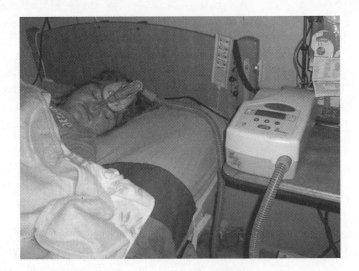

Figure 35.3   Michaela attached to her BiPAP machine. Reproduced with her kind permission.

Care of tubing

Weekly washing of connection tubing in warm soapy water is encouraged and it is rinsed in clear water and allowed to air dry as recommended. The tubing should be replaced yearly, or sooner if needed.

Care of filters

The BiPAP unit has white filters: the white ultra-fine filter should be changed monthly or sooner if dirty, and the grey pollen filter must be washed weekly in warm soapy water and towel dried completely before putting back into machine.

   Please adhere to manufacturer guidelines and community trust policies.

Question 4. Discuss the importance of communication by healthcare professionals when caring for Michaela, a young person with a life-limiting condition, in the community setting.

Activity of living: communication (Roper *et al*. 1996).
Effective communication is an essential professional competency that is developed over time. For parents to receive the news that their daughter may have a life-limiting condition must be a real nightmare. A diagnosis of SMA can create a mix of emotions, such as confusion and frustration. Indeed, the worry and fear must be overwhelming; therefore the family living with the consequences of such news need to know that cohesive supportive services are in place which will enable them as a family to 'live' a life that is as full and complete as possible. Ensuring the choice and opportunity of being cared for at home surrounded by loved ones is important within a multidisciplinary family-centred approach to their individual care needs (Casey 1995). Well-established multidisciplinary teamworking was seen

as instrumental in the smooth transition of moving Michaela, with complex needs, from hospital to home (RCN 2011).

Eighteen year old Michaela is considered to be in the 'formal operational' stage of her development (Bee & Boyd 2007). She can take several factors into account when making decisions and contributes to problem solving. Michaela can articulate her needs and opinions very well and has always been able to do so, as her family encourage and support her to do as much as possible and become involved with regional and national organisations. She is an ambassador for SMA and children with physical disabilities, representing Northern Ireland at House of Lords, London, launching a trail blazer for neuromuscular dystrophy and writes weekly articles in her local newspaper reporting cinema reviews. Michaela is robust in putting across her point of view about the lack of facilities in our everyday environment for young people with disabilities. For example, she was unable to access her local bank due to poor wheelchair access and requested that adaptations be made. Michaela's family have also expressed their concerns about the future, regarding the ongoing impact of care and what might happen should a change in family dynamics suddenly occur (Corkin 2007).

Furthermore, Michaela's parents and extended family should be able to concentrate on her needs and comfort, confident that the best possible care is available to them through the support of an experienced multidisciplinary team (see Figure 35.4). Young people and their parents are often frustrated when local healthcare organisations fail to share relevant

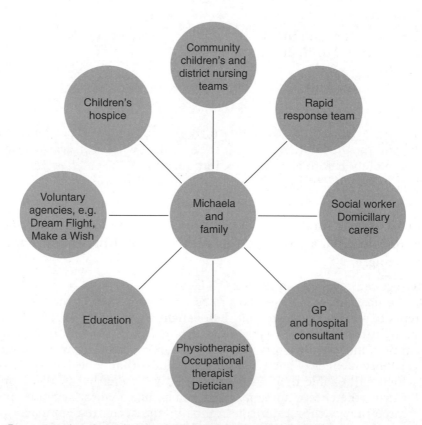

Figure 35.4   Demonstrating those involved in multidisciplinary teamworking.

information appropriately, particularly when a nursing care package is passed from children's to adult services. Healthcare professionals need to be actively engaged and involved with parents and carers in order to avoid a lack of co-ordination within the complexity of services. Parents may be the most powerful advocates for their young people, but they may need to strengthen their voice at times and should be offered the opportunity to speak of their experiences and needs (DH 2010).

The preferred location of caring for Michaela with her life-limiting condition is the family home, with her parents receiving adequate professional support. The ultimate aim is to ensure that Michaela and her family can establish a trusting relationship with healthcare workers and do not experience a lack of privacy in their home. Families of those affected by SMA may understand the financial hardship of living with SMA, so healthcare professionals should ensure these families do not feel isolated or abandoned in their hour of need.

All parents who take on the responsibility of providing complex care in their home need to feel competent, confident and well supported, as the availability of respite care is often very limited (Corkin *et al.* 2006). For many parents to remain the principle carers, they may have to learn complex nursing skills in order to assume 24-hour responsibility (Corkin & Chambers 2007). Community children's nursing services have gradually been transformed and local services are developing in order to support care packages in the home (DH 2011).

Question 5. Using the Roper, Logan & Tierney model in practice devise a care plan to address Michaela's personal cleansing and dressing.

Activity of living: personal cleansing and dressing.
Prior to devising a care plan to address Michaela's personal cleansing and dressing needs it is important to identify what issues need to be considered in relation to:

- Lifespan
- Dependence/independence
- Factors affecting personal cleansing and dressing

All individuals must be cared for 'holistically'; therefore the activity of living such as personal cleansing and dressing can be an issue, depending on the health problem of the individual.

Personal cleansing and dressing for an individual can be affected by the following: lifespan and dependence/independence. Factors influencing personal cleansing and dressing can be further divided into:

- Biological
- Psychological
- Socio-cultural
- Environmental
- Politico-economic

Roper *et al.* (1996)

Lifespan: Michaela is an adolescent/young person and therefore she needs her dignity and privacy to be considered at all times. All young people encounter problems with their personal care such as acne, greasy hair, dandruff and increased body perspiration. Menstruation following puberty may present further difficulties for Michaela both physically and psychologically.

Dependence/independence: historically Michaela's parents and sisters have undertaken her personal cleansing and dressing. But thought has to be given now to the fact that Michaela is attending college and that her parents are getting older and her father has recently suffered ill health himself.

Factors affecting personal cleansing and dressing: Michaela is having increasing episodes of chest infections which leads to further deterioration of her overall capabilities. While at school Michaela had a portable hoist which was used to transfer her over to a changing bench in the disabled toilet. However, since commencing college this facility is not available and Michaela has had to commence wearing incontinence products.

Young people's participation

The views of children, young people and their families should be actively sought and used in the planning, delivery and review of services (NICCY 2006). Children and young people have a right to participate in their care planning and healthcare professionals have a responsibility to facilitate this. Participation in decisions that affect children as individuals requires a child-centred approach with continuous dialogue, especially around good assessment, which is the foundation of effective care planning. A young person's perspective is crucial when assessing their needs, wishes and feelings. Care planning requires the involvement, participation and contribution of everyone involved in the child's life, including the child and his or her parents and should be based on an holistic assessment of the child's needs.

Based on professional experience, the authors feel it is important to note that when a parent wants to talk about a problem, they do not always want us to fix it – they may just want us to 'listen' and demonstrate we care. Community children's nursing has developed considerably in recent years and the future looks set for changes and developments, driven not only by a modernising workforce but also by professional and economic factors. Experiences and excellence in community care need to be shared, focusing on the identification, assessment and management of the life-limited child and young person.

Remember to tell parents and young people what they are doing right, as it will help them feel valued and strengthen partnership. Every child's life is a special gift – as parents we evolve, learn and change as our children teach us more than we will ever teach them.

References

Air Products (2009) *Your Guide to Non-Invasive Ventilation Therapy.* Ireland version, Dublin: www.airproducts.ie/homecare.

Bee, H. & Boyd, D. (2007) *The Developing Child,* 11th edn. London: Pearson.

Casey, A. (1995) Partnership nursing: influences on involvement of informal carers. *Journal of Advanced Nursing,* **22**, 1058–62.

Corkin, D. (2007) *A conceptual analysis: the 'burden' of caring in relation to children and young people with complex health needs.* Unpublished MSc dissertation.

Corkin, D. and Chambers, J. (2007) Community children's nursing in Northern Ireland. *Paediatric Nursing,* **19**(1), 25–7.

Corkin, D.A.P., Price, J. and Gillespie, E. (2006) Respite care for children, young people and families – are their needs addressed? *International Journal of Palliative Nursing*, **12**(9), 422–7.

Department of Health (2010) *Achieving Equity and Excellence for Children*. London: DH.

Department of Health (2011) *NHS at Home: Community Children's Nursing Services*. www.dh.gov.uk/ publications (accessed 10 May 2011).

Hockenberry, M.J., Wilson, D., Winkelstein, M.L. & Kline, N.E. (2003) *Wong's Nursing Care of Infants and Children*, 7th edn. St Louis: Mosby.

NICCY (Northern Ireland Commissioner for Children & Young People) (2006) *A Northern Ireland based review of children and young people's participation in the care planning process*. Belfast: NICCY.

Philips Respironics (2008) *My BiPAP Ventilator, My Helpful Guide*. Chichester: Philips Respironics.

Roper, N., Logan, W. & Tierney, A. (1996) *The Elements of Nursing*, 4th. edn. London: Churchill Livingstone.

Royal College of Nursing (2011) *Healthcare Service Standards in Caring for Neonates, Children and Young People*. London: RCN. www.rcn.org.uk/direct (accessed 10 May 2011).

www.fsma.org/FSMA *Community Families of Spinal Muscular Atrophy* (accessed 5 August 2010).

36

HIV/AIDS

Karen Salmon

Scenario

Bethlehem, now nine years old, lives in a single storey house with a caregiver, and nine other non-related children. At two years of age Bethlehem's mother became ill and died of HIV/AIDS, a year later her father took a new wife and she too became ill and died, 20 months later her father also died leaving Bethlehem and her brother in the care of their 18-year-old sister Magda.

Bethlehem was diagnosed as HIV antibody positive at age three; she began highly active antiretroviral therapy (HAART) at age four and is currently taking two nucleoside analogue reverse transcriptase inhibitors, lamivudine and zidovudine, and one non-nucleoside analogue reverse transcriptase inhibitor, efavirenz.

Activity 36.1

1. Define HIV/AIDS.
2. Describe the epidemiology of HIV/AIDS.
3. Discuss modes of transmission of HIV/AIDS.
4. Explain the natural course of progression of HIV.

Care Planning in Children and Young People's Nursing, First Edition.
Edited by Doris Corkin, Sonya Clarke, Lorna Liggett.
© 2012 Blackwell Publishing Ltd. Published 2012 by Blackwell Publishing Ltd.

The human immunodeficiency virus (HIV), which causes acquired immune deficiency syndrome (AIDS), is a retrovirus. There are two strains of HIV: HIV-1 and HIV-2. HIV-1 was first recognised in America in 1981; French scientists discovered the virus in 1983, and confirmed transmission routes. It is now acknowledged that cases of AIDS were first seen in central Africa in the 1970s, although at the time they were not recognised as such. HIV-1 is distributed worldwide, but HIV-2, discovered in 1987, is primarily found in West Africa (UNAIDS 2008). The most common route of HIV transmission is sexual. Methods of HIV transmission globally are: 80% unprotected sex (vaginal, anal and oral); 10% vertically from mother to child during pregnancy, labour or breastfeeding, 5% blood products and 5% IV drug contact (Adler 2001). Ninety per cent of those infected do not even know it and you cannot tell by their appearance who is infected. Ninety per cent of children with HIV/AIDS become infected by vertical transmission (UNAIDS 2002). There are many cultural factors that promote the spread of HIV/AIDS, including multiple sexual partners, use of commercial sex workers and harmful traditional practices like female genital mutilation, blood letting, tattooing, skin cutting and piercing practices (UNAIDS/WHO 2008).

How is HIV/AIDS not spread?

There is no evidence from multiple studies to show that HIV/AIDS is transmitted through:

- Touching or hugging
- Dry kissing (no exchange of saliva)
- Coughing or sneezing
- Shaking hands
- Telephones
- Sharing eating utensils or food cooked by an HIV antibody positive individual
- Toilet seats
- Bathtubs and swimming pools
- Mosquitoes or insect bites

Transmission through kissing with saliva exchange or through sweat or tears is considered very unlikely (Hubley 2002).

The impact of HIV/AIDS on children is overwhelming, including: prolonged illness of one or both parents, relatives, teachers or neighbours; death of a parent or parents; loss of financial resources due to illness or death and school drop-out or interruption to care for family members. Furthermore, there is the stigma or discrimination associated with HIV/AIDS and loss of caring adults to protect, teach, care for and love them (Tindyebwa *et al.* 2004; UN/AIDS 2008). Approximately 44 million children, in 34 developing nations severely affected by HIV/AIDS, had lost one or both parents to HIV or related complicating illnesses by 2010. In Ethiopia, AIDS was first reported in 1986. Since then infection rates have increased rapidly, with prevalence estimates ranging from 10–17%. Ethiopia has the third largest population with HIV/AIDS in the world after South Africa and India. Not all countries are affected equally; the burden of HIV/AIDS is heaviest in Sub-Saharan Africa (SSA). Comprising only one tenth of the world's population, SSA constitutes more than 70% of individuals living with HIV. Of the 2.1 million children under the age of 15 living with HIV worldwide, 90% live in SSA; also 90% of AIDS orphans live in SSA. It is predicted that by the year 2024 HIV/AIDS-related deaths will represent more than 70% of all deaths of 15–65 year olds in Ethiopia (MoH 2006). In 2007 it was estimated that over 1200 children and young people with HIV/AIDS were living in the UK and Republic of Ireland (RCOG 2007). In the UK, 50% of children with HIV/AIDS are ten years of age and over.

There is neither a cure nor vaccine to prevent HIV/AIDS. Hiding within the CD4 T lymphocyte, the virus can remain latent for years. Individuals infected with HIV appear healthy, are asymptomatic, and can remain so for years. AIDS is a progressive result of HIV infection and represents the late stage of HIV infection. AIDS is defined as a specific group of diseases or conditions, which are indicative of severe immune suppression related to infection with HIV. HIV causes AIDS by gradually destroying the body's immune system, specifically CD4 T lymphocytes, which allows common infections such as tuberculosis (TB), previously rare infections such as toxoplasma encephalitis, and cancers like Kaposi's sarcoma to flourish, and also causes neurological disturbances. Among individuals living with HIV/AIDS *Pneumocystis carinii* pneumonia (PCP) is common in the USA and Europe, is rare in African adults, but common among African infants. Also, these conditions rarely occur in children with healthy immune systems, and they are normally not serious. For children living with HIV/AIDS mild diseases frequently turn into fatal ones; reasons for this include less developed healthcare systems, poor nutrition and widespread infectious diseases.

Treatment

Highly active antiretroviral treatment (HAART), usually three or more drugs taken in combination, reduces the level of HIV in the blood, slows HIV disease progress, improves immunity and the patient's health and quality of life recover. Ethiopian guidelines recommend HAART for all HIV infected individuals with a CD4 count below 200 (normal CD4 counts are 600–1500 cells mm^3 of blood). The health impact is huge, with average CD4 counts increasing from 244 to 372 after 18 months of treatment. Antiretroviral therapy (ART), available in Ethiopia, includes nucleoside analogue reverse transcriptase inhibitors (NRTIs), which inhibit the replication of HIV by interfering with the enzyme transcriptase or non-nucleoside analogue reverse transcriptase inhibitors (NNRTIs), which block viral DNA. No protease inhibitors, nucleotide reverse transcriptase inhibitors or fusion inhibitors are available. Only 13% of those who need ART are accessing it (MoH 2006). Common side effects of NRTIs and NNRTIs include rash, nausea, diarrhoea, abdominal pain, headache and confusion (WHO 2006).

Stage 1: primary infection

This stage can last up to three months, often there are no symptoms, and no antibodies are found in the blood on testing; this is known as the *window period*. During the window period individuals are highly infectious and yet unaware of their condition. Flu-like symptoms, including fever, lymphadenopathy, pharyngitis, rash, myalgia, headache and diarrhoea are associated with sero-conversion, in adults, 2–4 weeks after HIV infection; these symptoms are unusual in children (Ammann 2004).

Stage 2: asymptomatic infection

Children have no symptoms, but do test positive for HIV antibodies. Antibodies may appear 2–4 weeks after infection, and are usually present after 3–6 months. The asymptomatic period is shorter in children. Thirty per cent of children are rapid progressors and will die by one year, 50% develop symptoms early in life followed by decline and death by 3–5 years; 20% are chronic non-progressors who remain well beyond eight years (Rich *et al.* 2000).

Stage 3: symptomatic infection

Children begin showing signs of HIV infection including persistent generalised lymphaden-opathy (PGL), oral and oesophageal candidiasis, and skin rashes, especially varicella zoster. Persistent generalised lymphadenopathy lymph node enlargement will be one centimetre or greater at two or more sites that persists for more than three months in the absence of a concurrent illness other than HIV to explain these findings. Up to 70% of HIV-infected individuals have PGL, which may be seen alone or in conjunction with systemic complaints like fatigue, fever and major sweats. Most children have some type of neurological involvement, such as developmental delay affecting motor or language skills and encephalitis. Hepatomegaly is also common in children infected with HIV/AIDS (Tudor-Williams & Gibb 2001).

Stage 4: AIDS

About 70% of vertically infected children with HIV/AIDS will have some signs or symptoms by 12 months of age. Without ART, children will advance to AIDS by age five and 80% have died by this age (see Table 36.1).

The median age of death is nine years; however, some children do not present with symptoms until their teens. With adults, WHO estimates that 50% develop AIDS within ten years of initial HIV infection. Symptoms of AIDS are those of opportunistic infections taking advantage of the damaged immune system. The WHO produced clinical case definitions for Africa in 1986 (see Table 36.2).

✎ Activity 36.2

Questions for reflection and discussion:

- Why is it important for nurses to educate people about how HIV is and is not transmitted?
- Why is important to understand the danger of HIV transmission during the 'window period'?

Table 36.1   Differences between children and adults with HIV/AIDS (modified from Tudor-Williams & Gibb 2001).

More rapid disease progression: 30% of children develop AIDS by age 12 months.
Higher viral loads at presentation.
Physiologically higher absolute CD4 counts.
Growth faltering common affecting height and weight.
Encephalopathy presents with developmental delay and hypertonic diplegia.
Opportunistic infections often more severe in children.
Poor primary responses to childhood immunisations.
Lymphoid interstitial pneumonitis common.
Malignancy uncommon less than 2% of children with HIV/AIDS.
More rapid clearance of ART requiring higher than adult equivalent doses, particularly in very young children.

Table 36.2 *WHO* Case definition of AIDS in Children under 13 years (modified from Tindyebwa 2004).

Major signs	Minor signs
Weight loss of more than 10% body weight in a short time or abnormally slow growth*.	Persistent cough for more than one month (in the absence of TB).
Chronic diarrhoea for more than one month.	Repeated infections, such as otitis media and pharyngitis.
Prolonged, intermittent or constant fever for more than one month.	Generalised pruriginous dermatitis.
Severe or recurrent pneumonia.	Oropharyngeal candidiasis.
	Generalised lymphadenopathy.
	Confirmed maternal HIV infection.

Note: there must be two major and two minor signs and confirmed maternal HIV infection, in the absence of immune-suppression by a known cause such as cancer or malnutrition.
*Downward crossing of at least two major percentile lines on height-for-age chart in a child of one year or older.

Although Roper *et al.* address 12 activities of daily living, this chapter will mainly address nursing care planning in relation to breathing, eating and drinking, maintaining a safe environment and elimination (Holland *et al.* 2008).

 Questions

1. Given Bethlehem's immuno-compromised status how would the children's nurse care for her breathing needs?
2. Reflecting on the nursing process and a model of care how would you care for Bethlehem's eating and drinking needs given the side effects of HAART treatment and risks of opportunistic infections?

Answers to questions

Question 1. Given Bethlehem's immuno-compromised status how would the children's nurse care for her breathing needs?

For the children's nurse, prevention of opportunistic infections is a priority in the care of children with HIV/AIDS. The World Health Organisation recommends that all children should receive the normal childhood immunisations, including diphtheria, polio, tetanus, measles and mumps, but those showing symptoms of HIV-related illness should not be given BCG or yellow fever (Gilbert *et al.* 2009). Children living with HIV/AIDS may have no immunity to infections that family members or friends carry; even relatively mild infections, like the influenza virus, may cause a child with HIV/AIDS to become very ill.

Box 36.1 Nursing care plan for breathing

Signs and symptoms	Nursing implementation	Nursing evaluation
Dyspnoea, tachyapnoea, cyanosis, wheezing, cough, inability to raise secretions, nasal flaring, use of accessory muscles.	Obtain sputum sample for diagnosis. Administer antibiotics or TB drugs as ordered, evaluate for side effects. Assist child with clearance of secretions by effective coughing (inhale slowly through nose, exhale and cough). Teach child to cover mouth when coughing. Prevent stasis of secretions by deep breathing, and ambulation. Encourage fluid intake to prevent dehydration.	Decreased symptoms of dyspnoea and air hunger, expectoration of secretions, relief of symptoms causing discomfort and improved respiratory function.

Optimal nursing care of children with HIV/AIDS requires prompt diagnosis and treatment of infections such as *Pneumocystis carinii* pneumonia (PCP), pneumococci or TB when they occur, as infectious diseases are the immediate cause of death in over 90% of children with advanced HIV/AIDS (Tindyebwa *et al.* 2004). Tuberculosis, a disease previously thought to be under control, may be primary, or a reactivation of latent TB (Hubley 2002). Children with HIV are ten times more likely to develop active TB than those not infected with HIV. Also, children may respond poorly to treatment and develop severe complications (Fielder 2010).

Question 2. Reflecting on the nursing process and a model of care how would you care for Bethlehem's eating and drinking needs given the side effects of HAART treatment and risks of opportunistic infections?

Children with HIV, who are well nourished, have fewer infections and progress more slowly from HIV to AIDS. Nutritional support is therefore important in the management of HIV infection in children. Although there are no special foods for children living with HIV/AIDS, good nutrition accompanied with vitamin A supplements help the immune system fight infections and diseases by increasing white blood cells. Vitamin A supplementation reduced overall mortality by 63%, AIDS-related mortality by 68%, and diarrhoea-associated mortality by 92% among HIV-infected children aged six months to five years (Fawzi *et al.* 2000). Both HIV and poor nutrition can damage the immune system. For the child with HIV/AIDS a balanced diet, particularly of carbohydrate, protein and vitamin and mineral groups of foods that are well cooked is important, as a high energy and protein diet reduces muscle wasting. A sick child has even greater food needs than a healthy one; it is important to encourage the child with AIDS to increase their food intake. Monthly growth monitoring is an appropriate way to monitor nutritional status; if growth falters additional investigations should be made to determine the cause.

Most children with HIV/AIDS develop mouth conditions at some point; candidiasis is the most common, followed by herpes zoster and other herpes viral infections. Infections of the mouth and throat may be painful and cause difficulty in swallowing.

Box 36.2   Nursing care plan for eating and drinking

Signs and symptoms	Nursing implementation	Nursing evaluation
Weight loss, anorexia, nausea and vomiting.	Assess severity and impact on activities of daily living (ADL). Monitor weight, growth, intake and output; increase calories 40–45 kcal/kg. Avoid punitive or judgemental statements about food intake or weight loss. Determine child's food preference and try small frequent feedings rather than fewer large meals. Avoid unpasteurised dairy products, unfiltered drinking water and foods that are undercooked, filling or gas forming. Encourage eating before taking medication. Teach carer to prepare and store food safely to decrease possibility of opportunistic infections from food.	Increase of nutritional intake, improved skin turgor and hair, nail, mucous membrane condition; verbalisation of satisfaction with diet, adequate energy for ADL.

Box 36.3   Nursing care plan for maintaining a safe environment

Signs and symptoms	Nursing implementation	Nursing evaluation
Painful, raw oral lesions, difficulty in swallowing.	Gently clean the mouth with a soft toothbrush and rinse with salt water (half a teaspoon in a cup of water), or lemon juice. Give soft, moist, easily digestible foods and plenty of fluids; avoid acidic and spicy foods. Prepare smaller quantities, but serve them often.	No or decreased areas of oral mucous membrane breakdown.

Chronic diarrhoea is very common, affecting up to 60% of children with HIV/AIDS at sometime in their illness. Stools may be mucoid and foul smelling with pus. The cause of the diarrhoea should be established and specific treatment provided, although in 50% of cases no specific aetiology is found. Symptoms of dehydration include thirst, irritability, tiredness, the skin going back slowly when pinched, and sunken eyes and fontanelle (in very young children).

Finally, children should not be passive recipients of nursing interventions. As they grow they should progressively be given opportunities to make decisions about their own care. Nurses must facilitate children's participation in those matters that affect them, including HIV. Carers also need to be involved in decision making and require support and care from

---

Box 36.4   Nursing care plan for elimination

Signs and symptoms	Nursing implementation	Nursing evaluation
Frequent diarrhoeal stools.	Monitor frequency, amount, colour and consistency of stools. Obtain sample for diagnosis. Assess hydration, encourage fluids like water, weak tea, or soup to prevent dehydration. Administer vitamin A supplement, rehydration solution or IV fluids as directed. Give low fat, low fibre diet, yoghurt, oat porridge and bananas. Cleanse and dry rectal area after each bowel movement and apply Vaseline® to prevent skin breakdown. Stress importance of good hand-washing technique.	Maintenance of stable bowel function, decrease in number of stools/day, balanced intake and output, expression of comfort and no skin breakdown.

---

the children's nurse, as burnout and anxiety are common experiences among those caring for the chronically ill. Alongside the nurse, friends and family members can provide recreational or shopping breaks and someone to talk things over with. Providing awards and honouring carers at community meetings is an effective way to motivate carers.

References

Ammann, A.J. (2004) Paediatric human immunodeficiency virus infection. In: Stiehm, E.R., Ochs, H.D. & Wikestein, J.A. (eds) *Immunological Disorders in Infants and Children*, 5th edn. Philadelphia: Saunders.

Adler, M.W. (2001) Development of the epidemic. In: Adler, M.W. (ed.) *ABC of AIDS*, 5th edn. London: BMJ Publishing Group.

Fawzi, W.W., Msamanga, G., Hunter, D., et al. (2000) Randomised trial of vitamin supplements in relation to vertical transmission of HIV in Tanzania. *Journal Acquired Immune Deficiency Syndrome*, **23**(3), 246–54.

Fielder, J.F. (2010) *Tuberculosis in the Era of HIV: A Clinical Manual for Care Providers Working in Africa and Other Resource-limited Settings*. Nairobi: Fielder Medical Assistance Foundation.

Gilbert, D.N., Moeliering, R.C., Eliopoulos, G.M., Saag, M.S. & Chambers, H.F. (2009) *The Sanford Guide to HIV/AIDS Therapy*, 17th edn. Virginia: Merck.

Holland, K., Jenkins, J., Solomon, J. & Whittam, S. (2008) *Applying the Roper Logan Tierney Model in Practice*, 2nd edn. London: Churchill Livingstone.

Hubley, J. (2002) *The AIDS Handbook: a Guide to the Understanding of AIDS and HIV*. London: Macmillan.

Ministry of Health (2006) *AIDS In: Ethiopia: Sixth Report*. Addis Ababa: HIV/AIDS Prevention and Control Office.

Rich, K.C., Fowler, M.G., Mofenson, L.M., et al. (2000) Maternal and infant factors predicting disease progression in human immunodeficiency virus type 1-infected infants. *Paediatrics*, **105**(1), 8.

Royal College of Obstetrics and Gynaecology (2007) National study of HIV in pregnancy and childhood. *Newsletter 72*. London: Royal College of Obstetrics and Gynaecology.

Tudor-Williams, G. & Gibb, D. (2001) HIV infection in children. In: Adler, M.W. *ABC of AIDS*, 5th edn. London: BMJ Publishing Group.

Tindyebwa, D., Kayita, J., Musoke, P., *et al.* (2004) *Handbook on Paediatric AIDS in Africa*, African Network for the Care of Children Affected by AIDS, Kampala.

UNAIDS (2002) *Paediatric HIV Infection and AIDS*. Geneva: UNAIDS Point of View.

UNAIDS (2008) *Report On The Global AIDS Epidemic*. Geneva: UNAIDS.

UNAIDS/WHO (2008) *Epidemiological Fact Sheet on HIV and AIDS: Core data on Epidemiology and Response: Ethiopia*. Geneva: UNAIDS/WHO.

World Health Organisation (2006) *Antiretroviral Therapy of HIV Infection in Infants and Children in Resource-limited Settings: Towards Universal Access*. Geneva: World Health Organisation.

37

Bereavement Support

Una Hughes and Breige Morgan

Scenario

Lucy was a two-year-old girl who died at home following a deteriorating illness. She was a third child born following an uneventful pregnancy, at term. When she was born her brother, Michael, was three years old and she had an 18-month-old sister, Annabel. Lucy's parents, Helen and Ian, began raising concerns about her developmental milestones and the fact that she was very slow to feed when she was nine months old. She developed absence seizures and her feeding difficulties increased. Lucy's condition remained undiagnosed, her seizures increased and there was a gradual deterioration in all developmental areas. Lucy's dad was working long hours to support the family and her mum had given up work to care for her and her siblings. Her swallow reflex decreased and Lucy required a gastrostomy. She had numerous hospital admissions and eventually her parents were informed that her condition was untreatable. Lucy's parents decided that there should be no further interventions. This was Helen's first experience of impending death and she was very worried about her own response to Lucy's death. Lucy's parents decided she should die at home and the community children's nursing (CCN) team and the specialist hospice community nurse worked together to facilitate a package of care.

Lucy's parents, her brother and sister and their extended family along with the CCN were present when Lucy died. Her parents had been able to plan and express their wishes for Lucy's funeral.

Helen appeared to cope well at the time of the funeral despite her fears about facing Lucy's death. The CCN and hospice nurse made a combined visit one week following Lucy's funeral as they had both been so closely involved with the family. Helen was very angry with Ian at this time.

Care Planning in Children and Young People's Nursing, First Edition.
Edited by Doris Corkin, Sonya Clarke, Lorna Liggett.
© 2012 Blackwell Publishing Ltd. Published 2012 by Blackwell Publishing Ltd.

He had had to return to work and she felt he was 'getting on with things'. Meanwhile she was trying to cope with her own grief, the escalating bad behaviour of Michael who was now five years old and 3½ -year-old Annabel, who had been toilet trained but was now requiring nappies, which was causing problems with her nursery placement. Helen was reassured by the CCN that regression was very common in young children when someone close to them dies, she offered advice on coping with their behaviours. The hospice nurse was able to offer examples of books which would help both the children at their different stages of development to come to terms with the death of their sister.

The CCN planned a visit when Ian would be home from work; he revealed the huge amount of pressure he felt he was under to support the family financially, as his job was not secure, and also that he felt that he needed to appear to be strong and protect Helen. Ian had not told Helen about his employment worries and when she heard about them she understood Ian's reasons for being so particular about getting back to work quickly. On subsequent visits over the next year the CCN witnessed the family becoming stronger and supporting each other and learning to live without Lucy. The hospice nurse specialist made contact over the two-year period following Lucy s death and the family were invited to the annual remembrance service. Cards were sent to the family on the anniversary of Lucy's death.

Questions

1. What is bereavement and who can offer bereavement care?
2. Discuss differences between the terms grief and mourning.
3. Explain the supportive role of the CCN following a child's death.
4. Could a care pathway provide co-ordinated bereavement support?

Answers to questions

Question 1. What is bereavement and who can offer bereavement care?

Although there are complex descriptions and definitions, the CRUSE booklet, *After Someone Dies: a Leaflet about Death, Bereavement and Grief for Young People*, puts this plainly and simply: 'Bereavement simply means losing someone through death' (Cruse Bereavement Care 2004).

Once a child has died, anyone can offer bereavement care, and it may come from unexpected sources, most people are not consciously thinking of their visits or chats as bereavement care. Family members, neighbours, friends, health professionals, teachers, funeral directors, any one of these people and more may be the catalyst who helps the parent through their grief. Very few people feel entirely comfortable talking to parents who are bereaved and most are not sure what to say. Most parents just appreciate that someone was there to listen and that they were 'allowed' to talk about their child openly and express their feelings regardless of the time since the child's death (Dominica 2006). Usually parents greatly appreciate the simple acts of kindness and thought, such as medical or nursing staff attending the funeral of their child or sending a sympathy card (MacDonald *et al.* 2005).

Bereavement care is seen as an integral part of palliative care (ACT 2009) and bereavement support should be offered to the service user at an appropriate level (DH & Children 2009). Therefore we should not avoid the bereaved and if it is difficult to find the words just being there is often enough (Dominica 2006).

A study by Dyregrov (2004), showed that just being able to talk about their bereavement experience helped parents. It should help to allay a professional's fear of a bereavement phone call or visit. Just listening can be enough. Building up good communication and trust, where parents can openly express their feelings will ultimately help to provide a better bereavement service (Price & Cairns 2009).

Activity 37.1

Explore the following websites for further understanding of bereavement:
   www.childbereavement.org.uk
   www.crusebereavementcare.org.uk

Question 2. Discuss differences between the terms grief and mourning.

Grief is the feeling experienced after a loss, and mourning is the outward expression of the loss. Grief is a universal reaction to the loss of someone, but the way different people and cultures mourn the loss of someone varies hugely. Therefore grief is what is felt, while mourning is what is done when someone dies (Payne *et al.* 2008).

The five stages of grief were first described by Kübler-Ross in 1969 and are still recognised today: denial, anger, bargaining, depression and acceptance. Grieving is a very personal experience, and for this reason can be a very lonely experience (Thomas & Chalmers 2009), as no one can tell someone how to grieve. People do not go through the stages at the same time, nor do they all follow an exact sequence, but most people complete the five stages, over time. Reactions to a child's death are altered by many things, including the relationship with the child, the type of death, whether it was expected or sudden, personality types, gender, culture, religious outlook, or past experience, to name but a few.

The task of mourning is to accept the reality of the loss, work through the pain and grief, adjust to a new 'normality', learn to live with the loss, develop new bonds and move on. Mourning often involves cultural customs and rituals to help the bereaved deal with their loss. The way people mourn will depend on their personal beliefs and experiences, their family customs and relationships, their religious affiliations and social rituals. Mourning rituals give the bereaved a focus and a structure to get them through a bewildering phase in the bereavement process.

Difficulties can occur when someone gets 'stuck' at one of the five stages of grief. This may lead to complicated grief or prolonged grief, which is a serious adverse outcome of bereavement, diagnosed by the individual experiencing four out of eight symptoms for at least six months. Hawton (2007) lists the eight symptoms as: 'trouble accepting the death, inability to trust others since the death, excessive bitterness related to the death, uneasiness about moving on with life, detachment from other people to whom the person was previously close, the feeling that life is now meaningless, the view that the future holds no prospect for fulfilment, and agitation since the death.' Most people can cope with their grief without specialist intervention (Worden 2003), only a small number will experience complicated grief and require specialist help from a GP, psychologists, psychiatrists, social workers and/or other specialists in the field of bereavement and grieving (Beardsmore & Fitzmaurice 2002; Davies *et al.* 2006; DH 2008, p34).

Question 3. Explain the supportive role of the CCN following a child's death.

Palliative care is about providing comfort rather than providing a cure. The aim of paediatric palliative care is to go on the journey with the child and family from diagnosis, through life, to death and beyond through bereavement (Pfund 2007). Unfortunately, it is often easier and more measurable to concentrate on the pre-death and actual-death side of paediatric palliative care, but, this is only a part of the care required. The emotional, social and spiritual elements of bereavement care are more difficult to quantify and provide. The care will depend on the individuals involved, the circumstances and the need for ongoing bereavement support following the death.

The way families deal with the death of their child is very individual, as their coping mechanisms for bereavement will vary. The way the CCN will support the family will depend on the family's reaction and ability to cope following the child's death. The CCN can play a pivotal role in coordinating bereavement care with other members of the multidisciplinary team, for example hospice nurse specialists, social workers and GPs.

The importance of bereavement follow-up cannot be underestimated and studies have shown that families were grateful for continued contact after their child's death and those who did not have follow-up contact felt disappointed, dismissed and abandoned (Contro *et al.* 2002; Field & Behrman 2003, p178). We inevitably will say things we regret or could have phrased better, but with reflective practice we can learn from our mistakes (McNeilly *et al.* 2006) and provide better support to parents and siblings who are bereaved.

The CCN delivering bereavement care will be documenting all the care, the decisions made, discussions with the family members and the plans for the future in the bereavement care plan. This will help to maintain good communication with the rest of the team and can help to highlight areas of concern, for example any family members who do not appear to be coping.

When a child dies, care for that child ends, but care for the family must continue (Field & Behrman 2003). Preparing the family for bereavement is an important part of the paediatric palliative care process. At times parents need someone who can 'take-over' but who will not 'over-take'. In other words, there are times when the professional needs to have the strength to carry the family through difficult times but also have the perception and understanding of the family to step back and allow the family to take the lead (Lewis & Prescott 2006). This, of course, can be draining on the health professional and good support is required to 'care for the carer' and enable them to continue supporting the child and family.

Question 4. Could a care pathway provide co-ordinated bereavement support?

Health professionals dealing with parents and children during bereavement care must take the plunge and be there for them. Rider (2003, p228) says: 'We only fail if we avoid our dying patients and their families'. Benner (1984) talks about 'presence' as the concept of being with a patient rather than doing something for them and lists it as one of the competencies of expert nurses. In bereavement care we can no longer help our patient and the focus shifts to helping their family. Rushton (2005) also looks at the nurse's presence and the act of being there even when it would be easier to run away or find an excuse to 'do' something else. The importance of being there for the family cannot be underestimated, but presence is not quantifiable and is not often factored into time and costing for nursing services. For this reason bereavement follow-up is often ad hoc and inconsistent, the needs of the living in our care take priority over the needs of the families of the children who have died.

One of the standards of the International Children's Palliative Care Network (ICPCN 2008) Charter is that support for the bereaved family should be available for as long as it is required (www.icpcn.org.uk). A bereavement service could provide the family with consistent support and help to guide them through the practicalities of what has to be done, while also providing someone 'neutral' to talk to in the months or years after the child's death.

In an ideal world a bereavement service would provide continuity to all bereaved families as there would be resources and time and staff who are adequately trained in bereavement care (Davies *et al.* 2006).

A care pathway, however, may be the way forward, a co-ordinated plan providing continuity and equality of care. It would provide a step-by-step format to aid practitioners in making decisions and recording variations and deviations from the expected. Care pathways assist with guiding the care families require on the journey through their child's palliative care and the evidence in the pathway guides choices and the best care children and young people should receive (Pfund 2007). This would help to highlight problems being encountered by grieving families whereby all the members of the multidisciplinary team work with them. The detailed guidance that a care pathway provides should help to support the staff involved in providing bereavement care as the aim of any care pathway is to strive for quality co-ordinated care. However, the difficulty with a care pathway is that it may become a perfunctory tick-list and the individuality required when dealing with a bereaved family could get lost in the process.

As a dedicated bereavement service or a bereavement care pathway is not always available, the following are some pointers to aid the professional when caring for a bereaved family. It is not a prescriptive or an exhaustive list, and nor is it in any particular order due to the differences in each grieving family's situation. The idea is that it will stimulate thought:

1. Familiarise yourself with the medical history and details of the child's death.
2. Liaise with the team providing end-of-life care, if you have not been involved.
3. Phone the parents and arrange a visit with them.
4. *Listen*, to parents and or siblings.
5. Always tell the truth, admit if you do not know something but offer to try to find out the information they are seeking.
6. Use the child's name when discussing them.
7. Think before you speak and be sensitive.
8. Do not use platitudes, for example 'she is in a better place'.
9. Judge each situation individually and be aware that some parents may wish to deal with the death of their child within their own circle of family and friends and may not want involvement from professionals.
10. Give information at the pace the family are ready to receive it.
11. Bring parents any written documentation about bereavement and support available in your locality and information about local support groups, if appropriate.
12. Be up to date with remembrance service details.

13. At times the professional may need to initiate the topic of the deceased child and then allow the parents to direct the conversation. They may wish to discuss some aspect of their child's care or how they or other family members are coping.
14. Reassure parents that the rollercoaster of emotions they are feeling is part of the normal grieving process.
15. Offer practical support and advice, for example registering the death, how to make funeral arrangements, etc.
16. Be sensitive when removing healthcare equipment from the home (if the child has had home care) when the parents want it done. Some parents may want it removed immediately on the child's death, others may need time before it is removed from their home.
17. Try to involve both parents, at times fathers can be reluctant to participate or can be forgotten about.
18. Be patient, you may need to repeat explanations many times.
19. Respect cultural and religious customs.
20. Remember to involve siblings and realise that they may be acting out of character after a traumatic loss.
21. Allow siblings space to vent their feelings; they may feel neglected. Bereaved parents may not be able to cope with their children's grief as well as their own.
22. Refer parents for further professional help if there are signs of complicated grief.
23. Keep in touch with the parents by phone and with follow-up visits as necessary.
24. Document all care in a bereavement care plan.

Summary

Today's health care is based on teamwork and nowhere more so than in the community setting. A multidisciplinary approach to paediatric palliative care has been increasingly experienced; unfortunately that progression has not reached bereavement care and it can fall between the cracks, with no one taking responsibility for it. Bereavement care is an essential part of palliative care, therefore it must be provided for as long as the family require it. Studies show that families appreciate support from health professionals.

Bereavement care is difficult and daunting, but if we avoid it we are not providing the best quality care that our patients and their families deserve. To prepare ourselves we must read around the subject and the frameworks and guidelines available and put it into practice. Anyone can give bereavement care, but developing and following a bereavement care pathway could provide a better service enabling healthcare professionals to ensure continuity and equality in the service they provide.

There are lots of ways for professionals to get help, to give themselves confidence and knowledge before embarking on bereavement care. It is not an exact science and although we learn through experience and reflective practice, some background information can help. Many bereavement charities have useful information for bereaved parents and the professionals working with them. They cover topics such as: sibling death, dos and don'ts lists compiled by bereaved parents, ways to support and guide the family and support for professionals themselves following a child's death. Books, publications and the Internet can be very useful for gaining an insight into the needs of the bereaved from different perspectives. Health professionals can increase their understanding, gain confidence and be better equipped to deal with bereaved families if they undertake some further education or study in relation to palliative care and bereavement.

References

Association for Children with Life Threatening or Terminal Conditions (ACT) (2009) *A Guide to the Development of Children's Palliative Care Services*, 3rd edn. Bristol: ACT.

Beardsmore, S. & Fitzmaurice, N. (2002) Palliative care in paediatric oncology. *European Journal of Cancer*, **38**(14), 1900–1907.

Benner, P. (1984) *From Novice to Expert: Excellence and Power in Clinical Nursing Practice*. Menlo Park, California: Addison-Wesley.

Contro, N., Larson, J., Scofield, S., Sourkes, B. & Cohen, H. (2002) Family perspectives on the quality of pediatric palliative care. *Archives of Pediatric Adolescent Medicine*, **156**, 14–19.

Cruse Bereavement Care (2004) *After Someone Dies: a Leaflet about Death, Bereavement and Grief for Young People*. www.childbereavementcare.org.uk.

Davies, B., Attig, T. & Towne, M. (2006) Bereavement. In: Goldman, A., Hain, R. & Liben, S. (eds). *Oxford Textbook of Palliative Care for Children*. Oxford: Oxford University Press. pp200–201.

Department of Health (2008) *Better Care: Better Lives. Improving Outcomes and Experiences for Children, Young People and their Families Living with Life Limiting and Life Threatening Conditions*. London: DH Publications.

Department of Health & Children (2009) *Palliative Care for Children with Life-Limited Conditions in Ireland – a National Policy*. www.dohc.ie/publications/pdf/palliate_care

Dominica, F. (2006) After the child's death: family care. In: Goldman, A., Hain, R. & Liben, S. (eds). *Oxford Textbook of Palliative Care for Children*. Oxford: Oxford University Press, 191–2.

Dyregrov K. (2004) Bereaved parents' experience of research participation. *Social Science and Medicine*, **58**(2), 391–400.

Field, M.J. & Behrman, R.E. (2003) *When Children Die, Improving Palliative and End of Life Care for Children and their Families*. Washington DC: The National Academies Press. p171.

Hawton, K. (2007) Complicated grief after bereavement, Editorial. *British Medical Journal*, **334**, 962–3.

International Children's Palliative Care Network (ICPCN) (2008) Charter. www.icpcn.org.uk

Kübler-Ross, E. (1969) *On Death and Dying*. New York: Macmillan.

Lewis, M. & Prescot, H. (2006) Impact of life-limiting illness on the family. In: Goldman, A., Hain, R. & Liben, S. (eds). *Oxford Textbook of Palliative Care for Children*, Oxford: Oxford University Press. p173.

McNeilly, P., Price, J. & McCloskey, S. (2006) Reflection in children's palliative care: a model. *European Journal of Palliative Care*, **13**(1), 31–4.

Macdonald, M.E., Liben, S., Carnevale, F.A., *et al.* (2005) Parental perspectives on hospital staff members' acts of kindness and commemoration after a child's death. *Pediatrics*, **116**(4), 884–90.

Payne, S., Seymour, J. & Ingleton, C. (2008) *Palliative Care Nursing: Principles and Evidence for Practice*, 2nd edn. Maidenhead, Berkshire: MacGraw-Hill Education, Open University Press.

Pfund, R. (2007) *Palliative Care Nursing of Children and Young People*. Oxon: Radcliffe Publishing Ltd.

Price, J. & Cairns, C. (2009) Communicating effectively. In: Price, J. & McNeilly, P. (eds). *Palliative Care for Children and Families, an Interdisciplinary Approach*, Basingstoke: Palgrave Macmillan. pp38–63.

Rider, E. (2003) Danny's mother – a lesson in humility. *Archives of Pediatric and Adolescent Medicine*, **157**(3), 228.

Rushton, C. (2005) A framework for integrated pediatric palliative care: being with dying. *Journal of Pediatric Nursing*, **20**, 311–25.

Thomas, J. & Chalmers, A. (2009) Bereavement care. In: Price, J. & McNeilly, P. (eds). *Palliative Care for Children and Families, an Interdisciplinary Approach*. Basingstoke: Palgrave Macmillan. pp192–212.

Worden, J.W. (2003) *Grief Counselling and Grief Therapy: a Handbook for the Mental Health Practitioner*, 3rd edn. East Sussex: Brunner-Routledge.

www.childbereavement.org.uk (accessed September 2010).

Appendix 1 Children's Nursing Care Plan

Please refer to Chapter 1.

Infant/Child/Young Person's Name: _____

DOB: _____

Date and time	A/L no	Potential/actual problems	Nursing objectives/ outcomes/goals	Nursing care plan (actions with rationale)	Review dates	Nurse's signature

Care Planning in Children and Young People's Nursing, First Edition.
Edited by Doris Corkin, Sonya Clarke, Lorna Liggett.
© 2012 Blackwell Publishing Ltd. Published 2012 by Blackwell Publishing Ltd.

Date	No	Problems	Nursing objectives	Nursing care plan	Review dates	Nurse's signature

Appendix 2 Bronchiolitis Integrated Care Pathway

Please refer to Chapter 7.

Patient name:	Date of admission:
Address:	Time of admission:
Hospital number:	Consultant:
DOB:	Contact telephone number:
Nursing assessment:	Expected date of discharge:

Temp: Pulse: Resp. rate: B/P:

O_2 Sat: % in room air: GCS: N/A

Weight: ____kg   Height: ____cm   Length: _____cm

Head circumference ___cm   Urinalysis: Y/N

Maintaining a safe environment:	Isolation required Y/N / N/A Oxygen Y/N Cot/bed/incubator Suction Y/N
Communication	Spoken language Speech/sight/hearing problems Y/N Interpreter required Y/N
Breathing	Breathing difficulties Y/N Cardiac problems Y/N Parent/carer smokers Y/N
Eating and drinking	Breastfed: Y/N Bottlefed: Y/N formula Spoonfed: one, two or three times a day?
Elimination	Nappies all the time Y/N Urinary problems Y/N Bowel problems Y/N
Personal cleansing and dressing	Skin problems Y/N Skin integrity Y/N
Controlling body temperature	History of high temperatures Y/N

Care Planning in Children and Young People's Nursing, First Edition.
Edited by Doris Corkin, Sonya Clarke, Lorna Liggett.
© 2012 Blackwell Publishing Ltd. Published 2012 by Blackwell Publishing Ltd.

Mobilising	Mobilising appropriate to age Y/N
	Mobility problems Y/N
Working and playing	Special toy Y/N
Expressing sexuality	Expression problems Y/N
Sleeping	Normal routine
	Disturbed patterns Y/N
	Special comforters Y/N
Dying	Any concerns noted Y/N

Medical assessment:
Presenting history:

_____

_____

_____

_____

_____

_____

Past medical history: _____

_____

_____

_____

_____

Birth history:
Term ☐   **Gestation:** ___ weeks   **Birthweight:**_____
Preterm ☐   **Delivery:** Vaginal ☐   Normal: ☐   Forceps: ☐
Caesarean section: Planned: ☐   Emergency: ☐

_____

_____

_____

_____

Neonatal problems:

_____

_____

_____

_____

Feeding:
Breast ☐   Artificial ☐   Mixed ☐

Immunisations: UTD/NUTD/none done   **Allergies:**
Family history:

_____

_____

Social history:

_____

_____

_____

_____

Assessment criteria and management guideline

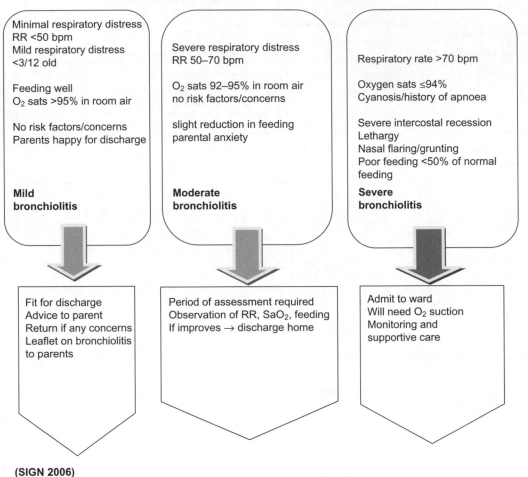

Minimal respiratory distress
RR <50 bpm
Mild respiratory distress
<3/12 old

Feeding well
O_2 sats >95% in room air

No risk factors/concerns
Parents happy for discharge

**Mild
bronchiolitis**

Severe respiratory distress
RR 50–70 bpm

O_2 sats 92–95% in room air
no risk factors/concerns

slight reduction in feeding
parental anxiety

**Moderate
bronchiolitis**

Respiratory rate >70 bpm

Oxygen sats ≤94%
Cyanosis/history of apnoea

Severe intercostal recession
Lethargy
Nasal flaring/grunting
Poor feeding <50% of normal
feeding

**Severe
bronchiolitis**

Fit for discharge
Advice to parent
Return if any concerns
Leaflet on bronchiolitis
to parents

Period of assessment required
Observation of RR, SaO_2, feeding
If improves → discharge home

Admit to ward
Will need O_2 suction
Monitoring and
supportive care

(SIGN 2006)

Bronchiolitis plan

Interventions	Clinical stage assessment: 1. Initial 2. Deteriorating 3. Improving 4. Discharge home								
	Assessor (initials only)								
	Date								
	Time								
Observations	Weight								
	Temperature								
	Respiratory rate (RR)								
	Heart rate (HR)								

Overall assessment	Normal								
	Mildly sick								
	Very ill								
Colour	Pink								
	Pale								
	Dusky/blue								
Resp. effort	Normal								
	Mild distress								
	Exhausted								
Resp. support	Oxygen saturation								
	% Oxygen/humified requirement								
Suctioning	No suction required								
	Suction pre- feed								
	Suction for respiratory distress								
Nutrition	Feeding normally								
	Feeding less than normal								
	Not feeding								
Intake	Oral feeds ___ mL/feed								
	IV fluids at ___ mL/hr								
Investigations: indicate if appropriate or completed Y/N/ N/A	Nasal aspirate								
	CXR								
	FBP								
	Blood gas								
	U+E								
	Blood culture								
Medications:									
Salbutamol	Frequency ___ hourly								
	Effective – Y/N								
Adrenaline	Frequency ___ hourly								
	Effective – Y/N								
Saline	Frequency ___ hourly								
	Effective – Y/N								
Other medications									
Education	Information leaflet given to and discussed with parents								
Discharge plan:	Resp. distress Y/N								
	Feeding satisfactorily Y/N								
	SaO$_2$ > 94% in room air Y/N								
	Family happy with home care Y/N								
	Review by GP in 1–2 days Y/N								

ICP Communication Sheet

Name: _____ **Hospital Number:** _____ **Date:** _____

Date	VARIANCIES	Signature

Appendix 3 RCN Recommendations and Good Practice Points

Please refer to Chapter 13.

From Royal College of Nursing (2010) The recognition and assessment of acute pain in children: clinical practice guideline. www.rcn.org.uk/childrenspainguideline

http://www.rcn.org.uk/__data/assets/pdf_file/0004/269185/003542.pdf

Quick reference guide (permission granted)

Full details of all the references cited in this appendix can be found on the RCN website at the link above.

Care Planning in Children and Young People's Nursing, First Edition.
Edited by Doris Corkin, Sonya Clarke, Lorna Liggett.
© 2012 Blackwell Publishing Ltd. Published 2012 by Blackwell Publishing Ltd.

6 Recommendations and good practice points

6.1 Recommendations

For each of the recommendations presented in this section, a summary of the evidence is presented together with full references to the research studies. The evidence of each study has been attributed a level of evidence using SIGN system (SIGN, 2008). This is followed by evidence statements based on the reviewed research and a brief overview of the GDG discussion and interpretation of the evidence.

> **RECOMMENDATION 1:**
>
> Be vigilant for any indication of pain.
>
> Pain should be anticipated in neonates and children at all times.

Summary of the evidence

There has been a traditional view that neonates, particularly preterm neonates, are less able to experience and interpret pain than older children and adults. The evidence does not support this view. The physiological and biochemical prerequisites for nociception are developed in utero, so from birth neonates are able to demonstrate physiological and behavioural responses to pain; this is supported by evidence from observational studies (Mathew and Mathew, 2003; Stevens and Franck, 2001; Duhn and Medves, 2004; Abu-Saad et al., 1998; Stevens and Koren, 1998; Franck and Miaskowski, 1997; Morison et al., 2001; Walden et al., 2001; Johnston et al., 1995). Like adults, responses to pain appear proportionate to pain severity (Porter et al., 1999), though this may not be the case with very preterm, sick, or exhausted neonates (Van Dijk et al., 2004). Surveys suggest that nurses use different cues to assess pain in preterm neonates and term babies. This might lead them to miss more subtle indicators of pain in preterm neonates, and so underestimate pain intensity in this group (Shapiro, 1993; Reyes, 2003). Immature motor capabilities, behavioural state, and clinical status may further complicate pain assessment in preterm babies (Duhn and Medves, 2004; Craig et al., 1993). These factors, combined with outdated views that neonates do not feel pain and a reluctance to prescribe and administer analgesia, may result in insufficient pain management in neonates (Shapiro, 1993; Purcell-Jones et al., 1988).

All studies cited are repeated cross-sectional studies (considered non-analytic studies) and have been attributed level of evidence 3 (SIGN, 2008).

Evidence statements

- A foetus acquires the physiological and biochemical prerequisites for nociception in utero. Following birth therefore, preterm neonates have the prerequisites for nociception. Observational studies have demonstrated physiological and behavioural responses to pain in all neonates.

- Repeated cross sectional studies before and after a painful event show that children and neonates experience pain in the same situations as adults.

GDG discussion

Given the evidence that neonates demonstrate physiological and behavioural responses to pain and that children and neonates experience pain in the same situations as adults, the GDG agreed that a fundamental principle for assessing pain in children is that practitioners should anticipate pain in any situation that an adult would consider painful. The GDG felt that it was important to recognise that pain should be anticipated at all times, especially (but not only) when painful situations occur.

> **RECOMMENDATION 2:**
>
> Children's self-report of their pain, where possible, is the preferred approach.
>
> For children who are unable to self-report, an appropriate behavioural or composite tool should be used.

Summary of the evidence

Children with CI who are non-verbal are unable to self-report reliably. Recent studies suggest that children with CI display predictable, observable behaviours that can be used to detect the presence and degree of pain. This has led to the development of observer-rated behavioural pain assessment tools specifically for use with children with CI (Breau et al., 2002a; Breau et al., 2002b; Voepel-Lewis et al., 2002; Hunt et al., 2004; Malviya et al., 2006; Hunt et al., 2007).

All studies cited are repeated cross-sectional studies (considered non-analytic studies) and have been attributed level of evidence 3 (SIGN, 2008).

Evidence statements

- The limited evidence available to date shows that, contrary to previous beliefs, children with cognitive impairment do demonstrate consistent, measurable patterns of pain behaviour, which allow for the use of standardised pain assessment tools.

- Evidence for pain assessment tools designed specifically for children with cognitive impairment shows that they are effective and reliable in a number of care contexts.

GDG discussion

The GDG recognised that children's self-report of their pain is considered the gold standard, where this is possible. As shown by the review of tools designed specifically for non-verbal children with CI, valid, reliable tools do exist for this population. The GDG agreed with this, while recognising that expertise needs to continue to be developed in this area. An important finding of this review was that children with CI display clear, measurable pain behaviours around which these specific assessment tools have been structured. The GDG also highlighted that there are other reasons why children are unable to self-report; for example, as they may be ventilated. Although self-report may not be possible in these cases, pain assessment should still be carried out.

RECOMMENDATION 3:

If pain is suspected or anticipated, use a validated pain assessment tool; do not rely on isolated indicators to assess pain.

Examples of signs that may indicate pain include changes in children's behaviour, appearance, activity level and vital signs.

No individual tool can be broadly recommended for pain assessment in all children and across all contexts.

Summary of the evidence

Both term and preterm neonates vary greatly in their physiological, biochemical and behavioural responses to pain (Franck and Miaskowski, 1997). Older children also show inconsistent behavioural and verbal responses that may be related to contextual and cultural factors (Stanford et al., 2005). Certain responses may be indicators of pain, though these responses should not be used in isolation and should cue formal assessment with valid, often composite, scales.

Biochemical and physiological responses

Studies have shown variable, undefined biochemical responses (for example, plasma or salivary cortisol and plasma catecholamine levels) to painful stimuli in neonates (Franck and Miaskowski, 1997). Similarly, although most studies in neonates show that heart rate increases and oxygen saturation decreases in response to procedures that are likely to be painful (Holsti et al., 2004; Grunau et al., 2001; Porter et al., 1999; Craig et al., 1993; Morison et al., 2003; Holsti et al., 2005; Gorduysus et al., 2002; Stevens and Johnston, 1994; Schwartz and Jeffries, 1990; Lindh et al., 1999) this is not always the case (Grunau et al., 2000; McIntosh et al., 1993). Gestational age, intensity and invasiveness of the pain stimulus (Porter et al., 1999), prior pain exposure (Grunau et al., 2001) and medical condition can all affect physiological response. In children aged 8 to 17 years, heart rate may not be a sensitive indicator of pain (Foster et al., 2003).

Behavioural responses

Many studies in term and preterm infants show increased frequency of limb flexion and finger splay in response to procedures that are likely to be painful (Holsti et al., 2004; Walden et al., 2001; Morison et al., 2003; Holsti et al., 2005; Grunau et al., 2000; Taddio et al., 2002; Stevens et al., 1993). But this is not always so. Startles and twitching do not seem to be useful indicators of pain (Grunau et al., 2000). Gestational age may affect the nature of behavioural response, though this is unpredictable. Some studies suggest that infants with a lower gestational age at birth respond more to pain (Holsti et al.,2004), while others suggest a dampened response (Grunau et al., 2001; Oberlander et al., 2000). Previous pain exposure may also affect behavioural response (Taddio et al., 1997; Taddio et al., 2002).

Facial expression and cry

Most studies assessing facial response to pain in neonates suggest that acute pain increases overall facial activity (Holsti et al., 2004; Craig et al., 1993; Grunau et al., 1990), in particular the brow-bulge, eye-squeeze, nasolabial furrow features and open mouth (Holsti et al., 2004; Holsti et al., 2005; Grunau et al., 1990; Rushforth and Levene, 1994). One repeated cross-sectional study suggests that newborn girls were more facially expressive than newborn boys in response to capillary puncture (Guinsburg et al., 2000). Again, these responses are variable and may be difficult to assess in some children. Another study found that, in some cases, no facial expression was observed although infants still mounted a cortical haemodynamic response, suggesting cortical response to painful stimulation may occur in the absence of facial expression (Slater et al., 2008). Short latency to cry and longer duration of first cry may be typical responses to acute pain (Grunau et al., 1990), but one cross-sectional study suggests that cry features are not a sensitive indicator of pain intensity in preterm neonates (Johnston et al., 1999). Relying on cry features to assess pain is inappropriate if all or some of the face is obscured, for example, in ventilated neonates, neonates with facial tapes, or eye patches (Van Dijk et al., 2004).

Research primarily in neonates suggests that neither physiological nor behavioural indicators of pain are highly sensitive. Studies demonstrating concordance between these cues lend support to a recommendation for the use of validated, multi-dimensional scales when assessing pain (Morison et al., 2001; National Association of Neonatal Nurses, 2001).

All studies cited are repeated cross-sectional studies (considered non-analytic studies) and having been attributed level of evidence 3 (SIGN, 2008).

Evidence statements

- Neonates, both term and preterm, and older children vary greatly in their responses to pain, be they biochemical, physiological, behavioural or verbal.

- Certain responses may be indicators of pain, but they should not be used in isolation to assess pain intensity.

- Studies demonstrate concordance between physiological and behavioural indicators of pain in neonates, which lends support to a recommendation for the use of validated, multi-dimensional scales when assessing pain.

GDG discussion

Principles given in these recommendations should be applied to all neonates and children, with or without CI, or critically ill children who are intubated and ventilated. All tools for all children should be chosen for the context in question and applied by appropriately trained people.

RECOMMENDATION 4:

Assess, record, and re-evaluate pain at regular intervals; the frequency of assessment should be determined according to the individual needs of the child and setting.

Be aware that language, ethnicity and cultural factors may influence the expression and assessment of pain.

Summary of the evidence

Evidence of the best time to assess pain is limited and based largely on expert opinion. Some experts recommend assessments and documentation of pain at least every four to six hours (Royal College of Nursing, 2002; Van Dijk et al., 2004; Anand, 2001; Agency for Health Care Policy and Research, 1992). An increase in pain severity, lack of response to pain management or worsening of a child's clinical condition may warrant more frequent assessment (Royal College of Nursing, 2002; Anand, 2001; Agency for Health Care Policy and Research, 1992). Pain assessments should also be used to evaluate the efficacy of management strategies (Anand, 2001). One RCT found that management within a framework including more regular pain assessments (every four hours compared with every six hours) in the 24 hours after surgery reduced the severity of post-operative pain and increased the use of post-operative analgesia (Stevens, 1990). One retrospective comparative study found that assessment every four hours using a self-report tool had no effect on analgesia, pain report, length of hospital stay or time and progress of ambulation when compared with chart review of children having no formal pain assessment (Boughton et al., 1998).

All studies cited are a body of expert opinion (level of evidence 3) with the exception of one randomised controlled trial (Stevens 1990; level of evidence 1-) and one case series with a retrospective control (Boughton et al., 1998; level of evidence 3).

Evidence statements

- Regular assessment of pain in a systematic framework improves outcomes for children.

- An increase in pain severity, a lack of response to a pain management intervention or a worsening of a child's clinical condition may warrant more frequent assessment.

- Both term and preterm neonates vary greatly in their physiological, biochemical and behavioural responses to pain.

- Older children also show inconsistent behavioural and verbal responses that may be related to contextual and cultural factors.

GDG discussion

The GDG agreed that a fundamental principle for assessing pain in children is that practitioners should anticipate pain in any situation that an adult would consider painful, and should be prepared to formally assess and manage pain using an appropriate tool. This principle applies to all children. The selection of an assessment tool, however, should be guided by the individual child's condition and circumstances to ensure that the most effective tool is chosen. For example, tool selection may be influenced by whether a child presents in acute pain or is pain free at the time of assessment and explanation of the tool. Cultural factors should be taken into consideration as necessary in the selection of an assessment tool. Pain assessment should not be seen as a one off, but rather as part of a cycle of assessment, management and reassessment. If a selected tool is not working, another appropriate tool should be selected in its place.

6.2 Good practice points

These good practice points are suggestions for best practice, based on GDG expertise in the absence of evidence. In terms of providing a complete, practical guideline, the good practice points are as important as the recommendations. These complement the evidence-based recommendations and are based on GDG members' clinical expertise, providing important guidance on the practice of assessing pain in children.

1. Acknowledging pain makes pain visible. Pain assessment should be incorporated into routine observations (as the fifth vital sign or 'TPRP' – temperature, pulse, respiration and pain).

2. Pain assessment is not an isolated element; it is an ongoing and integral part of total pain management. The other elements include implementation of appropriate interventions, evaluation and reassessment.

3. The child's pain assessment tool, written information and advice on pain assessment and treatment should be given to parents/carers as part of their preparation for discharge for continued use at home/other care settings.

4. Parents/carers may benefit from being taught to use pain assessment tools as part of the management of their child's pain.

5. Each organisation should appoint a dedicated lead facilitator to promote and support the implementation of pain assessment for all children, including those with cognitive impairment.

Appendix 4 Examples of Evaluation Tools

Please refer to Activity 14.2 in Chapter 14.

1. Accurate history taking – from witnesses of a 'seizure' and from the person can help medical staff to form an opinion. Very often the person will have little knowledge of the events which occurred as they may have been unconscious or confused following the seizure.
2. Physical examination and medical history – to rule out any physical cause particularly in infants and young children, for example cardiac arrhythmias, meningitis, involuntary movements, metabolic dysfunction such as hypocalcaemia or hyponatraemia, or an inherited genetic condition.
3. Diagnostic neuroimaging – CT, MRI, etc., to rule out presence of a physical abnormality, for example tumour, stroke or scarring.
4. Electroencephalograph (EEG) – to record and observe any abnormal electrical brain activity which might suggest a particular seizure type or syndrome. Could be in the form of video telemetry.
5. Blood and urine biochemistry – to rule out any underlying causes such as altered blood chemistry, drug /toxic levels, metabolic causes, for example diabetes.

Care Planning in Children and Young People's Nursing, First Edition.
Edited by Doris Corkin, Sonya Clarke, Lorna Liggett.
© 2012 Blackwell Publishing Ltd. Published 2012 by Blackwell Publishing Ltd.

Appendix 5 Sample Care Plan

Please refer to Activity 14.3 in Chapter 14.

Care Planning in Children and Young People's Nursing, First Edition.
Edited by Doris Corkin, Sonya Clarke, Lorna Liggett.
© 2012 Blackwell Publishing Ltd. Published 2012 by Blackwell Publishing Ltd.

A/L	Nursing assessment	Nursing problem	Goal/objective	Nursing interventions	Rationale
Maintaining a safe environment	Robert has had several seizures	Robert is at risk of injury during a seizure	Robert will remain safe during all seizures	• If possible, prevent Robert from falling, and remain with him. • Protect his head – place padding underneath. • Move objects in close proximity and make space. • Do NOT restrain Robert during seizure. • Loosen clothing around neck. • Do NOT place ANYTHING between his teeth. • When convulsing stops check airway and place in the recovery position. • Oxygen/suction should be available. • If seizure lasts longer than five minutes call for medical assistance. • Monitor vital signs and level of responsiveness until recovery.	• To reduce risk of injury at commencement of seizure. • To prevent further injury during seizure. • Could cause injury to limbs. • To reduce any airway obstruction. • Teeth can be broken, thus compromising his airway. • To maintain a patent airway. • To help clear airway and improve oxygen saturation when breathing becomes possible. • Robert's seizure may have developed into status epilepticus. • To observe recovery and return of normal vital signs.
	Robert is a newly diagnosed patient with epilepsy	Robert's seizure activity is uncontrolled	The frequency of Robert's seizures will reduce	• Administer prescribed AEDs. • Regular blood tests. • Observe Robert for seizures and document. • Educate Robert to ensure compliance with taking medication as prescribed. • Wear MedicAlert identification.	• AEDs help to control seizure activity. • To monitor therapeutic levels of ADEs. • To determine changes in seizure activity. • To prevent an increase in seizure activity. • To inform others in case of emergency.
	Robert and his family know little about epilepsy	Robert's family have a knowledge deficit related to epilepsy and its control	Robert's family will be able to identify appropriate care during a seizure and in relation to medication prior to discharge	• Educate the family regarding medication, to include side effects. • Teach family members how to place Robert in the recovery position and care for him during a seizure or status.	• Family aware of the need for compliance and to be able to observe for signs of increased seizure activity. • To ensure that family (and others) are able to prevent injury and airway obstruction.
Working and playing	Robert and his family know little about epilepsy	Robert and his family require information on living with epilepsy	Robert and his family will demonstrate adequate knowledge of possible lifestyle changes	• Inform Robert and his family regarding possible adjustments to lifestyle. • Provide appropriate literature. • Direct to a local support group for additional support.	• A diagnosis of epilepsy needs to be seen in the context of the patient's lifestyle and type of epilepsy. It may, in some instances, require some modification to the lifestyle, or introducing some additional safety precautions, but the general principle is to empower the patient to manage their condition.

Appendix 6 Management of Acute Asthma in Children

Reproduced from British Guidelines On The Management Of Asthma (May 2008, revised May 2011), with permission.
Please refer to Chapter 20.

Care Planning in Children and Young People's Nursing, First Edition.
Edited by Doris Corkin, Sonya Clarke, Lorna Liggett.
© 2012 Blackwell Publishing Ltd. Published 2012 by Blackwell Publishing Ltd.

Age 2-5 years

ASSESS ASTHMA SEVERITY

Moderate asthma

- $SpO_2 \geq 92\%$
- No clinical features of severe asthma

NB: If a patient has signs and symptoms across categories, always treat according to their most severe features

Severe asthma

- $SpO_2 < 92\%$
- Too breathless to talk or eat
- Heart rate > 140/min
- Respiratory rate > 40/min
- Use of accessory neck muscles

Life threatening asthma

$SpO_2 < 92\%$ plus any of:
- Silent chest
- Poor respiratory effort
- Agitation
- Altered consciousness
- Cyanosis

Oxygen via face mask/nasal prongs to achieve SpO_2 94–98%

- β_2 agonist 2–10 puffs via spacer ± facemask [given one at a time single puffs, tidal breathing and inhaled separately]
- Increase β_2 agonist dose by 2 puffs every 2 minutes up to 10 puffs according to response
- Consider soluble oral prednisolone 20 mg

Reassess within 1 hour

- β_2 agonist 10 puffs via spacer ± facemask or nebulised salbutamol 2.5 mg or terbutaline 5 mg
- Soluble prednisolone 20 mg or IV hydrocortisone 4 mg/kg
- Repeat β_2 agonist up to every 20–30 minutes according to response
- **If poor response** add 0.25 mg nebulised ipratropium bromide

- Nebulised β_2 agonist: salbutamol 2.5 mg or terbutaline 5 mg **plus** ipratropium bromide 0.25 mg nebulised
- Oral prednisolone 20 mg or IV hydrocortisone 4 mg/kg if vomiting

Discuss with senior clinician, PICU team or paediatrician

- Repeat bronchodilators every 20–30 minutes

ASSESS RESPONSE TO TREATMENT
Record respiratory rate, heart rate and oxygen saturation every 1–4 hours

RESPONDING

- Continue bronchodilators 1–4 hours prn
- Discharge when stable on 4 hourly treatment
- Continue oral prednisolone for up to 3 days

At discharge
- Ensure stable on 4 hourly inhaled treatment
- Review the need for regular treatment and the use of inhaled steroids
- Review inhaler technique
- Provide a written asthma action plan for treating future attacks
- Arrange follow up according to local policy

NOT RESPONDING

- **Arrange HDU/PICU transfer**

Consider:
- **Chest X-ray and blood gases**
- **IV salbutamol** 15 mcg/kg bolus over 10 minutes followed by continuous infusion 1–5 mcg/kg/min (dilute to 200 mcg/ml)
- **IV aminophylline** 5 mg/kg loading dose over 20 minutes (omit in those receiving oral theophyllines) followed by continuous infusion 1 mg/kg/hour

Age > 5 years

ASSESS ASTHMA SEVERITY

Moderate asthma

- $SpO_2 \geq 92\%$
- PEF > 50% best or predicted
- No clinical features of severe asthma

NB: If a patient has signs and symptoms across categories, always treat according to their most severe features

Severe asthma

- $SpO_2 < 92\%$
- PEF 33–50% best or predicted
- Heart rate > 125/min
- Respiratory rate > 30/min
- Use of accessory neck muscles

Life threatening asthma

$SpO_2 < 92\%$ plus any of:
- PEF < 33% best or predicted
- Silent chest
- Poor respiratory effort
- Altered consciousness
- Cyanosis

Oxygen via face mask/nasal prongs to achieve SpO_2 94–98%

- β_2 agonist 2–10 puffs via spacer
- Increase β_2 agonist dose by 2 puffs every 2 minutes up to 10 puffs according to response
- Oral prednisolone 30–40 mg

Reassess within 1 hour

- β_2 agonist 10 puffs via spacer or nebulised salbutamol 2.5–5 mg or terbutaline 5–10 mg
- Oral prednisolone 30–40 mg or IV hydrocortisone 4 mg/kg if vomiting
- **If poor response** nebulised ipratropium bromide 0.25 mg
- Repeat β_2 agonist and ipratropium up to every 20–30 minutes according to response

- Nebulised β_2 agonist: salbutamol 5 mg or terbutaline 10 mg **plus** ipratropium bromide 0.25 mg nebulised
  Oral prednisolone 30–40 mg or IV hydrocortisone 4 mg/kg if vomiting

Discuss with senior clinician, PICU team or paediatrician

- Repeat bronchodilators every 20–30 minutes

ASSESS RESPONSE TO TREATMENT
Record respiratory rate, heart rate, oxygen saturation and PEF/FEV every 1–4 hours

RESPONDING

- Continue bronchodilators 1–4 hours prn
- Discharge when stable on 4 hourly treatment
- Continue oral prednisolone 30–40 mg for up to 3 days

At discharge

- Ensure stable on 4 hourly inhaled treatment
- Review the need for regular treatment and the use of inhaled steroids
- Review inhaler technique
- Provide a written asthma action plan for treating future attacks
  Arrange follow up according to local policy

NOT RESPONDING

- **Continue 20–30 minute nebulisers and arrange HDU/PICU transfer**
- Consider: **Chest X-ray and blood gases**
- **Consider risks and benefits of:**
- **Bolus IV salbutamol** 15 mcg/kg if not already given
- Continuous **IV salbutamol infusion** 1–5 mcg/kg/min (200 mcg/ml solution)
- **IV aminophylline** 5 mg/kg loading dose over 20 minutes (omit in those receiving oral theophyllines) **followed by** continuous infusion 1 mg/kg/hour
- **Bolus IV infusion of magnesium sulphate** 40 mg/kg (max 2 g) over 20 minutes

Appendix 7 Activity of Living – Breathing

Please refer to Chapter 20.
(Based on Roper *et al.* (1996) model of care).

Problem	Goal	Nursing intervention	Date and sign ongoing review or as changes in condition dictate
George has been admitted following exacerbation of asthma.	To closely monitor George's condition for early detection of deterioration in condition and to assess for improvement in symptoms.	1. Nurse beside O_2 and suction point. 2. Record regular vital signs, observe George's respiratory rate and use of accessory muscles. Ensure observations are within normal limits in relation to age bracket. 3. Observe skin colour for signs of cyanosis or pallor. 4. If SpO_2 <93% administer O_2 therapy as prescribed by the doctor via O_2 mains supply. Administer humidified O_2 at correct rate and via correct device, i.e. nasal specs or Hudson mask. 5. George propped up in bed in a comfortable position to maximise breathing potential. 6. Administer treatment (oral/inhaled) as prescribed in accordance with NMC guidelines. 7. Nebulisers to be administered at a rate of 6l/min via correct nebuliser chamber for five minutes. 8. Observe for improvements or signs of deterioration in George's condition if side effects of medications noted, report and document to medical staff. 9. Explain procedures to George and his parents. Give reassurance and relieve any anxieties which George may have expressed. 10. Report changes to nurse in charge.	

Care Planning in Children and Young People's Nursing, First Edition.
Edited by Doris Corkin, Sonya Clarke, Lorna Liggett.
© 2012 Blackwell Publishing Ltd. Published 2012 by Blackwell Publishing Ltd.

Appendix 8 Asthma Treatment Card

Reproduced with permission from Dr Heather Steen, Consultant Paediatrician. Please refer to Chapter 20.

Care Planning in Children and Young People's Nursing, First Edition.
Edited by Doris Corkin, Sonya Clarke, Lorna Liggett.
© 2012 Blackwell Publishing Ltd. Published 2012 by Blackwell Publishing Ltd.

WHAT IS ASTHMA?

Asthma is the tubes of the lungs being irritated by things around them. Trigger factors cause them to narrow and become red and swollen.

SOME OF THE TRIGGER FACTORS IN YOUR CHILD MAY BE:

Common cold

Exercise

House dust mite

Cigarette smoke

Changes in weather

Pollen

Animals

Sprays, e.g. perfume, polish
NSAIDs, e.g. Junifen, Neurofen

YOU CAN HELP YOUR CHILD BY:

1) Making sure they take medication and use the devices prescribed.
2) Stop smoking and failing this, smoke outside. Do not smoke in cars.
3) Damp dusting followed by dry dusting.
4) Hoovering: floors, soft furnishings and mattress.
5) Washing bed linen and cuddly toys at 60°C.

THE SYMPTOMS OF ASTHMA ARE:

Cough – worse at night, after exercise or a cough that keeps coming back.

Wheeze – a whistling sound.

Shortness of breath especially after exercise.

Tight chest – some children may describe this as having a sore tummy or a pain in their heart.

Your child does not need to have all these symptoms to have asthma.

DANGER SIGNS

♦ Reliever lasts less than 3 hours
♦ Very distressed by wheezing or breathlessness
♦ Too breathless to feed or talk or walk
♦ Lips going blue
♦ Using abdominal muscles to help breathing

WHAT TO DO:

1) Allow child space to breath
2) No sudden change in temperature
3) Loosen tight clothing
4) Hold or sit child upright
5) Use reliever inhaler. Giving a high dose up to 20 puffs
6) If no improvement after 15 minutes
   Repeat high dose reliever and call for help.

EITHER:

A) Ambulance
B) Go to the nearest Casualty Department

TREATMENTS FOR ASTHMA

These fall into two main groups:
1a) Preventers
1b) Combined treatments
2) Relievers

PREVENTERS:

These are steroid based. They calm the tubes of the lungs and help prevent them from becoming red and swollen. They must be taken every day even if your child is well.

A drink must be taken after each treatment as they can sometimes cause a sore throat or thrush.

If using a mask, wipe the face afterwards with a damp cloth.

The main preventers are Budesonide, Beclomethasone, Fluticasone.

COMBINED TREATMENTS:

These are usually red or purple in colour. They contain steroid and long-acting relievers, to calm the tubes of the lungs and help keep them open for 12 hours. They can only be taken a maximum of twice daily. Seretide and Symbicort.

RELIEVERS:

Are usually blue in colour.

They open up the tubes of the lungs making it easier to breathe.

They should act quickly and give relief for up to four hours.

Take only when needed.
Main relievers: Ventolin, Bricanyl, Salamol and Salbutamol.

OTHER TREATMENTS

Name & Strength	Morning	Evening

HSC Belfast Health and Social Care Trust

ASTHMA INFORMATION & TREATMENT CARD

Child's Name: _____

Address: _____

DOB: _____

Weight: _____

Family Doctor: _____

Telephone: _____

Hospital/Clinic Consultant: _____

Telephone: _____

Contact Name: _____

YOUR CHILD'S ASTHMA

TREATMENT

PREVENTER

Give regularly even if your child is well
To calm lungs down

Name & Strength				
Times	AM	Lunch	Tea	Bed
Dose				
If Bad Give				

COMBINED TREATMENT

To calm lungs and keep airways open for 12 hours

Name & Strength		
Times	Morning	Evening
Dose		
If Bad Give		

RELIEVERS

To open up airways

Name & Strength	
If Bad Give	

LONG-ACTING RELIEVER

To keep airways open for 12 hours

Name & Strength	Morning	Evening
If Bad Give		

OTHER MEDICATIONS:

Your child may need some other medication to help control their asthma.

LONG-ACTING RELIEVERS

These work slowly by helping to keep the tubes of the lungs open for up to twelve hours.

The main long-acting relievers are:

* Volmax tablets * Serevent * Oxis

DECONGESTANTS

These help to dry up the secretions in your child's chest and nose.

The main decongestants are:

* Galpseud Plus * Sudafed

OTHER MEDICATIONS MAY INCLUDE:

* Singulair
* Granules or tablets, which help calm the tubes of the lungs down

This is to confirm that I have received information on the management of asthma, the potential side effects of steroids and the use and care of inhaler device.

Signature _____

Date _____

Index

Numbers in bold refer to tables; those in italics refer to figures.

Care Planning in Children and Young People's Nursing, First Edition.
Edited by Doris Corkin, Sonya Clarke, Lorna Liggett.
© 2012 Blackwell Publishing Ltd. Published 2012 by Blackwell Publishing Ltd.

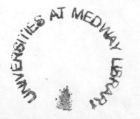